Behavioral Clinical Trials for Chronic Diseases

Lynda H. Powell • Kenneth E. Freedland •
Peter G. Kaufmann

Behavioral Clinical Trials
for Chronic Diseases

Scientific Foundations

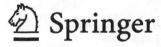

Lynda H. Powell
Department of Preventive Medicine
Rush University Medical Center
Chicago, IL, USA

Kenneth E. Freedland
Department of Psychiatry
Washington University in St. Louis
St. Louis, MO, USA

Peter G. Kaufmann
College of Nursing
Villanova University
Villanova, PA, USA

ISBN 978-3-030-39328-1   ISBN 978-3-030-39330-4   (eBook)
https://doi.org/10.1007/978-3-030-39330-4

This Springer imprint is published by the registered company Springer Nature Switzerland AG
The registered company address is: Gewerbestrasse 11, 6330 Cham, Switzerland

This book is dedicated to

Thomas A. Deutsch, MD,
former Dean of Rush Medical College.

In taking a leap of faith,
he inspired a pursuit of excellence.

Acknowledgments

The inspiration for this book came from the Fellows of the US National Institutes of Health Summer Institute on Behavioral Randomized Clinical Trials. Over its first 19 years, the Institute trained over 800 Fellows in behavioral clinical trial methodology. These Fellows contributed to the evolving methodology in behavioral trials with their questions. Although the diseases and treatments varied from Fellow to Fellow, and from year to year, their questions were much the same. They were less interested in *how* to do something than they were in *why* they should do it. These questions informed the choice of topics for each of the chapters as well as the style of presenting them. I want to acknowledge the leadership of Peter Kaufmann who conceived, founded, and led the Summer Institute from its beginning in 2000, and Kate Stoney who later assumed leadership and pulled it off with equal success. I also want to acknowledge the support provided by the US National Institutes of Health Office of Behavioral and Social Sciences Research, which was initiated by Peter Kaufmann and continued by Raynard Kington, David Abrams, Bob Kaplan, Bill Riley, and Christine Bachrach.

This book's focus on the integration of good science and good methods came from my inspirational sabbatical year at the Center for Advanced Study in the Behavioral Sciences at Stanford University. During that year, scientists from diverse areas of behavioral sciences, including philosophy, political science, law, psychology, sociology, evolutionary biology, anthropology, linguistics, economics, geography, history, public affairs, public health, and literature, presented their work. These diverse disciplines pursue behavioral problems from different perspectives, contribute a piece of a puzzle, and together progress knowledge. The Center encouraged us to look beyond the science of any single discipline in pursuit of excellence within our own. I would like to extend my sincerest admiration and gratitude to Margaret Levi, the charismatic Director of the Center, for her vision and for the many ways she encouraged discovery through cross-fertilization.

All chapters have been reviewed by at least two junior or senior investigators with interests and expertise in behavioral clinical trials. These reviews were not always easy, as is clear from such comments as – *"I have no idea what you are trying to say!" "You have completely missed the point."* But they helped us to see weaknesses and enhance strength. A special shout-out goes to Rachel Wu who reviewed and commented on every single chapter. Her basic science studies led her to make a creative leap to interventions. To do so, she needed to *"learn about this stuff."* All of these reviewers are listed in the Appendix. We thank them sincerely for their help.

On a more personal level, I would like to thank Bob Kaplan for his ongoing encouragement. He has written 21 books; this was my first. He never stopped asking for progress reports, providing tips, and normalizing the challenges. He expected success, and it was infectious. I would also like to thank Rick Reiss for his emotional support. After long hours at the computer on a beautiful summer day, he would describe what his day had been like on the outside, helping me to experience vicariously a post-book life. I am hoping that my family and friends, particularly Celeste Fraser, will now give me a second chance after several years of declining their many invitations.

And finally to Joyce Mack, my faithful Assistant, I give my heartfelt thanks. Joyce worked on every reference, figure, table, and formatting problem, obtained all the permissions, and served as a liaison between me and many moving parts of this book. She did this with a commitment to excellence, and a sense of ownership, that was equal to mine.

Lynda H. Powell
(On behalf of my coauthors, Ken Freedland and Peter Kaufmann)
October 2019

Contents

About the Authors

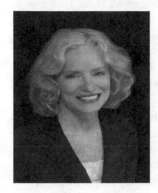

Lynda H. Powell, PhD is the Charles J. and Margaret Roberts Professor of Preventive Medicine, Medicine, Behavioral Sciences, and Pharmacology and Chair of the Department of Preventive Medicine at Rush University Medical Center in Chicago. She received her doctoral degree from Stanford University in counseling psychology and began her academic career in chronic disease epidemiology at Yale University's School of Public Health. She has been a past principal investigator of five major randomized behavioral trials and has served as a standing member of the NHLBI Clinical Trials Study Section. She co-developed the ORBIT model for behavioral treatment development. She is a founding faculty member and former co-director of the NIH/OBSSR Summer Institute on Randomized Behavioral Clinical Trials. She is interested in sustained lifestyle change and its impact on reduction of cardiometabolic risk and is recognized internationally as an expert in the design, conduct, analyses, and interpretation of behavioral clinical trials. She is a Fellow of the Academy of Behavioral Medicine Research, the American Psychosomatic Society, and the Society of Behavioral Medicine.

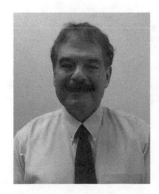

Kenneth E. Freedland, PhD is Professor of Psychiatry and Psychology at Washington University School of Medicine in St. Louis and the Editor-in-Chief of *Health Psychology*, the official journal of the Society for Health Psychology. He received his doctoral degree in clinical psychology from the University of Hawaii and began his academic career at Northwestern University Medical Center in Chicago. He has been on the faculty at Washington University since 1986 where his research has focused on depression, self-care, and other psychosocial and behavioral problems in patients with heart disease. He has served as a standing member of the NHLBI Clinical Trials Study Section and is the Program Director of the NIH/OBSSR Summer Institute on Randomized Behavioral Clinical Trials. He has published multiple papers on behavioral trial methodology, particularly the selection and design of comparators, and feasibility and pilot studies. Dr. Freedland is a past president of the Academy of Behavioral Medicine Research and a Fellow of the Society of Behavioral Medicine, the American Psychological Association, and the American Heart Association.

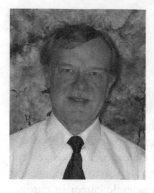

Peter G. Kaufmann, PhD is Professor and Associate Dean of Research at the Villanova University College of Nursing. He received his doctorate in psychology from the University of Chicago and conducted post-doctoral research in neuroscience at Duke University. After joining the National Heart, Lung, and Blood Institute of the National Institutes of Health, he led research on mechanisms through which behavioral factors influence cardiovascular risk, and developed a program of research on evidence-based behavioral medicine. He is an expert in the conduct of multisite randomized behavioral trials for cardiovascular risk factors such as stress, depressive symptoms, and health behaviors. He founded the NIH/OBSSR Summer Institute on Randomized Behavioral Clinical Trials and is widely known for his expertise in clinical trial methodology. Dr. Kaufmann is a Fellow of the Academy of Behavioral Medicine Research and past president of the Society of Behavioral Medicine.

Chapter 1
Introduction

*"You cannot solve a problem by continuing to use the same solutions
that created the problem in the first place."*

Albert Einstein

WINDOW OF OPPORTUNITY

The window of opportunity has never been opened wider for the integration of evidence-based behavioral treatments into clinical care. This opportunity has been created within the context of the current healthcare crisis and by the promise of behavioral treatments to cut, rather than to shift, costs.

The healthcare crisis is a problem of simple arithmetic. America and most other developed countries are graying in slow motion. Figure 1.1 presents a comparison of the distribution of ages in the American population in 1990, 2000, and as it is projected to be in 2025 [1].

The dark bars in Fig. 1.1 represent the baby boomer cohort, born between 1946 and 1964 and accounting for the largest segment of the population. In 1990 they entered the workforce, reaching their peak earning power in 2000. Their large numbers, compared to the relatively small number of retired elderly who have the greatest need for health care, made social programs such as Social Security and Medicare viable. Their large numbers also made it possible to develop a high-tech healthcare system that evolved into the most expensive, but not the most effective, in the world [2].

© Springer Nature Switzerland AG 2021
L. H. Powell et al., *Behavioral Clinical Trials for Chronic Diseases*,
https://doi.org/10.1007/978-3-030-39330-4_1

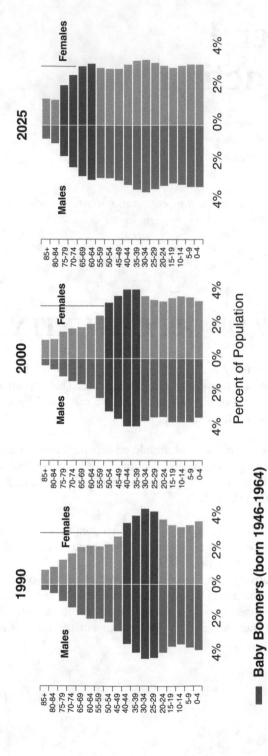

Baby Boomers (born 1946-1964)

Fig. 1.1 US age distribution in 1990, 2000, and as projected in 2025

This picture changes as the baby boomers reach the ages of 60–79 and retire. By 2025, a large majority of them will be drawing on, rather than contributing to, Medicare and Social Security. But more elderly baby boomers will need health care than contributions from smaller, younger, and healthier cohorts can support. When Social Security was first rolled out in 1940, there were 45 workers for every Social Security-eligible retiree. When Medicare was signed into law in 1965, this ratio had dropped to approximately five workers to every retiree. In 2030, this ratio is projected to be only two workers to every retiree [3].

This is a problem of supply and demand. It is being felt by patients who see their deductibles and co-pays in their health care plans rising faster than their incomes. It will not be neutralized by pumping more money into health care. Despite having the most expensive healthcare system in the world, the United States ranks only 31st among nations in life expectancy [2]. Various approaches to healthcare reform offer proposals for shifting costs, resulting in battles between red and blue states, federal and state governments, private and public coverage, and pro-regulation liberals and free-trade conservatives.

Within this context, the window of opportunity opens for preventive behavioral interventions if they can cut, rather than shift, costs. Regardless of the time in a person's life when a behavioral intervention is introduced—the prenatal period, infancy, childhood, adolescence, adulthood, or older adulthood—the fundamental goal is to extend health and compress morbidity into the short period immediately preceding a death at old age.

Interest in prevention is increasing. The Affordable Care Act mandates that private insurers provide evidence-based preventive services without shifting costs to patients. Third-party payers and employers offer financial incentives for healthy behaviors. Medical providers receive financial incentives for achieving control of cardio-metabolic risk factors that have fundamental roots in lifestyle. Quality improvement initiatives target the "triple threat" of improving patient experience, improving the health of populations, and reducing per capita costs [4], all of which require effective behavioral strategies.

THE EVIDENCE: OBSERVATIONAL STUDIES

People are living longer but not necessarily in good health. Morbidity and chronic disability now account for one-half of the healthcare burden in the United States [5]. The link between these problems and health behaviors is irrefutable. Large-scale American and international epidemiologic studies, with sample sizes ranging from 20,000 to 1.6 million, have consistently shown that engaging in at least three health behaviors, including such things as eating five servings of fruits and vegetables on most days, not smoking, and being physically active for 30 minutes on most days, is associated with 12–14 years of additional life expectancy, a 75% reduction in all-cause mortality, a 65% reduction in cancer mortality, an 82% reduction in cardio-vascular mortality, and a reduction in risk for Alzheimer's disease and dementia [2, 6–10].

Many believe that genes are the primary determinant of one's health. But studies of cardiovascular disease and dementia have challenged this assumption. When life-style and genetic predisposition are examined simultaneously, a healthy lifestyle provided protection for all people regardless of whether they are at low, medium, or high genetic risk [11, 12]. This means that people can overcome their inherent genetic risk for major chronic diseases by engaging in lifestyle behaviors that are neither extreme nor exceptional.

Despite the enormous value of healthy living, the percentage of the American popu-lation living a healthy lifestyle is low and decreasing. In 1996, only 8.5% of Americans reported engaging in at least four healthy behaviors. In 2007, this rate dropped to 7.7% [9]. A suboptimal lifestyle translates into an increase in cardio-metabolic risk. The prevalence of the metabolic syndrome, defined as having three out of five cardio-metabolic risk factors, all of which have fundamental roots in lifestyle, has increased over the past ten years from one-quarter to one-third of the American population [13].

Too many people lead unhealthy lifestyles. They are over-treated with tests, proce-dures, and medicines with high price tags and underwhelming results. The single greatest opportunity to improve health, reduce premature death, close the gap between health span and life span, and reduce healthcare costs lies in personal behavior.

THE EVIDENCE: INTERVENTION STUDIES

Many would argue that there is substantial and sound evidence to support the effi-cacy of behavioral interventions. But compared to the irrefutable link between behavior and chronic diseases in observational studies, evidence for the value of behavioral interventions to *reduce* chronic diseases is suboptimal. Admittedly, there is a large *quantity* of behavioral intervention studies. But they are often small refine-ment studies with a focus is on dimensions of a behavioral treatment, or they are small *Phase II* trials with a focus on improving behavioral or biomedical risk fac-tors. Both of these types of studies have limited clinical importance.

There is a vacuum of evidence from definitive behavioral trials with clinically impor-tant outcomes such as costly acute events, deaths, hospitalizations, remission, and recurrence. A powerful example of this vacuum comes from a review of all of the *Phase III* trials that have been conducted on either exercise or drug interventions for the secondary prevention of cardiovascular events. This review showed that 96% of the patients across all of these trials were enrolled in the drug trials, not the exercise trials, despite the equal efficacy of these two treatments in preventing mortality [14].

When a *Phase III* behavioral trial does find benefit, it is influential. The Diabetes Prevention Program showed that patients who were insulin-resistant and given a lifestyle intervention had a 58% lower incidence of diabetes than placebo and a 31% lower incidence than metformin [15]. These findings led to a new generation of effectiveness trials, third-party reimbursement for the lifestyle program, and implementation in community and clinical settings.

We do not need a greater *quantity* of evidence. We need a greater *quality* of evidence. The *Phase III* Diabetes Prevention Program trial provided the type of data that influenced clinical practice guidelines which, in turn, influenced third-party reimbursement, implementation into clinical practice, and a reduction in healthcare costs.

WHY WE WROTE THIS BOOK

We wrote this book because we are hoping to advance a culture of methodologically sophisticated PhD and MD investigators who have the vision, commitment, and depth of perspective to develop behavioral treatments and progressively test them using the standards that have come to be the norm in the medical sciences.

We wrote this book because we are experts in behavioral clinical trial methodology using the definition articulated by Niels Bohr, the Danish physicist and philosopher who won the 1922 Nobel Prize in Physics for his work on quan-

> *"An expert is a man who has made all of the mistakes which can be made, in a narrow field."*
> Niels Bohr
> Nobel Prize in Physics, 1922

tum theory (see box). We forgive Dr. Bohr for excluding women from this quote. Mistakes are certainly divided evenly across genders. But the point is that we have devoted, and continue to devote, our careers to behavioral trials and therefore have the dubious distinction of having made mistakes across all of their aspects—design, operations, oversight, and interpretation. These experiences have led to our humility in the face of the many challenges behavioral trials impose. We echo the more eloquent and moving words of Jadad and Enkin [16].

> *"Probably for too many years, we have designed, conducted, published, systematically reviewed, synthesized, taught, critiqued, lived with, and suffered with randomized controlled clinical trials. We have experienced the tremendous satisfaction ... the valuable contribution they have made to health care and human health ... and their potential and promise. ... But above all, we experienced humility."*

We wrote this book to provide some insight into the common questions with which investigators pursuing careers in behavioral trials struggle. We have mentored over 800 Fellows who have participated in the NIH-OBSSR Summer Institute for Behavioral Trials over the past 19 years. These Fellows conduct behavioral clinical trials for interventions ranging all the way from individual behavior to policy, and outcomes across the entire range of organ systems. Although the classes change from year to year, the questions they tend to ask are the same. These questions have informed the content of each of the chapters in this book.

Understanding principles, mistakes, consequences, and ways to avoid them can foster deeper insight into how to make the many difficult design decisions that are needed in behavioral trials. We do not want new investigators to follow in our footsteps. We want them to seek what we sought, but in ways that are better informed, more sophisticated, and more successful.

ORGANIZING PRINCIPLES

The chapters in this book focus on basic principles of behavioral clinical trial design. The choice of topics was based upon their fundamental importance, the challenges they present when a trial is behavioral in nature, and the dilemmas they can create for investigators. Each chapter features three organizing principles.

"Why Should You?" **Rather Than** *"How To"*

The clinical trial, and behavioral clinical trial, literature features papers and books that focus on *"how to"* use specific procedures to solve specific problems. The focused nature of this literature necessarily limits its ability to justify *"why should you?"* within the larger context of the competing decisions that characterize the design, conduct, and analysis of behavioral clinical trials.

We have tried to get at the *"why should you?"* by appealing to what constitutes good science. We begin each chapter with scientific principles derived from the scientific method. We present descriptions of the scientific process as articulated by the great philosophers

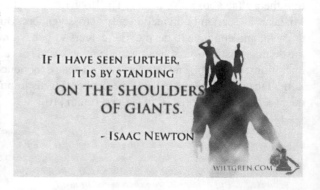

IF I HAVE SEEN FURTHER, IT IS BY STANDING ON THE SHOULDERS OF GIANTS.

- ISAAC NEWTON

WILTGREN.COM

of science, scientists, and statisticians whose innovations form the basis of how we practice science today. We describe the history of our struggles to answer the question of whether or not a treatment works, and the evolution of the clinical trial as the best solution. If we can, in Newton's words, "*stand on the shoulders of giants,*" we can see further.

Each chapter then continues with a presentation of one or more basic principles, how they can create a problem for behavioral clinical trials, an approach to solving the problems, and the consequences that have occurred when a principle was compromised. The idea is to foster a commitment to preserving the basic principle and an openness to considering new ways to do so. We hope that discussions of "*why should you?*" will, in turn, encourage a search for the right approach to "*how to,*" drawing on the extensive literature that now exists in papers and books on clinical trials and behavioral clinical trials.

Progressive Translational Science Model

This book focuses on behavioral clinical trials that seek to improve chronic disease outcomes. A progressive translational science model going all the way from discovery through to a confirmatory *Phase III* efficacy trial and beyond is well-suited to this purpose. Although translational science models extend to effectiveness, dissemination, and implementation studies, we do not focus on them here because we believe that the biggest roadblock to dissemination and implementation is the paucity of successful *Phase III* efficacy trials. Those with interests in these studies should consult the extensive literature that has developed in these areas.

A Comparison of Selected Design Elements in Behavioral Clinical Trials: The Status Quo and a Translational Model	
STATUS QUO	**TRANSLATIONAL MODEL**
Single comprehensive trial	Progression of studies and trials
Refinement studies and *Phase II* trials	Push to *Phase III* trials
Exploratory studies	Confirmatory trials
Effectiveness without efficacy	Efficacy precedes effectiveness
Statistical significance	Clinical significance
Miniature efficacy trials	Feasibility and plausibility
Fear of failure	Welcome failure
Representative participants	Targeted participants
"Hard sell" recruitment	Pros and cons of participation
Innovation	Replication
Moderators, mediators, mechanisms	Minimization of multiplicity in outcomes
Rugged individualism	Networks

The progressive translational model encourages a long-term commitment to a behavioral intervention where failure is expected, refinement is encouraged, and results from one study inform the design of the next. This model is consistent with the cultural movement that is evolving in the applied behavioral sciences, which has been energized by the need to enhance the uptake of behavioral treatments into clinical practice, and advanced by the emergence of a "metascience" of behavioral clinical trial methods [17]. *(See Chapter 12: Epilogue.)*

We do not simply present the status quo and what may be viewed currently as "best practices" in behavioral trial design. Instead, we seek to identify specific areas in a progressive translational science model where an alternative to the status quo exists. The box compares the status quo with a translational model on a sampling of specific design elements that will be found in more detail throughout this book.

Cross-Disciplinary Methods

When a behavioral treatment seeks to improve a chronic disease endpoint, its progressive evaluation is a cross-disciplinary undertaking. The most appropriate design and methods vary depending upon where in the treatment development process a study is placed. For example, refinement studies are often about exploring various treatment options such as the optimum mode, dose, and agent of change. The exploratory experimental design methods, embedded within the behavioral sciences, are well-suited to accomplishing such aims. Alternatively, confirmation of the value of a behavioral treatment on a chronic disease outcome often requires long follow-up periods for disease outcomes to accumulate. The methods of double-blind drug trials, developed within medicine and epidemiology, handle such data optimally. Beyond this, a behavioral clinical trial often faces challenges that cannot be solved within any particular discipline. The inability to double-blind a trial, and the difficulties in choosing an optimal comparator, pose unique problems for behavioral trial design that often need solutions that synthesize wisdom across many disciplines.

Each chapter features cross-disciplinary methods as they are brought to bear on specific challenges in behavioral clinical trial design. Since the application of these methods varies depending upon where in the treatment development process a study is placed, efforts have been made to distinguish among exploratory studies, refinement studies, *Phase II* trials that seek to confirm the value of a behavioral treatment on a behavioral or biomedical outcome, and *Phase III* trials that seek to confirm the value of a behavioral treatment on a chronic disease outcome. Once the phase of treatment development is defined, the optimal phase-specific methods are considerably easier to identify.

THE AUDIENCE

Anyone with an interest in the design, conduct, analysis, or interpretation of randomized behavioral clinical trials aimed at improving chronic disease endpoints would benefit from reading this book. Use of the term "behavioral"is for purposes of simplicity. This book applies to the design of trials for any non-drug treatment, including those at the behavioral, social, environmental, or policy level, where intervention development is needed, double-blinding is not possible, and progression to definitive clinical outcomes is anticipated.

We are especially interested in reaching junior scientists at the beginning of their research careers. Behavioral scientists are sophisticated in the treatment side of the behavioral clinical trial. They have expertise in developing behavioral treatments and can therefore design the kind of treatments that could actually improve definitive clinical outcomes. For this group, the topics found in this book can encourage a push beyond a sole focus on refinement and early testing, toward confirmatory trials with clinically important health outcomes.

Medical scientists are sophisticated in the chronic disease side of the behavioral clinical trial. A growing number have interests that go beyond finding the right medicine, device, or surgical procedure for their patients. They seek to find solutions to behavioral problems such as improving adherence to therapies, ability to communicate, quality of care, and proactivity in their patients. The topics found in this book can foster an appreciation of the developmental work that is needed to prepare a behavioral treatment for testing in a confirmatory behavioral trial.

Policy-makers, funders, and third-party payers who have interests in behavioral approaches for improving chronic diseases may find this book valuable. It could help them to identify ways to assess rigor in behavioral trials and thus assess the quality of the evidence they need to make good decisions.

And for those who do not work in any field of science, this book can be helpful in determining how much trust to place in a new behavioral trial evaluating a novel behavioral treatment, such as a new diet. Trust can be increased by knowing the specific aspects of a trial that determine its rigor. Rather than reading the technical descriptions within each chapter, an understanding of what to look for can be enhanced by the simple overview presented as the *Fundamental Points* which begin each chapter.

REFERENCES

1. Taylor P (2014) The next America: boomers, millennials, and the looming generational show-down. Public Affairs, New York
2. Organisation for Economic Cooperation and Development (OECD) (2013) OECD Health Data 2013: how does the United States compare? http://www.oecd.org/health/oecdhealthdata2013-countrynotes.htm.
3. Connelly M (2014) A changing shape in America's age distribution. https://www.nytimes.com/2014/05/13/upshot/a-changing-shape-in-americas-age-distribution.html
4. Berwick DM, Nolan TW, Whittington J (2008) The triple aim: care, health, and cost. Health Aff 27:759–769
5. US Burden of Disease Collaborators (2013) The state of US health, 1990-2010: burden of diseases, injuries, and risk factors. JAMA 310:591–606
6. Younus A, Aneni EC, Spatz ES, Osondu CU, Roberson L, Ogunmoroti O, Malik R, Ali SS, Aziz M, Feldman T, Virani SS, Maziak W, Agatston AS, Veledar E, Nasir K (2016) A systematic review of the prevalence and outcomes of ideal cardiovascular health in US and non-US populations. Mayo Clin Proc 91:649–670
7. Akesson A, Larsson SC, Discacciati A, Wolk A (2014) Low-risk diet and lifestyle habits in the primary prevention of myocardial infarction in men: a population-based prospective cohort study. J Am Coll Cardiol 64:1299–1306
8. Li Y, Pan A, Wang DD, Liu X, Dhana K, Franco OH, Kaptoge S, Di Angelantonio E, Stampfer M, Willett WC, Hu FB (2018) Impact of healthy lifestyle factors on life expectancies in the US population. Circulation 138:345–355
9. Ford ES, Li C, Zhao G, Pearson WS, Tsai J, Greenlund KJ (2010) Trends in low-risk lifestyle factors among adults in the United States: findings from the behavioral risk factor surveillance system 1996–2007. Prev Med 51:403–407
10. Loef M, Walach H (2012) The combined effects of healthy lifestyle behaviors on all cause mortality: a systematic review and meta-analysis. Prev Med 55:163–170
11. Khera AV, Emdin CA, Drake I, Natarajan P, Bick AG, Cook NR, Chasman DI, Baber U, Mehran R, Rader DJ, Fuster V, Boerwinkle E, Melander O, Orho-Melander M, Ridker PM, Kathiresan S (2016) Genetic risk, adherence to a healthy lifestyle, and coronary disease. N Engl J Med 375:2349–2358
12. Lourida I, Hannon E, Littlejohns TJ, Langa KM, Hyppönen E, Kuźma E, Llewellyn DJ (2019) Association of lifestyle and genetic risk with incidence of dementia. JAMA 322:430–437
13. Moore JX, Chaudhary N, Akinyemiju T (2017) Metabolic syndrome prevalence by race/ethnicity and sex in the United States, National Health and Nutrition Examination Survey, 1988–2012. Prev Chronic Dis 14:160287. https://doi.org/10.5888/pcd14.160287
14. Naci H, Ioannidis JPA (2015) Comparative effectiveness of exercise and drug interventions on mortality outcomes: metaepidemiological study. Br J Sports Med 49:1414–1422
15. Knowler WC, Barrett-Connor E, Fowler SE, Hamman RF, Lachin JM, Walker EA, Nathan DM, Diabetes Prevention Program Research Group (2002) Reduction in the incidence of type 2 diabetes with lifestyle intervention or metformin. N Engl J Med 346:393–403
16. Jadad AR, Enkin MW (2007) Randomized controlled trials. Questions, answers, and musings, 2nd edn. Blackwell/BMJ, Malden
17. Munafò MR, Nosek BA, Bishop DVM, Button KS, Chambers CD, Percie du Sert N, Simonsohn U, Wagenmakers E-J, Ware JJ, Ioannidis JPA (2017) A manifesto for reproducible science. Nat Hum Behav 1:0021. https://doi.org/10.1038/s41562-016-0021

Chapter 2
Quality of a Clinical Trial

"Knowing is not enough; we must apply.
Willing is not enough; we must do."
Goethe (1749–1832)

Fundamental Point

There is a mismatch between the standards for "evidence-based" treatments set by medicine and the evidence that exists for the value of behavioral treatments. In medicine, the highest-quality evidence comes from Phase III efficacy trials, with important clinical outcomes, and clinical trial methods. Evidence for behavioral treatments more often comes from Phase II efficacy trials, with outcomes that are behavioral or biomedical risk factors, and experimental methods. A progressive, translational model for behavioral treatment development and evaluation can encourage a push toward more high-quality Phase III behavioral trials that meet the standards expected by medical gatekeepers and third-party payers and enhance the potential for implementation of behavioral treatments into clinical practice.

To close the gap between evidence-based behavioral treatments for chronic diseases and their uptake in clinical practice, this book aims to encourage the development of evidence for the value of behavioral treatments that meets the standards for quality existing in medicine. Evidence for quality is strongest in *Phase III* efficacy trials which follow the agreed-upon "rules" for clinical trial methods. In the behavioral clinical trial literature, there are many more *Phase II* than *Phase III* trials. What is needed is not a larger quantity of such evidence, but a higher quality of evidence using the standards that exist in medicine. This book applies a progressive, translational science model to achieve that goal.

© Springer Nature Switzerland AG 2021   11
L. H. Powell et al., *Behavioral Clinical Trials for Chronic Diseases*,
https://doi.org/10.1007/978-3-030-39330-4_2

SCIENTIFIC PRINCIPLES

The overall aim of this book is to close the gap between evidence-based behavioral treatments for chronic diseases and their uptake in clinical practice. At least one reason for this gap is a discrepancy between what is meant by "evidence-based." What is evidence in one beholder's eye may not be evidence in another's. It could mean evidence from any randomized trial. It could mean evidence from a specific type of randomized trial. It could mean evidence from any well-designed and well-conducted systematic inquiry, including observational data, clinical reports, or pilot studies.

A basic premise of this book is that since the gatekeepers for chronic disease management are medical practitioners, the onus is on the behavioral trialist to conduct a trial using the same standards they use to evaluate any medical treatment. Positive trials that meet these standards for quality can become integrated into clinical practice guidelines [1, 2]. This is the pathway to reimbursement for a treatment by third-party payers [3] and implementation into clinical practice.

This premise makes it useful to examine the standards for high-quality evidence and high-quality clinical trials that have been set in medicine.

High-Quality Evidence

To understand what "high-quality" evidence means in medicine, consider the criteria used by national and international committees charged with grading the quality of evidence for medical treatments, as reported by the Institute of Medicine [4]. Table 2.1 summarizes the criteria used to achieve the highest-quality rating. The criteria are remarkably similar. Regardless of the specific committee doing the rating, they are consistent in judging the highest quality of evidence to be that coming from high-quality randomized controlled trials (RCT's). Although the existence of one well-designed clinical trial provides strong evidence, replication of results from several trials carried out by different investigators enhances the strength of the evidence and moves the rating from "strong" to "very strong."

High-Quality Trials

Since the above review committees consistently refer to "high-quality" randomized trials, it is of interest to consider what is meant by this. That is, what are the fundamentals that make a clinical trial one of high quality?

Table 2.1 Requirements for the highest quality of evidence for a treatment across a variety of international rating systems [4]

COUNTRY	SYSTEM	HIGHEST-QUALITY RATING	REQUIREMENTS
International	Grading of Recommendations, Assessment, Development, and Evaluation Working Group (2009)	High	RCT
United Kingdom	Centre for Evidence-Based Medicine (2009)	1a	Reviews of high-quality RCTs are consistent
		1b	Single RCT with narrow confidence interval
Scotland	Scottish Intercollegiate Guidelines Network (2009)	1++	Reviews of RCTs with very low risk of bias
		1+	RCT with low risk of bias
New Zealand	New Zealand Guidelines Group (2007)	A	≥ 1 review or RCT rated as 1++ and directly applicable to target population
Canada	The Canadian Hypertension Education Program (2007)	A	RCT with blinded assessment, intent-to-treat analysis, follow-up and sample size sufficient to detect clinically important difference
United States	Institute for Clinical Systems Improvement: 157 Medical Groups in Minnesota (2003)	A	RCT which is free of doubts about bias, design flaws, generalizability
	Strength of Recommendation Taxonomy, American Family Physicians (2004)	Level 1	Consistent good-quality patient-oriented RCTs or a high-quality individual RCT
	US Preventive Services Task Force (2008)	High	Consistent results from well-designed and conducted studies in representative primary care populations
	American College of Cardiology/American Heart Association (2009)	A	Data derived from multiple RCTs
		B	Data derived from single RCT
	American Academy of Pediatrics (2004)	A	Well-designed RCTs on relevant populations
	American Academy of Neurology (2004)	Class I	Prospective RCT with masked outcome, representative population, clear primary outcome, defined inclusions/exclusions, low rate of dropouts and crossovers, baseline characteristics equivalent across arms
	American College of Chest Physicians (2009)	High	RCTs without important limitations
	National Comprehensive Cancer Network (2008)	High	High-powered RCTs or meta-analyses
	Infectious Disease Society of America (2001)	I	Evidence from >1 properly randomized trial

Most of what we know about the fundamentals of clinical trials comes from the design of double-blind drug trials. This topic has been the focus of an extensive literature, much of which has been summarized in a large number of papers and a wide range of books [5–28]. These fundamentals developed rapidly since the 1950s when clinical trials became more popular, missteps became more common, and the need to prevent these missteps rose. These fundamentals are now referred to as the "rules" of clinical trials and have wide acceptance in the medical community. One of the classic texts for these basic principles is the *Fundamentals of Clinical Trials* [20] now in its 5th edition. Table 2.2 presents a selection of some of the fundamental principles of clinical trials presented in this classic text. They pertain primarily to *Phase III* double-blind drug trials and focus on maximizing internal validity and minimizing alternative explanations for results. These rules are articulated by reviewers of clinical trial papers submitted to high-quality journals. If they are not followed, the paper is often rejected, and it generally ends up in journals with less visibility and lower impact.

Table 2.2 Selected fundamental "rules" of clinical trials [20]

TREATMENT DEVELOPMENT	Well-defined progression: *Phase I* (dose), *Phase II* (biologic activity), *Phase III* (efficacy), *Phase IV* (effectiveness)
PURPOSE	Single primary question with secondary questions carefully justified and surrogate measures evaluated primarily in early-phase studies
POPULATION	Well-defined with high likelihood of detecting hypothesized results by having high risk for the primary outcome, high likelihood of adhering to the treatment protocol, and no competing adverse events
DESIGN	Randomized allocation to treatment or control to minimize confounding and invalid statistical tests
SAMPLE SIZE	An approximation, derived from conservative assumptions
ADHERENCE TO TREATMENT	Select participants who will adhere to treatment. Maximize adherence by careful participant selection, simple treatment protocols, intensive monitoring, and a variety of remediation strategies
RETENTION IN TRIAL	Estimated rate of withdrawal from the trial is pre-specified and minimized by careful participant selection, simple trial protocols, intensive monitoring, a variety of retention strategies, and, if needed, reduction of final assessment battery to the primary endpoint only
PRIMARY OUTCOME	One clinically relevant primary endpoint, often an event rate with a long follow-up
MONITORING	Independent monitoring of data quality, safety, and adherence, with a limited number of pre-planned tests to detect early harm, benefit, or futility
ANALYSES	Intent-to-treat with no exclusions for any reason to avoid bias of unknown magnitude and direction resulting from compromised random assignment. Minimal missing data which is generally not at random
REPORTING	Obligation to report not only results but also whether trial worked as planned

Another window into what constitutes quality in a clinical trial has been presented by the Cochrane Collaboration. This group has published a series of papers presenting guidelines for reporting clinical trials. Although these guidelines reflect best practices for reporting and stop short of judging what constitutes a high-quality trial directly, they are an indirect measure of the criteria others should use in making a judgment of the quality of any particular trial. A selected summary of the guidelines for reporting parallel group randomized trials [29] and the extension for trials of social and psychological interventions [30] is presented in Table 2.3.

Table 2.3 Selected CONSORT reporting criteria for parallel group randomized trials [29] and trials of social and psychological interventions [30]	
Population	Number of losses [29]
	Number of losses included in analyses [29]
Design	How sample size was determined [29]
	Unit of randomization [30]
	How the intervention is hypothesized to work [30]
Primary Outcome	Pre-specified [29]
Analyses	Describe any subgroup analyses [29]
	Distinguish between pre-specified and exploratory hypotheses [29]
	Provide details on how missing data are handled [30]
Adherence to Treatment	Provide details on delivery and implementation of treatment(s) [30]
Blinding	Provide details on who was blinded and how [29]

These guidelines recommend increased visibility in the reporting of clinical trials in important areas such as the number of losses and how missing data are treated, pre-specification of a primary endpoint, distinction between hypothesized and exploratory aims, the extent of blinding, and how a treatment is hypothesized to work.

CHALLENGES FOR BEHAVIORAL TRIALS

Clinical trials in medicine that are rated of the highest quality share specific features. They are:

- *Phase III* efficacy trials with a single, pre-specified, clinically relevant outcome;
- Conducted in a population at risk, selected because they are likely to remain in the trial and implement the treatment;
- Conservative, preserving the randomization by analyzing results on all participants who were randomized regardless of their response and, in the case of missing data, using conservative approaches to account for it;

- Objective, minimizing the adverse effects of preferences with double-blind designs and, when they are not possible, pushing to extend the blind to as many entities as possible.

There is often a mismatch between these quality indicators and the large number of behavioral intervention studies that exist in the literature. *Phase II* behavioral trials examining the impact of treatment on behavioral, biomedical, or surrogate outcomes are more common than *Phase III* efficacy trials examining impact on definitive chronic disease endpoints. The behavioral literature is characterized by trials with multiple endpoints, liberal approaches to missing data, and primary analyses based upon responders only.

Many of these design choices are well justified. The point here is not to say the choices are wrong within the context of the research aims. But rather they are inconsistent with the quality standards common in medical research.

Not Enough *Phase III* Behavioral Efficacy Trials

One frequently hears the statement that the evidence is overwhelming that behavioral treatments can improve health. Indeed, there are literally thousands of behavioral randomized trials listed in clinicaltrials.gov. But a closer look reveals that the majority are *Phase II* behavioral trials where the aim is to evaluate the impact of a behavioral treatment on a behavioral risk factor, mechanism, or surrogate endpoint. There are comparatively few *Phase III* behavioral trials that evaluate the impact of a behavioral treatment on a definitive chronic disease outcome.

When the aim is to integrate behavioral treatments into clinical practice, it is imperative to make the distinction between *Phase II* and *Phase III* evidence. Outcomes such as physical activity, diet, and stress are not of great interest to medical gatekeepers and third-party payers. Outcomes that reduce costs, such as remission of the metabolic syndrome, control of blood pressure, and incidence of diabetes are of greater interest. There are now quality metrics in place which provide fiscal rewards to practitioners who achieve control of chronic disease outcomes. If behavioral treatments can help practitioners achieve quality metrics, their value as an option in clinical care is enhanced.

In the absence of compelling data from *Phase III* behavioral trials that show improvement in a chronic disease endpoint, there is uncertainty in the medical community about the value of behavioral treatments. Indeed, the reality may be that there is not simply uncertainty. There may be no uncertainty because behavioral treatments are not even considered. This point of view is dramatically different from the point of view within the behavioral sciences about the overwhelming evidence that exists.

Evidence for an "Evidence-Based" Behavioral Treatment

There are many who believe that data generated from any randomized design provides the "evidence base" for a treatment. This is based upon the elegance of random assignment in being able to establish cause-and-effect relationships. But there are different reasons for using a randomized design. And these different purposes do not carry equal weight in providing the evidence base for a treatment [31].

Table 2.4 compares four different types of studies using the randomized design—experiments, *Phase II* efficacy trials, *Phase III* efficacy trials, and effectiveness trials. It can be seen that the aims are quite different, going all of the way from establishing covariation between a behavioral factor and a biomedical risk factor to assessing the ability to implement a behavioral treatment in clinical practice. As the aim evolves, so too do the methods for design and analysis.

The highest quality of evidence for a behavioral treatment comes from the *Phase III* efficacy trial aimed at improving a clinical outcome. Other types of randomized designs contribute important preliminary data but do not carry the same weight in assessing the quality of evidence, influencing clinical practice guidelines, and encouraging implementation in clinical practice.

Take, for example, the impact of anger on blood pressure. A randomized design may be used to conduct an *experiment* to test the hypothesis that change in anger results in reduction of blood pressure. Here the focus is on covariation and the use of an established treatment that would guarantee a reduction in anger is an essential part of the design. A randomized design may be used to *optimize* an anger treatment. Here the focus would be on identifying active treatment components by comparing an anger treatment to a non-specific attention control. A randomized design may be used to *improve outcomes*. Here an anger intervention combined with drug therapy would be compared to drug therapy alone on blood pressure control. A randomized design may be used to *assess impact*. Here the approach would be to randomize clinics to offer or not offer an anger management intervention for the purpose of determining whether or not anger management helps practices to achieve quality metrics associated with blood pressure control.

All of these randomized studies are important in understanding the role of anger on blood pressure control. The convergence of the results across different types of studies increases confidence that this association is real. When they lead to the *Phase III* efficacy trial, the potential evidence is that anger treatment enhances blood pressure control, over and above standard approaches. This is the evidence that influences clinical practice guidelines.

Table 2.4 Comparison of characteristics of four types of randomized designs

CATEGORY	ELEMENT	EXPERIMENT	PHASE II EFFICACY	PHASE III EFFICACY	EFFECTIVENESS
AIM		Establish covariation	Reduce behavioral or biological risk	Improve clinical outcome	Implement in practice
POPULATION	Setting	Artificial settings, often laboratories	Ecologically valid	Ecologically valid	Ecologically valid
	Participants	• Often volunteers who respond to ads • Incentives for adherence	• High behavioral risk • Selected to adhere to treatment and complete the trial	• High risk for primary endpoint • Selected to adhere to treatment and complete the trial, and at low risk for competing event	Represents diversity in age, illness severity, comorbidities, and adherence
INTERVENTION	Flexibility	• Strict protocol • Trained interventionists	• Strict protocol • Trained interventionists • Strategies for improvement in adherence • Co-interventions prohibited	• Strict protocol • Trained interventionists • Strategies for improvement in adherence • Co-interventions prohibited	• Flexibility in implementing protocol • Adherence is an outcome • Co-interventions permitted
	Comparator	Control for non-specific elements (e.g., passage of time)	Control for non-specific treatment elements (e.g., attention)	Compare to usual, enhanced, or standard of care	Compare to clinically relevant option
OUTCOME	Primary	Surrogates or mechanisms	Behavioral, biomedical risk factor	Clinical endpoint	Patient-centered, disease relevant
	Duration of follow-up	Often cross-sectional or short-term	Time needed to change behavioral risk factor	Time needed to change clinical endpoint	Time needed to detect effect in practice
ANALYSIS	Primary	Responders	Intent-to-treat	Intent-to-treat	Available data
	Subgroup	None	Pre-planned	Pre-planned	None
	Safety	Not relevant	Short-term	Short-term	Long-term

Need for Progressive Science

In contrast to drug development which is supported by industry, has an average duration of 6.8 years, and costs approximately $1.3 billion [32], behavioral treatments tend to be developed by individuals who rely upon local and federal support that is comparatively small and often transitory. It is not surprising, therefore, that the culture that has emerged in applied behavioral science is not one of a progressive testing of questions but rather one of "one fell swoop" trials where all relevant questions are attempted to be answered with one trial. This approach is not only difficult from a design perspective, but it maximizes the risk of inconclusive findings and therefore minimizes progression to *Phase III* trials.

Nowhere is this problem more apparent than the tension between internal and external validity. Classic experimental design is progressive. Internal validity is a prerequisite for external validity. A concern about whether or not a causal relationship holds across different persons, settings, and treatment variables becomes a non-issue if the relationship has not first been demonstrated to be causal [33]. The rationale for this progression is based

> ### Infanticide
>
> *"A new treatment is born into a hostile environment. It needs to be kept alive in infancy. It needs to mature until it reaches a point at which it can be brought into contact with the abundance of problems that could undermine it. Scientists should protect early development; not contribute to premature death."*
>
> Feyerabend [34]

upon signal to noise. Early tests under ideal circumstances minimize background noise and maximize treatment signal. If a signal exists under optimal conditions, its erosion in the face of increasing levels of noise can direct attention toward targets for refinement. Too rigorous a test too soon in the developmental process is similar to committing infanticide (see box) [34].

Attempting to design a trial with both strong internal and external validity poses a dilemma. Pursuit of internal validity may compromise generalizability when participants with a high likelihood of dropping out of the trial are excluded. Pursuit of generalizability may compromise internal validity when participants with the high likelihood of dropping out are included.

One way to resolve the dilemma is to jump directly to conducting trials with strong external validity even though efficacy has not been established. The popularity of effectiveness trials [35, 36], paired with the paucity of efficacy trials, suggests that this is an attractive option. But the problem with this approach is how to make causal inferences about a treatment when the equivalence between randomized arms is not preserved. The methodology for this does not now exist. Even a huge sample size cannot overcome this problem.

Another way to resolve the dilemma is to reject it. Many behavioral trials feature elements of both efficacy and effectiveness. This point is made persuasively by the RITES (Rating of Included Trials on the Efficacy-Effectiveness Spectrum) criteria [36] which describe where any single behavioral trial falls on a continuum of efficacy/effectiveness on each of four criteria: participants, setting, flexibility of interventions, and clinical relevance. Although appealing, the problem of "robbing Peter to pay Paul" remains. That is, the ability to establish causality can be undermined by a premature introduction of noise.

A progressive, translational approach resolves the dilemma by encouraging a progression of studies where efficacy precedes effectiveness. All questions are valued but they are not all answered at once. Strong, internally valid results provide the springboard to understanding diversity of impact.

OVERCOMING THESE CHALLENGES IN A BEHAVIORAL TRIAL

Overview of the Book

What is needed is not a larger quantity of evidence, but a higher quality of evidence. The gap in behavioral clinical trials research is the evidence that a behavioral treatment can improve a clinically important chronic disease outcome. The basic theme of this book is to apply a progressive, translational science model to fill that gap.

The logic of a *Phase III* trial is deceptively simple. Figure 2.1 presents this structure in its simplest form, the two-arm parallel group design. In keeping with any randomized

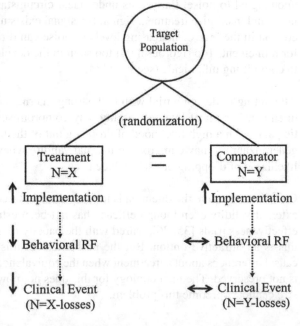

Fig. 2.1 Structure of a *Phase III* behavioral clinical trial

design, there is a treatment group and a comparator which are randomly equivalent at the time of randomization. Treatment is implemented with fidelity, and its strength is determined by whether or not the behavioral risk factor target of treatment was improved. The comparator arm is implemented with fidelity, and its strength is determined by a lack of change on the behavioral risk factor target. Follow-up continues as long as needed to detect potential benefit on a clinical endpoint. Losses are kept to a minimum in both arms to preserve the equivalence achieved at randomization and permit causal inferences between the treatment and the clinical event.

To achieve a high-quality *Phase III* behavioral trial, the same set of "rules" as those established for drug trials and summarized in Table 2.2 are followed. But above and beyond this, behavioral treatments pose unique challenges. As the importance of behavioral clinical trials grows and experience cumulates, these unique challenges are increasingly recognized, and there is now a growing literature, including a number of excellent books [37–41] aimed at summarizing this experience and providing recommendations. Those with interests in such related areas as experiments, effectiveness trials, community-based participatory research, and dissemination and implementation research are encouraged to consult the focused literature that is growing in these areas.

The chapters in this book are loosely organized in the chronological order in which the topic is encountered in practice. But each pertains to one of three general fundamentals of behavioral efficacy trials: progression of questions, strong behavioral treatments, and protection of internal validity. Each chapter reviews the elements of good science and good clinical trials, challenges faced by behavioral clinical trials, and ways to enhance quality in the face of these challenges. The focus is on "why" a design element is important rather than "how" to implement it.

An overview of these chapters follows.

Progression of Questions

Science is a progressive process. Insights from one study feed progression to a new study with new questions and new methodologies to answer them. The choice of design elements varies depending upon the evolving questions posed.

Link Between Stage of Development, Question, and Comparator
As an understanding of a treatment grows, the choice of a comparator in a randomized design evolves. *Chapter 6: Choice of a Comparator* encourages close links among the stage of development of a behavioral treatment, the stage-specific question of interest, and the decision about the appropriate comparator.

Link Between Question and Outcome

Selecting a single, clinically meaningful and objectively assessed primary outcome is essential to a rigorous evaluation of whether or not a behavioral treatment improves health. *Chapter 9: Outcomes* reviews several options for primary endpoints and encourages a minimization of multiple secondary outcomes to avoid unintended adverse consequences. Pursuit of moderators, mediators, and mechanisms is encouraged in earlier phases of treatment development.

Range of Designs

A progressive understanding of the value of a behavioral treatment draws heavily on the randomized design but includes a progression of questions that may be answered better by designs that are simpler, less costly, and less time intensive. *Chapter 3: Behavioral Treatment Development* encourages versatility in the use of a range of designs to answer a range of questions, the value of "tinkering" to enhance treatment strength, and the importance of low-cost failures to the achievement of innovation and success. Pilot and feasibility studies have come to be vague terms with a variety of different interpretations. *Chapter 7: Feasibility and Pilot Studies* aims to reduce this vagueness, focus their purpose on feasibility and readiness to conduct a trial, and identify methodologies that are well-suited to accomplish their purpose.

Strong Behavioral Treatments

To justify a *Phase III* behavioral clinical trial, the treatment under investigation must be promising. It must have supporting data that it can improve a behavioral risk factor at a level that is sufficient to produce an effect on an important chronic disease endpoint. The treatment must be delivered with fidelity and understood and implemented by participants.

Progressive Development

Chapter 3: Behavioral Treatment Development articulates the process of developing a behavioral treatment, going all of the way from ideas generated by insights from basic science and medical practice to a proof-of-concept test of plausibility. It highlights the chain of evidence needed to justify readiness for a *Phase III* behavioral trial and the steps in a progressive process that are directed toward achieving it.

Hypothesized Pathway

In the early phase of developing a behavioral treatment, decisions are enhanced by the existence of a quantified pathway by which a behavioral treatment is hypothesized to improve a chronic disease endpoint. *Chapter 4: Hypothesized Pathway and Bias* shows the power of an a priori pathway in testing hypotheses and in facilitating decisions after a study about progressing to more rigorous testing or moving back to refine or optimize. It presents an integration of biases from the behavioral sciences, epidemiology, and biostatistics that can undercut the ability to test a hypothesis.

Clinical Significance

Chapter 5: Clinical Significance encourages greater use of clinical, over statistical, significance throughout all phases of treatment development and evaluation. Use of clinical significance as a criterion for success provides freedom from the need for large sample sizes in early treatment development and makes it easier to use a variety of small sample designs to conduct preliminary tests. If the strength of a behavioral treatment is judged by whether it is strong enough to move a clinical endpoint, it justifies the decision to move to a *Phase III* behavioral efficacy trial.

Protection of Internal Validity

Behavioral trials are at unique risk for compromising internal validity largely because of the problem that investigators, staff, and participants are aware of the different treatments being tested. In double-blind drug trials, there is design control for this problem because neither investigators, staff, or patients know which drug a patient is on. Such design control is uncommon in behavioral trials. Thus unique procedures are needed to prevent bias.

Protection of Random Assignment

Chapter 8: Protection of Random Assignment provides a strong rationale for protecting the equivalence created by the random assignment. When this equivalence is altered, the potential for confounding undercuts causal interpretations and raises the possibility that results were due to some extraneous third factor and not to treatment. The important link between the target population and the ability to protect the random assignment is discussed, encouraging careful consideration of who the target population is, how to recruit them, and how to retain them in the trial for its duration.

Objectivity

Investigator, staff, and patient preference for a particular trial outcome can be an independent source of bias in a behavioral trial. *Chapter 10: Preferences, Equipoise and Blinding* describes expectancy bias as a creation of investigators who have a preference for, and certainty about, a particular result. It has adverse implications such as differential adherence and retention, treatment contamination, and ascertainment bias. The rigor of the trial depends upon an attitude of investigator equipoise coupled with trial procedures aimed at extending the blind in as many ways, and to as many players, as possible.

REFERENCES

1. Jensen MD, Ryan DH, Apovian CM, Ard JD, Comuzzie AG, Donato KA, Hu FB, Hubbard VS, Jakicic JM, Kushner RF, Loria CM, Millen BE, Nonas CA, Pi-Sunyer FX, Stevens J, Stevens VJ, Wadden TA, Wolfe BM, Yanovski SZ, Jordan HS, Kendall KA, Lux LJ, Mentor-Marcel R, Morgan LC, Trisolini MG, Wnek J, Anderson JL, Halperin JL, Albert NM, Bozkurt B, Brindis RG, Curtis LH, DeMets D, Hochman JS, Kovacs RJ, Ohman EM, Pressler SJ, Sellke FW, Shen WK, Smith SC Jr, Tomaselli GF, American College of Cardiology, American Heart Association Task Force on Practice Guidelines, Obesity Society (2014) 2013 AHA/ACC/TOS guideline for the management of overweight and obesity in adults: a report of the American College of Cardiology/American Heart Association Task Force on Practice Guidelines and the Obesity Society. Circulation 129:S102–S138
2. Eckel RH, Jakicic JM, Ard JD, de Jesus JM, Houston Miller N, Hubbard VS, Lee IM, Lichtenstein AH, Loria CM, Millen BE, Nonas CA, Sacks FM, Smith SC Jr, Svetkey LP, Wadden TA, Yanovski SZ, Kendall KA, Morgan LC, Trisolini MG, Velasco G, Wnek J, Anderson JL, Halperin JL, Albert NM, Bozkurt B, Brindis RG, Curtis LH, DeMets D, Hochman JS, Kovacs RJ, Ohman EM, Pressler SJ, Sellke FW, Shen WK, Smith SC Jr, Tomaselli GF, American College of Cardiology, American Heart Association Task Force on Practice Guidelines (2014) 2013 AHA/ACC guideline on lifestyle management to reduce cardiovascular risk: a report of the American College of Cardiology/American Heart Association Task Force on Practice Guidelines. Circulation 129:S79–S99
3. Centers for Medicare & Medicaid Services (2014) Decision memo for cardiac rehabilitation (CR) programs – chronic heart failure (CAG-00437N). www.cms.gov/medicare-coverage-database/details/nca-decisionmemo.aspx?NCAId=270
4. Institute of Medicine, Committee on Standards for Developing Trustworthy Clinical Practice Guidelines: Graham R, Mancher M, Miller Wolman D, Greenfield S, Steinberg E (eds) (2011) Clinical practice guidelines we can trust. National Academies Press, Washington DC
5. Schwartz D, Flamant R, Lellouch J (1980) Clinical trials. Academic Press, New York
6. Pocock SJ (1983) Clinical trials: a practical approach. Wiley, New York
7. Shapiro SH, Louis TA (1983) Clinical trials: issues and approaches. Marcel Dekker, New York
8. Meinert CL (2013) Clinical trials handbook: Design and conduct. Wiley, Hoboken
9. Ascione FJ (2001) Principles of scientific literature evaluation: critiquing clinical drug trials. American Pharmaceutical Association, Washington DC
10. Chin R (2005) Principles and practice of clinical trial design. A textbook of clinical research medicine. Boston Academic Publishing, Boston
11. Alves WM, Skolnick BE (2005) Handbook of neuroemergency clinical trials. Academic Press, Cambridge
12. Piantadosi S (2017) Clinical trials: a methodologic perspective, 3rd edn. Wiley, Hoboken
13. Matthews JNS (2008) Introduction to randomized controlled clinical trials, 2nd edn. Chapman & Hall/CRC, Boca Raton
14. Wang D, Bakhai A (2006) Clinical trials: a practical guide to design, analysis, and reporting. Remedica, London
15. Jadad AR, Enkin MW (2007) Randomized controlled trials. Questions, answers and musings, 2nd edn. Blackwell/BMJ, Malden
16. Machin D, Day S, Green S (2006) Textbook of clinical trials, 2nd edn. Wiley, Chicester
17. Woodbury-Harris KM, Coull BM (2009) Clinical trials in the neurosciences. Karger, Basel
18. Hackshaw AK (2009) A concise guide to clinical trials. Wiley Blackwell/BMJ, Hoboken
19. Domanski M, McKinlay S (2009) Successful randomized trials. A handbook for the 21st century. Lippincott Williams & Wilkins, Philadelphia
20. Friedman LM, Furberg CD, DeMets D, Reboussin DM, Granger CB (2015) Fundamentals of clinical trials, 5th edn. Springer, Cham

21. Machin D, Fayers PM (2010) Randomized clinical trials: design, practice, and reporting. Wiley Blackwell, Hoboken
22. Chin R, Bairu M (2011) Global clinical trials. Effective implementation and management. Academic Press, Cambridge
23. Peace KE, Chen DG (2010) Clinical trials methodology. Chapman & Hall/CRC, Boca Raton
24. van Belle G, Kerr KF (2012) Design and analysis of experiments in the health sciences. Wiley, Hoboken
25. Ventegodt S (2012) Randomized clinical trials & placebo: can you trust the drugs are working and safe? Nova Science, New York
26. Harrington D (2012) Designs for clinical trials. Perspectives on current issues. Springer, New York
27. Hulley SB, Cummings SR, Browner WS, Grady DG, Newman TB (2013) Designing clinical research, 4th edn. Lippincott Williams & Wilkins, Philadelphia
28. Chow SC, Liu JP (2014) Design and analysis of clinical trials: concepts and methodologies, 3rd edn. Wiley, Hoboken
29. Moher D, Hopewell S, Schulz KF, Montori V, Gotzsche PC, Devereaux PJ, Elbourne D, Egger M, Altman DG (2010) CONSORT 2010 explanation and elaboration: updated guidelines for reporting parallel group randomised trials. BMJ 340:c869. https://doi.org/10.1136/bmj.c869
30. Montgomery P, Grant S, Mayo-Wilson E, Macdonald G, Michie S, Hopewell S, Moher D, on behalf of the CONSORT-SPI Group (2018) Reporting randomised trials of social and psychological interventions: the CONSORT-SPI 2018 extension. Trials 19:407. https://doi.org/10.1186/s13063-018-2733-1
31. Freedland KE (2020) Purpose-guided trial design in health-related behavioral intervention research. Health Psych 39:539–548
32. Schuler P, Buckley B (2015) Re-engineering clinical trials. Best practices for streamlining drug development. Academic Press, London
33. Shadish WR, Cook TD, Campbell DT (2002) Experimental and quasi-experimental designs for generalized causal inference. Houghton Mifflin, Boston
34. Feyerabend PK (1981) Problems of empiricism. Philosophical papers, volume 2. Cambridge University Press, Cambridge
35. Gartlehner G, Hansen RA, Nissman D, Lohr KN, Carey TS (2006) Criteria for distinguishing effectiveness from efficacy trials in systematic reviews. AHRQ Publication No. 06-0046, Rockville
36. Wieland LS, Berman BM, Altman DG, Barth J, Bouter LM, D'Adamo CR, Linde K, Moher D, Mullins CD, Treweek S, Tunis S, van der Windt DA, Zwarenstein M, Witt C (2017) Rating of included trials on the efficacy-effectiveness spectrum: development of a new tool for systematic reviews. J Clin Epidemiol 84:95–104
37. Gitlin LN, Czaja SJ (2016) Behavioral intervention research. Designing, evaluating, and implementing. Springer, New York
38. Areán PA, Kraemer HC (2013) High-quality pyschotherapy research: From conception to piloting to national trials. Oxford University Press, New York
39. Boutron I, Ravaud P, Moher D (2012) Randomized clinical trials of nonpharmacological treatments. Chapman & Hall/CRC, Boca Raton
40. Nezu AM, Nezu CM (2008) Evidence-based outcome research: a practical guide to conducting randomized controlled trials for psychosocial interventions. Oxford University Press, Oxford
41. Torgerson DJ, Torgerson CJ (2008) Designing randomised trials in health, education and the social sciences. An introduction. Palgrave Macmillan, New York

Chapter 3
Behavioral Treatment Development

Derived from the Dutch verb quacken (to boast), "quack" is a word people use to describe medical charlatans. Quacks peddled adulterated and mislabeled medicines throughout the United States without penalty until 1906 when the Congress passed the Food and Drug Act that outlawed the practice [1]. In the United States, the Food and Drug Administration (FDA) regulates a vast array of products, including drugs, medical devices, and some dietary supplements, foods, and cosmetics. However, there is no regulation for medically indicated behavioral treatments for chronic diseases. Thus, it is difficult for consumers to distinguish between behavioral treatments that work and ineffective treatments promoted by behavioral "quacks."

> ### Fundamental Point
>
> *Development of behavioral treatments for chronic diseases is a cross-disciplinary, translational process featuring a progression of questions, a variety of study designs linked to them, and lots of tinkering. The aim of this process is to provide the evidence needed to determine if it is plausible that a behavioral treatment can improve an important clinical outcome, and it is feasible to answer this question in a rigorous, randomized efficacy trial.*

This chapter proposes a progressive, translational model for developing behavioral treatments for chronic diseases. It begins by describing the long-standing, evolving, and widely accepted process of drug development. It then draws on basic elements of this process to present the revised ORBIT model for developing behavioral treatments for chronic diseases. This model pushes toward *Phase III* behavioral efficacy testing in three progressive phases: (1) *Discovery* of an important clinical problem and a basic science underpinning for a behavioral treatment that could solve it; (2) *Design* of the treatment by first assembling basic elements and then refining them to enhance efficiency without sacrificing efficacy; and (3)

© Springer Nature Switzerland AG 2021 27
L. H. Powell et al., *Behavioral Clinical Trials for Chronic Diseases*,
https://doi.org/10.1007/978-3-030-39330-4_3

Preliminary Testing of a fixed protocol using proof-of-concept studies, feasibility studies, and *Phase II* behavioral trials with behavioral and biomedical outcomes. Recommendations for fostering translational behavioral treatment research are suggested for funding agencies, publication practices, and investigators.

SCIENTIFIC PRINCIPLE

The Drug Development Model

The process of drug development has evolved in response to public health need and is now widely accepted and well regulated. It provides an excellent model for a process of developing a behavioral treatment for a chronic disease, a process which is considerably less well understood and accepted.

Regulations Protect Consumers

US federal regulations are intended to protect consumers from falling victim to fraud and misrepresentation (Table 3.1) [1–3]. Regulations respond to the evolving need for consumer protection. In the early 1900s, the goal was to insure drug *purity* to protect consumers from the proliferation of medicinal products of unknown composition. In the late 1930s, the goal was *safety* to protect consumers from accidents such as the deaths of 107 persons from sulfanilamide, an antibiotic drug whose toxicity had been known. In the early 1960s, the goal was to insure *efficacy* and to put the burden of proof on the manufacturer to support the claim that a drug was safe and efficacious. This was triggered by the epidemic of birth defects and deaths in infants that resulted from the drug thalidomide. Since the burden of proof was now on the manufacturer, throughout the 1970s and 1980s, *guidelines for scientific quality* were issued by the FDA. In the late 1980s and 1990s, *acceleration* of the process of approval was demanded by consumers who were facing urgent threats to life in the face of the AIDS epidemic [4]. Since AIDS was an international problem, *harmonization of standards* for the drug approval across countries was facilitated by the formation of the International Congress on Harmonisation [5].

Public health crises and the need for consumer protection triggered regulatory actions to insure the purity, safety, efficacy, and rapid dissemination of drugs. Behavioral treatments for chronic diseases have not been heavily regulated, possibly because they are unlikely to be used in the face of acute public health crises to save lives. This leaves the purity, safety, efficacy, and standardization of behavioral treatments unregulated.

Table 3.1 History of drug legislation

Goal	Public Health Crisis	Legislation	Actions
Ensure Purity	Proliferation of drugs of unknown composition	Food and Drug Administration Act (1906)	Drug was required to meet standards for strength and purity. Burden of proof on the regulators.
Assure Safety	Accidental deaths from the antibiotic sulfanilamide	Federal Food, Drug, and Cosmetic Act (1938)	Drug was required to be safe, with penalty for fraudulent or misleading claims. Burden of proof on the regulators.
Promote Efficacy	Deaths and birth defects from thalidomide	Kefauver-Harris Amendment (1962)	Drug was required to be safe and efficacious. Burden of proof on the manufacturer.
		FDA Guidelines (1970s–1980s)	Guidelines for quality of scientific data including: investigator qualifications, trial management, patient safeguards, and adherence and protocol monitoring.
Encourage Dissemination	Need for rapid response to AIDS epidemic	FDA Regulation (1987)	"Accelerated" approval if drug provides benefit over existing treatments on surrogate endpoints.
		FDA Modernization Act (1997)	"Fast-track" approval if drug concerns a serious or life-threatening condition.
		International Congress on Harmonisation (1995–present)	A forum for harmonizing standards for drug approval across countries.

The Process of Drug Development

Table 3.2 summarizes the widely accepted process of drug development [6]. It begins with a period of *Discovery* during which a link is made between a therapeutic need and a drug candidate. Promising compounds progress to a *Non-clinical* phase characterized by testing in vitro and in animals for biologic activity and safety. These studies form the basis for the case made to the FDA to obtain approval to test the drug in humans. *Human Pharmacology* studies focus on closely monitored healthy volunteers to evaluate human safety and pharmacology. Success in healthy subjects justifies progression to patients. *Therapeutic Exploratory* studies focus on a small number of highly selected and closely watched patients to provide a preliminary understanding of safety and efficacy. The cost of high failure rates in these early studies of humans is minimized by keeping them small and studying accessible subjects, often in quasi-experimental pre-post designs. These small studies do,

Table 3.2   The process of drug development

Phase: Objective	Central Goal	Common Methods	Milestone
Discovery	Identify a promising candidate	Integration of clinical need with advances in pathophysiology, pharmacology, computer science, and chemistry	Drug has desired biologic activity
Non-Clinical	Non-human safety and biological activity	Animal and laboratory studies in vitro, ex vitro, in vivo	FDA permission to test drug in humans
Phase I: **Human Pharmacology**	In healthy volunteers, short-term safety, tolerability, pharmacokinetics, pharmacodynamics	Short-term studies of a small number of healthy subjects who serve as their own controls and are monitored carefully for dose-response and drug interactions	Drug is safe and has biologic activity in healthy humans
Phase II: **Therapeutic Exploratory**	In patients, short-term safety, tolerability, and efficacy	Short-term studies of a small number of well-defined patients who serve as their own controls and are carefully monitored on surrogate endpoints	Drug is safe and has biologic activity in patients
Phase III: **Therapeutic Confirmatory**	In diverse patients, safety and efficacy on clinical endpoints over long-term use	Randomized efficacy trial with morbidity/mortality outcomes	FDA permission to market the drug as therapy for an important clinical endpoint
Phase IV: **Therapeutic Use**	Refine risk/benefit and implementation in general populations and in special populations and environments	Registries, electronic medical records, randomized trials, pharmacoeconomic studies	Ongoing optimization and refinement

however, provide the clinical evidence needed to justify a *Phase III Therapeutic Confirmatory* efficacy trial which investigates the impact of the drug on clinically meaningful endpoints in a larger, more diverse sample of patients using a rigorous, randomized design. These *Phase III* trials are the key to FDA approval and introduction into the commercial market [3, 6]. *Therapeutic Use* studies conduct ongoing monitoring to identify rare side effects and need for optimization for special populations or real-world conditions. Since these studies often draw on big data sources such as registries and electronic medical records, they are likely to become increasingly common in the future.

General Features of the Drug Development Process

The drug development process has several features that are known, accepted, and expected in the effort to bring a drug to market.

Multidisciplinary Collaboration

The time, cost, and range of studies needed to bring a drug to market make it obvious that this is a multidisciplinary effort. Close connections between clinical medicine and basic science are forged by the "clinician-scientist" training model which features didactic instruction at the intersection of basic and clinical research with forward and backward translation from clinic to lab and vice versa [7]. Sophistication in solving emerging problems is enhanced by, among other things, computer science, information technology, and bioinformatics. Standards for quality of evidence have been set by methodologists in basic science, epidemiology, and biostatistics, are accepted by scientists and stakeholders throughout the world, and serve to regulate industry's profit-oriented goals.

High Failure Rates

Drug development is an uphill battle that is costly in time and money. The Tufts Center for the Study of Drug Development Research reported an average clinical phase duration of 6.8 years across all types of drugs [8]. Price Waterhouse Coopers estimates that the cost to bring a single drug to market now exceeds $1.3 billion [8]. This is due, in large part, to high failure rates which are increasing over time [9] and are most common in *Phase III* efficacy trials and in drugs for chronic diseases [10]. Among drugs that survive long enough to be tested in humans, 80% fail to receive FDA approval [8]. Calls for reform include more intensive surveillance in early phase studies to reduce later, and more costly, failures [8].

Progressive Development

Drug development is a logical, but not necessarily linear, progression of small early studies that are used to support and plan for larger, more definitive trials. International guidelines proposed by the International Conference of Harmonisation [5] encouraged a shift away from classifying studies by phases (e.g., *Phase I, Phase II*) and toward their classification by purpose (e.g., *Exploratory, Confirmatory*) because a study with the same purpose may occur at several different phases. The goal is for approval to market the drug, which generally requires at least one well-designed *Phase III* clinical trial with additional supporting evidence. Marketing of the drug is planned well before the drug is introduced into the market by studying need, demand, pricing, appeal, and accessibility.

Progressive development has two important features. First, it *minimizes the costs of failure*. In the face of suboptimal results, there is relatively low risk in refining and trying again if the study, and its budget, is small. Second, it studies *signal under a progression of noise*. A weak signal under highly controlled conditions may lead to a judgment of futility. But a strong signal under highly controlled conditions fosters interest in progressing to less controlled conditions to study erosion of the signal and explore refinements that may potentiate it. An understanding of the range of signal-to-noise ratios can inform decisions about whether any gain in disease management is worth the effort needed to optimize use.

CHALLENGES FOR BEHAVIORAL TRIALS

Some have come to believe that there would be distinct advantages if regulatory approval was required for medically justified behavioral treatments for chronic diseases [11]. They argue that while a number of official documents describe criteria for evidence-based treatments, there is no regulatory system for introducing these treatments into practice. Thus, advances made in prevention research in the past decades are not reflected in a parallel improvement in practice, and there is a proliferation of ineffective preventive treatments available to patients. Allocation of resources for the delivery of ineffective treatments is of particular concern in the context of overstretched healthcare systems. A regulatory system that evaluates behavioral treatments in a way that is logically consistent with the evaluation of drug therapies could enhance the translation of behavioral treatments from research into practice.

Multiple Perspectives on Behavioral Treatment Development

A number of investigators have proposed processes for developing evidence to support a behavioral treatment [12–23]. These efforts to standardize have two general characteristics.

Discipline-Specific Models

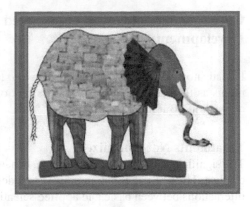

In the metaphor of the blind men and the elephant, the blind men attempted to figure out what they were observing by focusing on only one particular part of the elephant. Those who examined the ear said it was a fan, and those who examined the tail said it was a rope (see box). This is an apt metaphor for current attempts to standardize the process of behavioral treatment development. Each effort examines a different part of this complex process. Some are specific to the problem, focusing on treatments for obesity [16] or drug abuse [17]. Some are specific to the treatment, focusing on psychotherapy for mental health problems [18]. Some are specific to the disease, focusing on cancer [19] or chronic diseases [15]. Some focus on early treatment development, including intervention mapping [20, 21], multiphase optimization [22], or mixed methods [23], while others focus on later phases of treatment development [13, 14]. Basic elements of these discipline- and time-specific models are fundamentally compatible. But there have been no efforts directed toward harmonization of them.

Culture-Specific Models

Scientific understanding is embedded within cultural traditions which have their own unique spirit of inquiry [14, 24]. In behavioral treatment development, two traditions predominate. Translational research focuses on health outcomes and develops treatments progressively. Efficacy is a prerequisite for effectiveness. Without knowing if a treatment works under optimum conditions, a null result in real-world conditions could be explained either by an inefficacious treatment or by an implementation failure [14]. In contrast, social program evaluation focuses on a variety of health and social outcomes embedded in dynamic, real-world systems. Although randomized designs are preferred, they can be foregone in the face of complex interventions, poorly understood causal mechanisms, difficulties in reaching widely dispersed target populations, and the fact that many social programs have already been implemented before any evaluations have been conducted [13].

Consequences of Not Being Guided by a Model for Treatment Development

Investigators have the freedom to develop, test, and implement behavioral treatments as they see fit. This freedom is part of what makes an academic career so compelling. But it comes at a price.

Treatments Not Optimized

The significance and sophistication of a behavioral treatment is a cross-disciplinary product. The popular clinician-scientist model in the biomedical sciences cultivates interactions between basic and applied scientists. But it is uncommon in the behavioral sciences, thus making crosstalk difficult. Without an in-depth understanding of pressing medical problems faced in clinical practice, the significance of a behavioral treatment in solving these problems may be underestimated. Without an awareness of fundamental processes underlying maintenance, motivation, emotion, self-regulation, and decision-making, the strength and sophistication of behavioral treatments may not be optimized.

Progressive development maximizes strength. Observation leads to hypothesis formation, testing, refutation, and then a new, more refined hypothesis [25]. The culture that has emerged in behavioral treatment development is less progressive and more consistent with "one fell swoop" research. Funders, reviewers, and investigators all converge on the strategy of answering all relevant questions in one trial with one standard design. New treatments are often tested in noisy real-world settings with stringent control groups, stacking the odds against their success and running a high risk of abandonment in the face of failure. Promising treatments are untested in rigorous and influential *Phase III* efficacy trials. Without incentives to push toward *Phase III* efficacy trials, the behavioral treatment has not been subjected to the ultimate gold standard in medicine, the ticket to publication in high-visibility medical journals, and the key to implementation in clinical practice.

Variable Standards for "Evidence Based"

Standards for the quality of the scientific evidence for a new drug are consistent across regulatory agencies, professional societies that set practice guidelines, and third-party payers. But the quality of evidence to support a new behavioral treatment is often "in the eye of the beholder." Standards for the quality of a single behavioral trial have been established [12, 13, 26]. The US Preventive Services Task Force issues guidelines for elements of effective treatments (www.ahrq.gov). The National Registry of Evidence-Based Programs and Practices provides a list of programs for mental health and substance use interventions rated by the quality of the evidence (https://knowledge.samhsa.gov/ta.centers/national-registry-evidence-based-programs-and-practices). But there remains a vagueness about what is, and what is not, an "evidence-based" behavioral treatment. To say that a behavioral treatment is "evidence-based" can mean that it has support from several high-quality *Phase III* clinical trials, one low-quality *Phase II* clinical trial, a quasi-experimental community study, a pilot study, or an observational study.

Vulnerable Patients

The absence of an accepted chain of scientific evidence supporting the safety and efficacy of a behavioral treatment leaves patients vulnerable on several fronts. They are vulnerable to "quacks" who offer treatments that sound attractive but lack evidence to support their claims (see box). Half of the recommendations made on popular medical talk shows such as *"The Doctors"* and *"Dr. Oz"* have either

Vulnerable Patients
A "quick-fix" weight loss product called Sensa Weight Loss Crystals was fined and forced off of the market for "false and deceptive advertising" but not before the company turned a $4.6 billion profit [27].

no evidence to support them or are contradicted by the best medical evidence, and conflicts of interest are rarely disclosed [28]. On the *"Dr Oz"* show, 43.2% of the advice offered is for such behavioral risk factors as diet or weight loss [28]. Without regulation, these claims can be made without fear of legal ramifications. Patients are vulnerable to harms which could range from a serious adverse event, such as mortality, to the time and money wasted for an ineffective treatment. But the ultimate vulnerability for patients is the need to make decisions based upon inadequate data. They must decide, on their own, whether or not to try a behavioral treatment on the faith that its claims are valid, it is safe, and its costs in time and money will be justified by its benefits for health.

OVERCOMING THESE CHALLENGES IN A BEHAVIORAL TRIAL

The ORBIT Model for Developing Behavioral Treatments for Chronic Diseases

Background

When the purpose of a behavioral treatment is to improve a chronic disease outcome, treatment development is well suited to a translational research tradition, and the Obesity-Related Behavioral Intervention Trials (ORBIT) model is useful as a guide for the process [15]. Like all of the comparable models for behavioral treatment development, ORBIT is specific rather than general. Because a defining feature is the focus on chronic disease as a primary outcome, it has been aligned closely with the process of drug development, using similar basic principles and terminology. Because the biggest gap in knowledge exists in the pre-efficacy phases of behavioral treatment development, this is the primary focus. Although the model was developed within the context of obesity, the process can be applied to any behavioral treatment aimed at improving any chronic disease outcome.

Development of the ORBIT model was a collaboration between multidisciplinary academic researchers and program officers at the National Institutes of Health (NIH). (*See Appendix at the end of this chapter*.) The rationale for this collaboration was that issues in behavioral treatment development are fundamentally multidisciplinary, requiring infrastructure support that is typically provided at the federal level. Recognizing the importance of behavioral treatment development, the NIH Office of Behavioral and Social Sciences Research (OBSSR), in collaboration with the National Heart, Lung, and Blood Institute (NHLBI), the National Cancer Institute (NCI), the National Institute of Diabetes, Digestive and Kidney Diseases (NIDDK), the *Eunice Kennedy Shriver* National Institute of Child Health and Human Development (NICHD), and investigators from the U01 ORBIT consortium organized, in 2010, a cross-disciplinary conference of experts in fields related to the development and early testing of behavioral treatments for chronic diseases. An important goal of this conference was to propose guidelines for developing behavioral treatments to prevent or manage chronic diseases. Areas of emphasis included the identification of innovative approaches to solving important clinical problems based on basic behavioral science theory and research, the design and preliminary testing of promising treatments, and readiness to conduct a *Phase III* behavioral efficacy trial. Conference participants included members of the ORBIT consortium, NIH program officers, and experts in discoveries, designs, methodologies, and infrastructures needed to develop and test innovative, health-related behavioral treatments (Conference information can be found at http://www.nihorbit.org/ORBIT%20 Content/Workshops%20and%20Conferences.aspx?PageView=Shared).

Overview

Figure 3.1 presents the revised ORBIT model for behavioral treatment development. It is a progressive approach characterized by purpose-guided phases. The intent is to guide the collection of a chain of evidence needed to support the case that a behavioral treatment could improve a chronic disease endpoint.

The purpose-guided phases are modeled after the widely-accepted phases of drug development [6]. The *Discovery* phase encourages creative insights about significant questions, and strong treatments through multidisciplinary crosstalk among medical clinicians, basic scientists, applied scientists, and theoreticians. The *Design* phase is characterized by a focus on the dimensions of a treatment. It features a fluid, exploratory define phase where tinkering (i.e., fiddling or playing with a treatment) during the course of systematic observation is at a premium, followed by a refine phase where the goal is to maximize the efficiency with which a treatment is delivered without losing efficacy. The milestone for completion of the *Design* phase is a fixed treatment ready to begin efficacy testing accompanied by a quantified pathway by which the treatment is hypothesized to translate into a chronic disease outcome. The *Preliminary Testing* phase features progressive testing, moving from small and inexpensive early tests to larger, more expensive, and conclusive later tests.

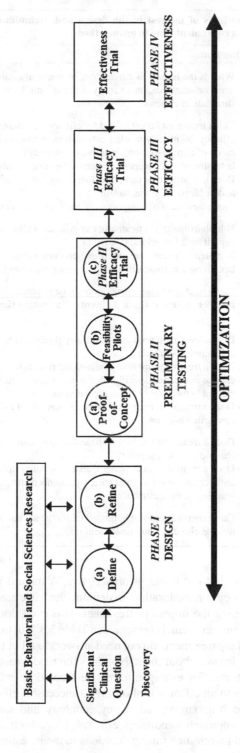

Fig. 3.1 The revised ORBIT model for development of behavioral treatments for chronic diseases

Table 3.3 Progressive questions of interest in the design and preliminary testing of a behavioral treatment and a convenient time to answer them

Timing	Questions
Exploratory studies *Phase Ia*	– What is the impact of a treatment, or potential treatment components or strategies, on a variety of behavioral, biomedical, and/or surrogate endpoints?
Refinement studies *Phase Ib*	– Can a treatment be optimized for efficiency, without losing efficacy, by modifying elements such as number of components, mode of administration, duration, or intensity? – Is treatment effectiveness moderated by diverse subgroups? – Does a treatment or component affect hypothesized behavioral and/or biomedical mechanisms? – Can a treatment or component be implemented with fidelity?.
Proof-of-concept studies *Phase IIa*	– Is it plausible that a treatment can produce a clinically significant benefit on a behavioral risk factor? – Is it plausible that a treatment can produce a clinically significant benefit on a chronic disease or surrogate endpoint?.
Feasibility and Pilot studies *Phase IIb*	– Can a treatment and/or trial protocol be implemented with fidelity in different settings or at different collaborating sites?
Phase II efficacy trials *Phase IIc*	– Does a treatment produce a clinically significant benefit on a behavioral risk factor? – Does a treatment improve a behavioral risk factor better than chance alone, non-specific attention, passage of time, and/or current behavioral or biomedical treatments? – Does a treatment improve a relevant biomedical risk factor or surrogate endpoint?.
Phase III efficacy trials *Phase III*	– Does a treatment produce a clinically significant benefit on a chronic disease endpoint? – Does a treatment work better than a clinically important comparator such as the standard of care, an enhanced standard of care, a placebo, or no treatment?
Effectiveness trials *Phase IV*	– Can a treatment be implemented with efficacy and fidelity in diverse clinic or community settings?.

This model is progressive but not linear or proscriptive. A natural progression of questions evolve from a focus on exploration, to defining the basic elements of treatment, and then to evaluating the impact of treatment. This evolution of questions, and a convenient time to answer them, is presented in Table 3.3. But this is not necessarily a linear process. Many treatments do not need answers to all of these questions because much is already known about them. Nor does the model restrict the timing for asking specific questions. For example, a treatment could be refined and optimized *before* progressing to an efficacy trial or *after* a successful efficacy trial. The former "building" approach maximizes efficiency, economy, and scalability, while the latter "dismantling" approach maximizes efficacy. Since both approaches are sound, the ORBIT model leaves such timing decisions to the investigative team.

This model encourages continuous refinement and the freedom to fail. The bidirectional arrows between all phases are intended to expand investigator options, in light of results, from only "progress" or "abandon" to include the third option of "refine." In many cases, refinement in the face of failure is the seedbed for innovation rather than a cause for abandonment. Regardless of the stage of development, each new study provides an opportunity to refine. The existence of a hypothesized pathway shows where in the pathway goals might not have been met and refinement might be needed.

The ORBIT model has been refined to include *Phase II* efficacy trials among the activities of Preliminary Testing (Fig. 3.1). In the previous version of this model [15], *Phase II* efficacy trials were subsumed under the category of *Phase III* efficacy trials. This revision distinguishes *Phase II* trials, those with behavioral, biomedical, or surrogate outcomes, from *Phase III* trials which have a chronic disease outcome. This is an important and intentional distinction. The majority of trials that have been conducted on behavioral treatments are *Phase II* trials, but the standard of evidence that is required to incorporate a treatment into clinical practice is *Phase III* trials. It is hoped that this distinction will provide a rationale for encouraging progression to *Phase III* trials.

Details of the questions and methods that are characteristic of each of the purpose-guided phases follow and serve as an extension and elaboration of the original presentation of the ORBIT model [15].

Discovery

At its earliest stages, behavioral treatment development begins with the discovery that a behavioral strategy might solve an important clinical problem. Unexpected creative insights and recognition of potential are right-brain processes. This is different from the left-brain mindset of attention, focus, concentration, and linear development within which most academics live.

Discovery is propelled by the drive for exploration, the thrill of the chase, and an openness to experience. In Proust's words,

> **Creative Discovery and the Birth of Behavioral Medicine**
>
> Meyer Friedman, a respected San Francisco cardiologist practicing in the 1960s, noticed that the fabric on the seats of the chairs in his waiting room was worn out only at the front. Why? After pondering this for some time, he made the creative leap that this was a sign of time urgency. The patients were literally fidgeting on the edge of their seats when having to wait for the doctor. This gave birth to the hypothesis that coronary disease was caused, in part, by stress, one component of which was time urgency. This discovery, called Type A behavior, marked the beginning of the field of behavioral medicine.

"The real voyage of discovery is not in traveling to new lands, but in seeing old lands with new eyes."

Discovery is a non-linear, disorganized, and chaotic process with unexpected twists and turns in thinking. It is precipitated by the discomfort of a prolonged impasse in left-brain activity. A change in activity can activate the murky but infinite library of associations in the brain where the magic of right-brain processes happen [29]. Insight comes as an unexpected epiphany, in the shower or during a walk, with a remarkable degree of confidence in the rightness of the solution. This moment of sudden insight "just seems obvious" [30].

What Sparks Creativity in Entrepreneurs [31]
"A 3-mile walk. My head de-clutters and I think clearly."
"Preparing food. I get lost in the process. My brain rests and I have my best ideas."
"Reading in bed before sleep. I float into another world and my imagination flows."
"Diving in the ocean. No phone, no internet, no talking, no noise. Just the sound of my breathing and the calming lull of the ocean."
"Walking my dog. I credit him with some of my best ideas."
"Driving."
"When I am on the move, usually in the air at 30,000 feet. I consider conversations I have just had and the brand new perspectives they invite."
"Mowing the grass with a push mower. The combination of the outdoors, strength, cardio, and repetitive motion frees my mind."
"When my head is buried in data and I am exercising my brain. Sometimes something that was lying dormant inside pops out. May be unrelated… it's very funny."
"A quiet milkshake shop with a comic book. The carb boost and the creative reading give me positive energy and motivation."

Most academic environments inhibit these creative connections by placing more value on product than process. But for those inclined toward process, discovery of innovative ideas is a skill that can be nurtured [32]. It is an essential part of the earliest stages of behavioral intervention development. It is essential to the creative connection between a significant clinical problem and the possibility that it could be solved with a behavioral treatment. It is essential to the creative connection between a principle of human behavior and the application of that principle in the service of enhancing the focus, strength, and sophistication of a behavioral treatment.

Discovery of a Significant Clinical Problem

The ORBIT model encourages a close connection between applied behavioral scientists and clinicians in medical practice. Face-to-face connection is better than simply reading the medical literature. The unpredictable and uncontrollable creative process needs to be stimulated. Becoming a participant observer within a clinical context makes it possible to see the world through the eyes of a clinician and of a patient. Discovery may include the following.

- The first step in the clinical algorithms for management of blood pressure, lipids, and prediabetes is lifestyle change [33–36]. But providers often go right to the second step—drug management—because neither they, nor their patients, have much faith in, or access to, lifestyle change programs.

- Regardless of the nature of the disease, patient adherence to prescribed drug therapy hovers around only 50% [37, 38]. Provider adherence to evidence-based guidelines for drug therapy is not much better [39].

- Orthopedic surgeons are becoming interested in obesity management. Even though it is a major risk factor for hip or knee replacements, their interest is based upon the fact that obesity undercuts both peri- and postoperative surgical outcomes.

- Many neurosurgeons would welcome an effective pre-surgical smoking cessation program since smoking is associated with worse outcomes following neurosurgery.

Table 3.4 presents a way to identify a significant clinical problem. A disease may be important because of the breadth of its impact, its cost, and/or its unfavorable trends over time. There may be no current treatment for this disease. The current treatment may not be potent or durable enough to change an important clinical outcome. The current treatment may be effective, but adherence to it is poor, it has too many side effects, or is too costly for routine use. These problems could be solved by the new treatment. It targets a novel pathway or a novel risk factor. It is less costly and/or has fewer side effects than the current treatment.

Table 3.4 The argument for a significant clinical problem	
Disease	• Affects many • Affects a subgroup • Is increasing • Is increasing in a subgroup • Is not decreasing • Is costly
Current treatment	• No current treatment • Not very effective • Uncertain effectiveness (clinical equipoise) • Effective but adherence is poor • Effective but side effects are serious
New treatment	• Shows promise in preliminary work • Targets novel risk factor • Targets novel pathway • Less costly than standard • Fewer side effects

Early identification of a significant clinical problem provides an ultimate goal for a program of research. Framing the problem from a medical perspective encourages early focus on several important priorities.

- It sets sights on a *Phase III* efficacy trial to provide a conclusive test of whether or not a behavioral treatment can solve an important medical problem.

- It encourages consideration early in the developmental process of what a clinically meaningful medical outcome would be.

- It makes it possible to judge success of intermediate steps in treatment development on the ability of the behavioral treatment to improve surrogate markers of the clinically meaningful medical outcome.

- It encourages commitment to achieving a clinically significant level of behavioral change from the treatment that is potent enough to produce meaningful change on the clinically meaningful medical outcome.

Discovery of a Basic Science Basis for Treatment

A *Phase III* behavioral efficacy trial is based upon the assumption that change in a behavioral risk factor following an intervention will be potent enough to produce a clinically significant improvement on a chronic disease endpoint. The ORBIT model encourages close connections between basic and applied behavioral and social science to maximize the potency of the intervention. Traditionally, theory has formed the foundation of applied behavioral treatments. A number of theories of behavioral change exist, but they are often nonoverlapping, imprecise, not coherent with one another, not falsifiable, and not widely accepted within or across disciplines [40, 41]. Basic experimental studies, upon which theory is often based, identify specific mechanisms that drive behavior and thereby provide a more precise basis for choosing components and techniques that influence these mechanisms. Research aimed at identifying mechanisms of initiation, personalization, and maintenance of behavior change is the foundation of the NIH Science of Behavior Change (SOBC) Common Fund program [42].

Following are some examples of how the basic science of fundamental human processes can maximize the strength, integrity, sophistication, innovation, and promise of behavioral treatments.

- Neuroscience experiments show that mobilization of executive function can serve as a "brake" on impulsive eating [43]. This could form the basis of an intervention aimed at reducing impulsive eating by enhancing executive function with self-management skill training in such areas as planning and problem-solving.

- Neuroscience studies of the area of the brain engaged while making food choices have shown that patients with anorexia nervosa who choose low-calorie foods engage the dorsal striatum, the center for automatic behavior. Thus, rather than previous explanations for anorexia which focus on single-minded self-control [44], it may be firmly entrenched automatic habits that override primary hunger drives [45, 46]. A novel treatment for eating disorders would cultivate the development of new, automatic habits [47], using the principles of habit formation [48].

- Behavioral economics experiments show that people disproportionately respond to immediate rather than distal incentives [49]. Thus, motivation to engage in physical activity may be strengthened by the rationale to improve mood, rather than the rationale to lose weight or prevent a heart attack.

- Basic studies of infant cognitive development have identified six aspects of the environment that foster accelerated learning [50]. But the learning environments of older adults are often deficient in these six environmental factors. An intervention for older adults that creates an optimized learning environment featuring these six characteristics could be an innovative way to enhance learning, improve brain health, and challenge the belief that *"You can't teach old dogs new tricks"* [50].

- The DARE (Drug Abuse Resistance Education) program to prevent drug abuse in teens by having police lecture to kids in elementary school was the cornerstone of prevention between 1980 and 2009, offered in 75% of American schools, and cost taxpayers between $200 million and $2 billion. A series of meta-analyses evaluating both short- and long-term effects showed no benefit on drug abuse and the possibility of a "boomerang" effect of *encouraging* drug abuse in teens [51, 52]. Prevention scientists revised the program using a translational research model that drew on the basic science principle of interactive "learning by doing." This revision resulted in dramatic reductions in substance use, replaced the original DARE curriculum, and is now offered throughout the United States and in 44 other countries [53].

In summary, the key feature of the *Discovery* phase is crosstalk among practitioners in clinical medicine, basic behavioral and social scientists, and applied behavioral scientists. While a clinical problem can foster a search for relevant basic science guidance, basic science discoveries can inspire an application of those insights to the solution of a pressing clinical problem. Several relevant but independent basic science findings can justify a multi-component treatment, each component of which has its own treatment target and methods of accomplishing change. If early testing shows that a treatment approaches, but does not achieve, clinically significant milestones, avenues for optimization may be informed by going back to basic science insights.

The Design Phase: *Phase I*

The overall goals of the Design phase are to assemble and refine the basic features of a behavioral treatment. Subjects can be a small number of highly selected individuals who are studied intensively, rather than a more representative group. Protocols can be fluid, rather than fixed, permitting ongoing adjustments while in the course of observing, in response to evolving findings. Tinkering with a treatment to try to boost its strength, even when in the middle of systematic observation, is encouraged. Failures present opportunities to refine, at minimal cost, rather than to abandon treatments. Milestones for judging success are based upon achievement of pre-specified, clinically significant goals which are deliberately set to be ambitious in early studies to provide a needed cushion for subsequent testing in more diverse samples. This phase is divided into two parts: defining the basic elements of the treatment and refining it to improve efficiency without reducing strength.

Define the Basic Elements: *Phase Ia*

Purpose. One of Steven Covey's *7 Habits of Highly Effective People* [54] is *"Begin With the End In Mind."* To illustrate this habit, consider undertaking a road trip from Washington DC to San Francisco. The "end" is San Francisco. To get to it, the trip would most likely be guided by a GPS or some other type of roadmap. Without a map, following the sun would achieve

Tinkering	
Definition	Attempt to repair or improve something in a casual or desultory way, often to no useful effect
Usage	They tinkered endlessly with the car
Synonyms	adjust, fix, mind, play with, fiddle with mess with, trifle with, dabble, muck about, take apart

eventual success, but a roadmap would be more efficient. The implication for behavioral treatment development is to define the "end," and the roadmap for arriving at it, early in the developmental process to promote direction and efficiency. This roadmap is the hypothesized pathway. It is the essential product of the Define phase. Table 3.5 summarizes the goal, common questions, selected methods, and milestone for progression that characterize this phase.

Common Questions and Selected Methods. Some of the common questions of concern in the early Define phase of treatment development follow.

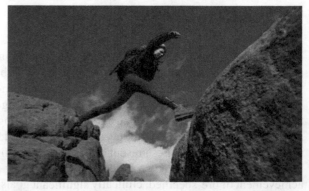

Question: What is the ultimate clinical endpoint and how much improvement on it would be clinically relevant? If the goal is to push toward a *Phase III* efficacy trial, the ultimate endpoint will likely be a disease. Rena Wing, the architect of the successful and now famous Diabetes Prevention Program [55, 56], was faced with this question early in her career. She showed this photo in her presentation, *Development of a Behavioral Clinical Trial:*

Table 3.5 Define the basic elements *(Phase Ia)*

Central Goal	Common Questions	Selected Methods	Milestone
A priori specification of the structure and goals of treatment	What is the ultimate clinical endpoint and how much improvement in it would be clinically relevant?	Clinical guidelines Meta-analyses Advice from clinicians	A quantified, hypothesized pathway by which a behavioral treatment could solve a pressing clinical problem
	What is the behavioral risk factor target that could improve the clinical endpoint and what level of improvement in it is needed to move that clinical endpoint?	Epidemiologic studies Meta-analyses Experiments Cross-sectional studies of covariation between a behavior risk factor and a surrogate disease endpoint	
	What are promising components, and strategies for change in them, that could improve this behavioral risk factor?	Basic behavioral/social science studies Theory Experiments Ecologic studies [57–59]	
	What level of implementation of these strategies is needed to achieve clinically significant improvement in the behavioral risk factor?	Small N studies [60–65]	

The Road from Discovery to Action, at the NIH-sponsored ORBIT Workshop on Treatment Development: From Ideas to Interventions. After pursuing a career studying weight loss interventions, she was told by her advisors "*You need a disease.*" This would both maximize impact on medical care and enhance funding potential within the disease-specific NIH Institutes. Because of the strong connection between obesity and diabetes, she chose diabetes. This is when she jumped from one rock (weight loss studies) to the other (weight loss for diabetes management). Her investigations shifted from studying strategies for weight loss to studying the implications of weight loss on diabetes and its biomarkers.

Specifying a disease of interest, developing sophistication on why it is a problem, and understanding the current state of the art in managing it provide the context within which a new behavioral treatment will be offered. Could the new behavioral treatment be better than existing treatments? Could it do as well as existing treatments but at less cost? Clinically relevant milestones for success in improving a disease endpoint can be identified by referencing the success rate achieved by current state-of-the-art treatments. (*See Chapter 5: Clinical Significance.*)

Question: What is the behavioral risk factor target of treatment and how much improvement in it is needed to move the clinical endpoint? The behavioral target of treatment should have a known association to a clinical endpoint; that is, it should be a *behavioral risk factor* for a chronic disease. If it is not an established risk factor, then preliminary work showing such an association, usually accomplished with epidemiologic studies, would be indicated before setting sights on a clinical trial.

A trickier task is identifying the level of change on the behavioral risk factor that is needed to move the clinical endpoint. This is a categorical, not a continuous, undertaking because improvement that is statistically significant on continuous scale may be an inadequate level of improvement to move a clinical endpoint. A target for the level of behavior change needed to reduce clinical risk is key to evaluating the success of a behavioral treatment in early developmental studies. Clinically significant cutpoints exist for established behavioral risk factors such as smoking, weight, alcohol/drug abuse, fat intake, sodium intake, physical inactivity, depression, and low social support. For example, weight loss of ≥5% of body weight in obese adults with cardiovascular disease risk factors has been shown to result in clinically meaningful cardiovascular and metabolic benefits [66]. However, in the case of novel behavioral risk factors where such an evidence base may not exist, observational studies examining covariation between the behavioral factor and a relevant biomedical risk factor would be justified. For example, a cross-sectional study of the covariation between different levels of a measure of stress and a cardio-metabolic biomarker such as blood pressure would be an important way to determine the cutpoint on a stress scale that is associated with a normal blood pressure. (*See Chapter 5: Clinical Significance.*)

Question: What components, strategies for change, and level of implementation are needed to improve the behavioral risk factor? Promising strategies for change are informed by understanding controlling antecedent conditions which can include biological, psychophysiological, psychological, neuropsychological, behavioral, social, cultural, environmental, and policy-level factors. Informant interviews and focus groups can elicit beliefs about factors that affect behavior. But watching people unobtrusively make choices as they go about their day in their naturalistic settings may be an even more powerful approach. Human-centered design [57–59] aims to make the healthy choice the easy choice by first watching people behave in their natural settings and then manipulating some aspect of that naturalistic context in the service of changing a behavior. Involvement of the consumer in the design and testing of a product was developed and refined in the field of marketing [67, 68] and then adapted to the field of behavioral medicine to foster user-centered strategies which place a premium on strength, acceptability, and feasibility [23, 69]. New applications of this approach have been made possible by advances in the technologies for connecting with people throughout their day, including ecological momentary assessment [70] and "just-in-time" adaptive interventions [71]. These methodologies facilitate the identification of treatment components, strategies for change, and critical time points for treatment delivery and outcome assessment.

The very early phases of treatment development feature intensive studies of small numbers of highly selected subjects. There has been renewed interest in small N studies, and recent investigations have shown their versatility in use, range of designs (e.g., time series, ABA, and multiple baseline), and analytic techniques [60–64]. A series of small, early phase, easy to implement studies which inform the design of a treatment is the essence of Stevens' concept of "evidentiary studies" [16]. An example would be a naturalistic observational study of physical activity in children before and after their teacher was given specialized training.

Milestone. The milestone for progression is the existence of a "roadmap" for the forthcoming program of research. This takes the form of a quantified pathway by which a new behavioral treatment is hypothesized to improve a clinical endpoint. (*See Chapter 4: Hypothesized Pathway and Bias.*)

Refine for Strength and Efficiency: *Phase Ib*

Purpose. As healthcare resources tighten, treatments that are *both* efficacious and efficient become increasingly desirable. This can be a problem of particular concern for behavioral treatments which may be strong but overly complex, or simple but too weak. The central goal of the Refine phase is to streamline a promising but complex treatment to promote efficiency while at the same time retaining sufficient strength to accomplish a clinically significant improvement on a behavioral risk factor

Common Questions and Selected Methods. Table 3.6 summarizes the goals, milestones, common questions, and selected methods that are common in the Refine phase. These types of studies are relatively common in applied behavioral science. The general format is to study dimensions of the treatment such as the optimal dose, mode, or agent of delivery, the minimum number of components needed, and adaptations to the treatment to maximize efficacy in subgroups or for non-response. In some areas, such as adapting treatment to heterogeneous response, the methodology is well-established [72]. In others, such as determining the optimum dose (i.e., the duration, frequency, and amount of treatment needed), a methodological literature is emerging [73]. If a treatment is well-established but there is interest in applying it to a new population, setting, or mode of delivery, refinement studies are ideal.

Several of the questions in Table 3.6 deserve special comment because they are important, but understudied, in refinement studies.

Question: What is the optimum timing of intervention? Finding a time to intervene when the subject is most likely to be receptive maximizes the ability of the treatment to be received and acted upon. For example, a peak learning moment can occur when a patient has "a new lease on life" after receiving a coronary artery stent that unblocks an artery. Learning moments occur during daily life when faced with repeating cues that trigger habits which, when summed over a lifetime, influence

Table 3.6 Refine for strength and efficiency *(Phase Ib)*

Central Goal	Common Questions	Selected Methods	Milestone
Refine treatment to preserve strength while maximizing efficiency	What is the optimum – Number of components? – Dose? – Duration? – Mode of delivery?	• Factorial, fractional factorial designs [74, 75] • Experiments [76] • Bayesian estimation [77, 78] • Single-case designs [60–64, 79]	Investigator satisfaction that treatment package is complete and a fixed protocol is now ready for preliminary testing
	What is the optimum timing of delivery?	• "Just-in-time" adaptive interventions [71, 80–82]	
	What is the optimum timing of assessment?	• Single-case designs [60–64, 79] • Time series designs [83]	
	How can acceptability be maximized to reduce dropouts and improve adherence?	• Randomized comparative effectiveness designs [84] • Qualitative studies [69, 85] • Human-centered design [57–59]	
	How can heterogeneity in response be reduced?	• Personalized behavioral treatments [86–88] • SMART designs [72, 89] • Adaptive interventions [90, 91] • Signal detection [92]	
	What is the impact of treatment on the complex system within which it is embedded?	• Modeling complex systems [93–95]	

health. "Just-in-time" adaptive interventions make use of mobile technology to deliver interventions when the need arises [71]. With mobile sensing technology, it is possible to track individuals as they go throughout their day, identify environmental cues that trigger unwanted behaviors, intervene in real time, and replace old habits with new ones in real time [71]. An excellent example is provided by Gustafson and colleagues [80] who track the location of young addicts who have just emerged from rehabilitation and, when they approach the place where their addicted friends congregate, deliver a series of smartphone interceptions that bolster the will to pass the temptation by.

Question: What is the optimum timing of outcome assessment? The sustainability of effects of behavioral treatments is a question at the forefront of behavioral medicine. The "checkmark" phenomenon in which short-term change is followed by a longer-term return to baseline is the rule rather than the exception. The problem is that treatments that produce powerful short-term effects which are not sustained over time are unlikely to be powerful enough to affect chronic disease endpoints which accumulate over long periods of time. Long-term studies of small numbers of subjects to describe patterns of change during and after an intervention are well suited to providing insight into this important question. Figure 3.2 portrays an array of effects that could occur after an intervention (I) is concluded. Analytic procedures drawn from engineering can quantify these patterns over time to determine the appropriate timing for outcome assessment [96]. More importantly for the treatment developer, understanding that the effects of treatment are either short-term, delayed, or variable can encourage interest in refining for the purpose of producing more enduring effects. Single-case designs [60–64] and time series designs [83] offer low-cost options for studying evolution of effects over long periods of time in small numbers of subjects.

Question: How can heterogeneity in response be reduced? Identification of moderators of treatment is an aim for a refinement study, not a confirmatory clinical trial. A significant moderator indicates that treatment worked better for one sub-

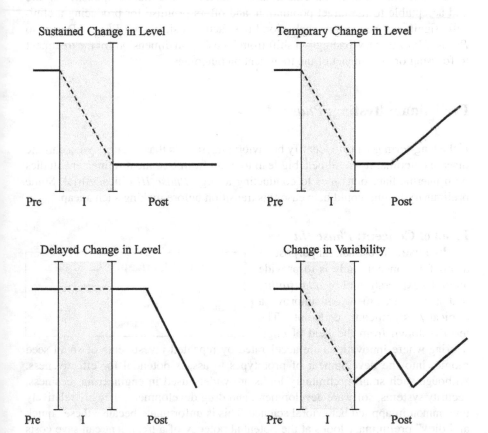

Fig. 3.2 Varieties of intervention (I) effects

group than it did for another. This jeopardizes efficacy in a clinical trial which is usually powered on the assumption that on average all treated participants will respond and, at best, considers only the effect of dropouts, not non-adherers, in the determination of sample size. If moderator effects are identified in refinement studies, they provide the basis for tailoring treatment to improve subgroup response. Readiness for a confirmatory *Phase II* or *Phase III* behavioral efficacy trial is signaled when treatment has been optimized for all important subgroups. The methods for studying heterogeneity in response to treatment are developing rapidly. Signal detection methods can identify subgroups for whom tailoring of treatment could optimize outcomes [92]. Adaptive designs provide the methodology for identifying decision rules for potentiating treatment in the face of non-response, giving rise to adaptive treatments which go beyond a "one-size-fits-all" approach to behavioral treatments [72].

Milestone. The essential milestone for moving to *Phase II* Preliminary Testing is the satisfaction of the investigative team that it has a fixed treatment package that needs no further refinement. This treatment includes essential components, is safe and acceptable to the target population, and offers promise for producing a clinically significant benefit on a behavioral risk factor. A shift from *Phase I* Design to *Phase II* Preliminary Testing is a shift from focusing on dimensions of the treatment to focusing on the impact of the treatment on outcomes

Preliminary Testing: *Phase II*

If the long-term goal is to identify behavioral treatments that can improve a chronic disease outcome, it would be a big leap to jump from treatment refinement studies with intermediate outcomes to conducting a large *Phase III* efficacy trial. Some preliminary testing could help ease this transition before making such a leap.

Proof of Concept: *Phase IIa*

Purpose. The essential purpose of a proof-of-concept study is to provide an initial exploration of the *plausibility* that a fixed treatment can improve a clinically significant endpoint. The term is drawn from the field of engi-

> **Proof of Concept: Rationale**
>
> A comparator is useless when a behavioral treatment is too weak to warrant any comparison.

neering where innovations are accelerated by repeated investments of small seed monies into the development of prototypes to assess potential for effectiveness. Although such small preliminary looks are widely used in engineering, business, security systems, software development, and drug development, they are relatively uncommon in applied behavioral science. This is unfortunate because these "quick and dirty" preliminary looks at the potential potency of a treatment can save costs and foster innovation through refinement. Indeed, if the end game is to improve a chronic disease endpoint, it is a waste of time and resources to conduct a randomized study of a treatment that is too weak to affect such an endpoint. A comparator is useless when a treatment is too weak to warrant any comparison.

A common design for a proof-of-concept study is a small, quasi-experimental, pre-post comparison where the outcome is whether or not a clinically significant goal was met. Sample size calculations are unnecessary because no statistical hypothesis testing is conducted. Proof-of-concept studies are not intended to provide solid "proof" that the intervention works. It is acceptable for threats to internal validity to be present. Small select samples limit generalizability of results. Absence of a comparator leaves unanswered such questions as whether participants would get better over time on their own. Clinical, rather than statistical, tests are used to judge results, raising the possibility that any changes were due to chance alone.

But the goal of this design is not to answer any of these questions. It is simply to determine whether or not there is any merit in going forward with a more rigorous randomized study to answer them. Since the resources needed to conduct these small studies are minimal, they provide an ideal bridge between early studies aimed at designing and refining a treatment and rigorous testing using randomized designs.

Common Questions and Selected Methods. Table 3.7 summarizes the goal, question, methods, and milestone for proof-of-concept studies. The key goal is to determine whether or not it is plausible that a treatment can achieve a clinically significant improvement in a behavioral risk factor target of treatment or a surrogate clinical outcome.

Table 3.7 Proof of concept (*Phase IIa*)

Central Goal	Common Questions	Selected Methods	Milestones
Clinically significant signal	In a small, highly selected sample, is it plausible that a fixed treatment package can produce a clinically significant improvement in a behavioral risk factor or clinical endpoint?	• Quasi-experimental treatment-only pre-post design [97] • N-of-1 time series [98].	Clinical significance justifies proceeding to a randomized trial

Question: In a small, selected sample, can this treatment produce a clinically significant improvement on a behavioral or biomedical risk factor? There are four basic elements of a proof-of-concept test: (1) a pretreatment baseline; (2) a post-treatment follow-up; (3) a clinically significant cutpoint on the behavioral or clinical target of treatment; and (4) a small number of accessible subjects. In quasi-experimental, within-subjects designs, subjects act as their own controls in a pre-post treatment comparison. The sample size can be small since clinical, not statistical, benefit is sought, thus obviating the need for sample size calculations. The sample can be selected from accessible subjects, rather than representative subjects, because this initial test will determine only whether the treatment merits further, more rigorous testing. The focus is placed *only* on the treatment and whether it can produce clinically significant change. The question of *why* any change might have occurred (e.g., the passage of time; non-specific attention, etc.) is dealt with in subsequent randomized designs.

Figure 3.3 provides an example. The aim of this study was to determine if it was plausible that a smartphone intervention could produce clinically meaningful adherence to asthma controller medication in inner-city teens with asthma [99]. The study was supported by a very small institutional grant permitting the assessment of only four subjects in a pre-post,

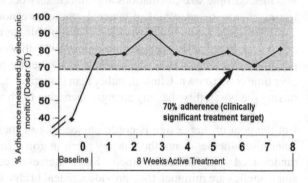

Fig. 3.3 Adherence to drug therapy during run-in and after introduction of treatment, in four subjects

quasi-experimental design. The milestone for judging success was provided by clinical guidelines in allergy and immunology, which indicate that ≥70% adherence to controller medication for asthma is needed to achieve a clinical benefit. It can be seen that compared to a run-in baseline of only 40% adherence, the introduction of the smartphone treatment was associated with a clinically significant benefit of >70% adherence.

This small study can be criticized on a variety of fronts. Perhaps this dramatic benefit was an historical trend that had nothing to do with the actual treatment under investigation. This was not a representative sample. It may have been a highly-selected and highly-motivated sample, unlike most inner-city teens. Because there was no statistical analysis, it is unclear whether the results could have occurred by chance alone. Because there was no control for attention, results may be due to non-specific attention. These are legitimate questions that need to be answered. But the point here is that this small study increased interest in answering them. Under further investigation, the treatment *might* work again, but maybe it would not. To answer this question, a larger, more diverse sample using a randomized design is needed. Alternatively, had this intervention not demonstrated a clinically significant effect, it would be a waste of time and money to test it in a larger randomized trial without further refinement.

Studies such as this one can be embedded into treatment development or career development grants and can serve as part of preliminary studies that justify support for a randomized study. The study presented in Fig. 3.3 provided the basis for receipt of an NIH career development K-award to the investigator.

Milestone. If a behavioral treatment achieves clinically significant benefit on a behavioral risk factor, this provides the milestone for moving forward for more preliminary testing of this fixed protocol. If this milestone was approached, but not achieved, all that may be needed might be small adjustments to justify forward movement to randomized pilot testing. If the clinical criterion was not even approached, return to earlier developmental studies (*Phase I*) or a decision to abandon the treatment may be indicated.

Feasibility and Pilot Studies: *Phase IIb*
The term "pilot study" has come to be a vague term, meaning a variety of different things ranging from a miniature efficacy trial to a feasibility study. The importance of preparatory work before undertaking a *Phase II* or *Phase III* efficacy trial makes it imperative to reduce confusion and promote clarity. Thus, a chapter in this book has been devoted to this important topic. (*See Chapter 7: Feasibility and Pilot Studies.*)

Phase II Efficacy Trials: *Phase IIc*
Purpose The ORBIT model in Fig. 3.1 presents an important revision to the original model [15]. It now includes *Phase II* behavioral efficacy trials among the activities in the Preliminary Testing phase. The *Phase II* behavioral trial is the concomitant of the *Phase II* drug trial. On the drug side, the aim is to determine if the drug has its intended biologic effect on a surrogate endpoint [100]. On the behavioral side, the aim is to determine if the behavioral intervention has its intended effect on a behavioral risk factor, biologic mediator, or relevant surrogate endpoint.

Common Questions and Selected Methods. It is easiest to understand ORBIT *Phase II* efficacy trials by comparing them to *Phase I* refinement studies and *Phase III* efficacy trials (Table 3.8)

Table 3.8 Comparison of three types of randomized behavioral studies			
	Phase I Refinement	*Phase II* Efficacy	*Phase III* Efficacy
Aim	Relative value of various treatment elements	Efficacy in reducing behavioral or biological risk	Efficacy in improving a definitive clinical outcome
Outcome	Behavioral risk factor or biological mediator	Behavioral risk factor, biological mediator, or surrogate endpoint	Chronic condition or disease
Comparator	Compares different treatment elements	Controls for non-specific factors or compares to existing treatments	Compares to existing practice
Function	Optimization of treatment to enhance efficiency while preserving efficacy	Prerequisite for *Phase III* trial	Prerequisite for effectiveness trial or introduction into clinical practice

Refinement studies focus on treatment. Efficacy trials focus on outcome. Refinement studies aim to identify optimum elements of treatment by comparing such things as different components, modes of administration, durations, and intensities. *Phase II* efficacy trials aim to determine whether a behavioral treatment can produce a clinically significant improvement in behavioral or biomedical risk, and whether or not it is better than non-specific factors or other existing treatments. *Phase III* efficacy trials aim to determine whether or not a behavioral treatment can produce a clinically significant improvement in a chronic disease endpoint and whether or not it is better than some current standard of care.

A *Phase II* efficacy trial can function as a prerequisite for a *Phase III* trial or an end unto itself. It can be an end unto itself when improvement in a behavioral risk factor has such a strong and consistent association with improvement in a chronic disease that a *Phase III* trial is unnecessary. A good example of this is in the area of smoking. Since the association between smoking and lung cancer is irrefutable, a behavioral trial showing that a reduction in smoking reduces lung cancer incidence is unnecessary. A more pressing need may be to identify treatments that can produce *sustained* smoking cessation. Here, the state of the science has obviated the need to document the value of a behavioral treatment on a chronic disease and moved toward the need for more powerful behavioral treatments. If, instead, interest was in testing the value of smoking cessation on some other chronic disease where associations were less well established, a *Phase III* efficacy trial would be needed.

Phase II and *Phase III* behavioral efficacy trials face similar challenges in such areas as bias from unblinded designs, choice of comparators, and protection from confounding. Thus, the methods proposed in various chapters of this book pertain to both types of trials. Where there are differences, they are noted.

Although *Phase I* refinement studies, *Phase II* efficacy trials, and *Phase III* efficacy trials all share a randomized design, the ORBIT model makes a point of distinguishing among them. This is to encourage progressive translational science that is characterized by a progression of phase-specific questions linked to a progression of phase-specific methods, and a push toward testing in *Phase III* trials with chronic disease endpoints rather than settling with the *Phase II* trial in the belief that the work has been done and the case has been made. The fundamental promise that behavioral treatments can help to reduce the burden of chronic diseases remains largely unfulfilled [101]. To make this case, convincing evidence from *Phase III* trials that shows that chronic disease endpoints are improved by a behavioral treatment is needed.

Milestones. When a *Phase III* trial is the end game, support from a *Phase II* trial is a milestone. Here, the *Phase II* trial would be conceptualized as a preliminary study showing that the behavioral treatment is strong enough to reduce behavioral risk to a level needed to improve a chronic disease endpoint. When a *Phase II* trial is the end game, effectiveness or implementation studies would be reasonable next steps.

SELECTED EXPERIENCE FROM A BEHAVIORAL TRIAL

Scientific Progression in the Diabetes Prevention Program

Scientific progression in developing a behavioral treatment is a key to success. An excellent example of this is the development of the Diabetes Prevention Program (DPP) [55, 56], one of the most successful *Phase III* behavioral efficacy trials to date. The DPP showed that lifestyle was 30% better than the best drug available and 60% better than placebo in preventing conversion to diabetes in patients who were insulin resistant. This lifestyle treatment was developed progressively and systematically over 40 years. Table 3.9 reconstructs this development using the basic elements of the ORBIT model.

Extensive development such as that described in Table 3.9 would be a daunting task for any single investigator. But it is evident that the DPP was based upon the work of a wide range of multidisciplinary investigators who were, at best, loosely connected. To borrow the analogy of building a house, the director of the DPP lifestyle treatment, Rena Wing, served in the role of "architect." She and her team created the "design" for the "house" relying upon a large number of "contractors" to inform such specialty tasks as "painting, plumbing, and electrical wiring." Becoming an "architect" and drawing on the skills of "contractors" makes treatment development less daunting for any one individual.

RECOMMENDATIONS

The healthcare crisis demands a cut, not a shift, in healthcare costs. This presents an opportunity for behavioral treatments, which have the potential to cut costs by targeting fundamental behavioral roots of chronic diseases. But to do this, behavioral treatments must be well-developed, tested with rigorous methods, successful in improving clinically significant endpoints, and visible in publications in top medical journals and clinical practice guidelines. Funding agencies, publication practices, and investigators can help to achieve this end.

Funding Agencies

More support for behavioral treatment development is needed. By way of comparison, industry spends approximately 7 years developing a drug and $1.3 billion to bring it to market [8]. The NIH, a major funder for behavioral treatment develop-

Table 3.9 Treatment development in the Diabetes Prevention Program [55, 56]

Goal (*Phase*)	Observation/Decision	Evidence
Discovery		
Clinical question	Overweight is a key risk factor for diabetes	Weight gain is associated with substantial increase in risk for diabetes [102].
Fundamental process	Behavior controls overeating	Operant conditioning resulted in 1 lb./wk. weight loss over 1 year [103].
	Behavior modification is an effective treatment for obesity	Behavior modification was twice as effective at weight loss as psychotherapy, or the average achieved in the medical literature [104].
Define (*Phase Ia*)		
Clinical endpoint	Diabetes	Improvement in lifestyle reduces diabetes [105].
Clinical cutpoint	33%	Lifestyle change produced 33% reduction in diabetes in non-randomized studies [106–108].
Behavior risk factor targets	Overweight/obesity	– Reduction in weight reduces diabetes [105]. – Modest reduction in weight reduces fasting glucose [109].
	Physical activity	Increase in physical activity reduces diabetes [108, 110].
Behavioral cutpoints	Overweight/obesity: 7% reduction in body weight	– Behavioral weight loss studies achieve ~ 6% reduction in weight at 18 months [111, 112]. – Multi-center trials achieve ~5% reduction in body weight [113–115]. – 3–7 kg weight loss (5–10% reduction in body weight) associated with 33% reduction in diabetes [116].
	Physical activity: 150 min moderate activity/week	150 min of moderate physical activity/week improves outcomes; can be maintained for 10 years [117–119].
Hypothesized pathway	(Chap. 4, Fig. 4.5)	
Refine (*Phase Ib*)		
Number of components	2	Weight loss is sustained over 2 years if physical activity is added to diet [120].
Length of treatment	6 months	Longer treatments are associated with greater weight loss [120].
Maintenance	Continues for duration of follow-up	Ongoing contact during maintenance promotes sustained change [121].
Diversity in response	Toolbox, as needed	Set common goals but individualize method of achieving them [56].
Time needed to achieve goals	6 months	In first 6 months, individuals achieve maximum weight loss [122].
Mode of treatment	Both individual and group	Both individual and group treatment optimize outcomes [115].
Proof of Concept (*Phase IIa*)	Can a lifestyle program achieve a clinically significant improvement in diabetes?	In non-randomized studies, lifestyle treatment produced a 33% reduction in diabetes [106–108].

ment, allocates only a small proportion of its budget to behavioral research. In 2016, NIH invested 57.7% of its extramural research budget on genetic studies [123] compared to a 2013 expenditure of only 3.0% of its budget on any type of behavioral research [124]. The NIH spent approximately $350 million to fund Clinical and Translational Science Awards (CTSA's) which have not typically supported behavioral research at the T0-T1 phase [7]. It is not surprising that this difference in expenditures translates into a clinical trial literature that overrepresents drug treatments for chronic diseases which have fundamental lifestyle roots. A recent report reviewed drug and exercise treatments for the secondary prevention of coronary heart disease. Despite equal efficacy, 81% of trials found for the review were drug trials, and when all of the patients in these trials were combined, 96% of them were in the drug trials [125].

Dedicated Funding
The NIH is recognizing the need to correct the imbalance in funding by directing more resources toward behavioral treatment development [7]. Transdisciplinary translational behavioral (TDTB) research refers to the early development of behavioral treatments that are the fruit of diverse perspectives [7]. Dedicated funding opportunities for TDTB research are growing and include a variety of funding, center, network, institute, meeting, and workshop opportunities. By providing these opportunities, the NIH is promoting a culture within the behavioral community to pursue TDTB research. Czajkowski and colleagues [7] provide an excellent review of this evolution and its associated funding opportunities.

Dedicated Review Groups
A dedicated standing study section is needed for early behavioral treatment development studies. Within the behavioral sciences, significantly more resources have been directed toward dissemination and implementation research than early phase treatment development research [7]. This is a huge gap given that dissemination and implementation are built upon the existence of "evidence-based behavioral treatments" and that few behavioral treatments are supported by the *Phase III* efficacy trial standards that exist in the biomedical sciences. The enthusiasm in the behavioral community for dissemination and implementation research is obvious from the fact that at least 61 models for this process have been created [126] and the NIH now has a dedicated standing study section for dissemination and implementation research [7]. A dedicated standing study section for behavioral treatment development would encourage establishment of unique criteria for judging grant applications and enhance the overall quality of grant reviews.

Training Opportunities
Workshop and institute opportunities provide training in early behavioral treatment development research which is ideal for postdoctoral and junior faculty. These opportunities exist within specialized institutes dedicated to specific diseases and within trans-institute programs such as those offered by the Office of Behavioral

and Social Science Research, the Roadmap, and the Common Fund. Since specialized training in translational research and behavioral treatment development does not generally exist within most PhD or MD training programs, existence of postdoctoral training opportunities is essential to the growth and sophistication of this process. NIH training opportunities in the "clinician-scientist" model common in medicine [7] should be extended to behavioral medicine. This would foster forward and backward translation among applied behavioral medicine, basic behavioral and social science, and clinical medicine.

Publication Practices

Academic progression requires a consistent publication record. Thus, opportunities to publish results of early phase behavioral treatment development studies are crucial to academic success and sustained interest. Journal editors and reviewers often criticize the small, quasi-experimental studies needed to develop behavioral treatments, reinforcing instead fully developed randomized designs. This culture is changing on several fronts.

Dedicated Journals
Journals specifically directed toward early treatment development now exist. Examples include the journal *Pilot and Feasibility Studies* which is specifically directed toward early phase studies and the journal *Translational Behavioral Medicine* which is directed toward transdisciplinary, translational behavioral research.

Articulated Missions
Journal editors have the opportunity to create a vision for how their science should proceed, and to change existing publication practices through the articulation of this vision and its translation into policies for accepting papers. An example of this has been presented by the appointment of Ken Freedland as editor-in-chief of *Health Psychology*. He articulated his vision in an editorial [101] and then worked to implement it with special issues directed toward specific aspects of translational research and with a specially-selected editorial board and reviewers. These changes have resulted in the successful publication of early phase behavioral treatment development studies such as that published by Powell et al. [97] which featured a treatment-only, proof-of-concept design, no statistical testing, and an articulation of failures and proposed solutions.

Investigators

Pursue Scientific Progression

The success of behavioral clinical trials that aim to improve chronic diseases relies upon the development of strong behavioral treatments that can produce clinically significant change in behavioral risk factors. To achieve this, a translational program of research with long-term lofty goals, an interest in discovery, a willingness to fail and refine, and an ability to integrate and synthesize the wisdom that exists across disciplines is needed. Progressive, translational research needs focus and persistence. It needs commitment to a program of research with long-term and "big picture" thinking. It needs a big problem to solve and a passion for solving it that mobilizes focus, persistence, and progression. Not everyone needs or wants this. But those who do want it, and are not daunted by the roller coaster of successes and failures that are part of the ride, could be the "architects" of a *Phase III* behavioral efficacy trial that changes clinical practice.

Communicate Scientific Progression to Reviewers

Small studies, such as treatment-only proof-of-concept studies, take on greater significance when they are viewed as a crucial step within an integrated program of treatment development. Communication of this "big picture" plan to reviewers of grants and papers can enhance the significance of any single small study and potentially maximize a successful review. Figure 3.4 presents a description of the "big picture" in a program of treatment development. This figure has the greatest impact when placed up front on the Specific Aims page of a grant proposal.

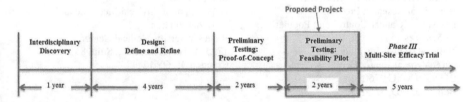

Fig. 3.4 Example of presentation of a program of behavioral treatment development in a grant proposal

Pursue Foundation, Center, and Institutional Support

Early phases of behavioral treatment development are fluid and focus on exploration, discovery, tinkering, high failure rates, and refinement in the face of failure. This process requires time but generally not much money. Many foundation, center, and institutional grants are specifically designed to provide support for exploratory studies that will ultimately translate into larger federal funding. One reason for committing to a disease of interest early is that many of these grant opportunities are linked to diseases; not treatments. Philanthropy offices, which exist in most academic institutions, can help connect investigators with closely-aligned potential funders. Centers frequently have funding that is earmarked for exploratory studies and can offer opportunities for a team-based approach to treatment development.

APPENDIX
Obesity-Related Behavioral Treatment Intervention Trials (ORBIT) Consortium

Nancy Adler, PhD
Professor of Medical Psychology
Department of Health Psychology
University of California, San Francisco
3333 California St., Suite 465
San Francisco, CA 94143

David Cella, PhD
Ralph Seal Paffenbarger Professor
Chair
Department of Medical Social Sciences
Director, Institute for Public Health and Medicine
625 N. Michigan, 21st Floor
Chicago, IL 60611

Susan M. Czajkowski, PhD
Chief
Health Behaviors Research Branch
Behavioral Research Program
Division of Cancer Control and Population Sciences
National Cancer Institute
9609 Medical Center Drive
BG 9609 MSC 9760
Bethesda, MD 20892

Elissa Epel, PhD
Professor
Vice-Chair
Department of Psychiatry
UCSF Weill Institute for Neurosciences
University of California San Francisco
3333 California Street
San Francisco, CA 94118

Josephine Boyington, PhD
Program Director
Clinical Applications and Prevention Branch
Division of Cardiovascular Sciences
National Heart, Lung, and Blood Institute
6701 Rockledge Drive
Suite 10224
Bethesda, MD 20892

Mary E. Charlson, MD
The William T. Foley Distinguished
  Professor of Medicine
Weill Cornell Medical College
1300 York Ave, Box # 46
New York, NY 10065

Sheila A. Dugan, MD
Professor
Interim Chair
Department of Physical Medicine and
  Rehabilitation
Rush University Medical Center
1725 W. Harrison Street, Suite 855
Chicago, IL 60612

Leonard H. Epstein, PhD
SUNY Distinguished Professor
Division Chief, Behavioral Medicine
Department of Pediatrics
Jacobs School of Medicine and Biomedical
  Sciences
State University of New York at Buffalo
3435 Main Street, G56 Farber Hall
Buffalo, New York 14214

Lynne Haverkos, MD, PhD
(retired)
National Institute of Child Health and Human
  Development
BG 6710B Rm 233 LB
6710 Rockledge Drive
Bethesda, MD 20817

Imke Janssen, PhD
Associate Professor
Department of Preventive Medicine
Rush University Medical Center
1700 W. Van Buren St., Suite 470
Chicago, IL 60612

Barbara Laraia, PhD, RD, MPH
Professor
Community Health Sciences
School of Public Health
University of California, Berkeley
2121 Berkeley Way, Room 5302
Berkeley, CA 94720

Deborah H. Olster, PhD
Senior Advisor
Office of the Assistant Director
Directorate for Social, Behavioral, and
  Economic Sciences
National Science Foundation
2415 Eisenhower Avenue
Alexandria, VA 22314

Janey C. Peterson, Ed.D, MS
Associate Professor
Division of General Internal Medicine
Weill Cornell Medical College
525 East 68th Street, Room 2011
New York, NY 10065

Kim D. Reynolds, PhD
Professor
School of Community & Global Health
Claremont Graduate University
675 W. Foothill Blvd., Suite 200
Claremont, CA 91711

Christine Hunter, PhD, ABPP
Deputy Director
Office of Behavioral and Social Sciences
  Research
National Institutes of Health
Building 31, Room B1C19
31 Center Drive
Bethesda, MD 20892

Kai-Lin Catherine Jen, PhD
Professor
Department of Nutrition and Food Science
Wayne State University
3009 Science Hall
Detroit, MI 48202

Sylvie Naar, PhD
Distinguished Endowed Professor in
  Behavioral Health
Director, Center for Translational Behavioral
  Science
Department of Behavioral Sciences and
  Social Medicine
Florida State University
1115 West Call Street
Tallahassee, FL 32306

Frank Perna, EdD, PhD
Program Director
Health Behaviors Research Branch
Behavioral Research Program
Division of Cancer Control and Population
  Sciences
National Cancer Institute
9609 Medical Center Drive
BG 9609 MSC 9760
Bethesda, MD 20892

Lynda H. Powell, PhD
The Charles J. and Margaret Roberts
  Professor of Preventive Medicine
Chair
Department of Preventive Medicine
Rush University Medical Center
1700 W. Van Buren St., Suite 470
Chicago, IL 60612

Rena R. Wing, PhD
Professor of Psychiatry and Human Behavior
Director, Weight Control and Diabetes
  Research Center
Warren Alpert Medical School of Brown
  University
The Miriam Hospital
196 Richmond St.
Providence, RI 02903

REFERENCES

1. Thaul S (2012) How FDA approves drugs and regulates their safety and effectiveness. FDA drug approval, elements, and considerations. Nova Science, Hauppauge
2. Ascione FJ (2001) Principles of scientific literature evaluation: critiquing clinical drug trials. American Pharmaceutical Association, Washington DC
3. Lipsky MS, Sharp LK (2001) From idea to market: the drug approval process. J Am Board Fam Pract 14:362–367
4. Friedman MA, Woodcock J, Lumpkin MM, Shuren JE, Hass A, Thompson LJ (1999) The safety of newly approved medicines: Do recent market removals mean there is a problem? JAMA 281:1728–1734
5. ICH Expert Working Group (1997) ICH Harmonised Tripartite Guideline. General considerations for clinical trials E8. www.ich.org/fileadmin/Public_Web_Site/ICH_Products/Guidelines/Efficacy/E8/Step4/E8_Guideline.pdf
6. Turner JR (2010) New drug development. An introduction to clinical trials, 2nd edn. Springer, New York
7. Czajkowski SM, Lynch MR, Hall KL, Stipelman BA, Haverkos L, Perl H, Scott MS, Shirley MC (2016) Transdisciplinary translational behavioral (TDTB) research: opportunities, barriers, and innovations. Transl Behav Med 6:32–43
8. Schuler P, Buckley B (2015) Re-engineering clinical trials: best practices for streamlining drug development. Academic Press, Cambridge
9. Munos B (2009) Lessons from 60 years of pharmaceutical innovation. Nat Rev Drug Discov 8:959–968
10. DiMasi JA, Feldman L, Seckler A, Wilson A (2010) Trends in risks associated with new drug development: success rates for investigational drugs. Clin Pharmacol Ther 87:272–277
11. Faggiano F, Allara E, Giannotta F, Molinar R, Sumnall H, Wiers R, Michie S, Collins L, Conrod P (2014) Europe needs a central, transparent, and evidence-based approval process for behavioural prevention interventions. PLoS Med 11:e1001740. https://doi.org/10.1371/journal.pmed.1001740
12. Campbell M, Fitzpatrick R, Haines A, Kinmonth AL, Sandercock P, Spiegelhalter D, Tyrer P (2000) Framework for design and evaluation of complex interventions to improve health. BMJ 21:694–696
13. Craig P, Dieppe P, Macintyre S, Michie S, Nazareth I, Petticrew M (2013) Developing and evaluating complex interventions: the new Medical Research Council guidance. Int J Nurs Stud 50:587–592
14. Flay BR (1986) Efficacy and effectiveness trials (and other phases of research) in the development of health promotion programs. Prev Med 15:451–474
15. Czajkowski SM, Powell LH, Adler N, Naar-King S, Reynolds KD, Hunter CM, Laraia B, Olster DH, Perna FM, Peterson JC, Epel E, Boyington JE, Charlson ME (2015) From ideas to efficacy: the ORBIT model for developing behavioral treatments for chronic diseases. Health Psychol 34:971–982
16. Stevens J, Taber DR, Murray DM, Ward DS (2007) Advances and controversies in the design of obesity prevention trials. Obesity 15:2163–2170
17. Rounsaville BJ, Carroll KM, Onken LS (2001) A stage model of behavioral therapies research. Getting started and moving on from stage I. Clin Psychol Sci Pract 8:133–142
18. Arean PA, Kraemer HC (2013) High-quality psychotherapy research: From conception to piloting to national trials. Oxford University Press, New York
19. Greenwald P, Cullen JW (1985) The new emphasis in cancer control. J Natl Cancer Inst 74:543–551
20. Bartholomew L, Parcel G, Kok G, Gottlieb G, Fernandez ME (2011) Planning health promotion programs: intervention mapping. Jossey-Bass, San Francisco

21. Michie S, van Stralen MM, West R (2011) The behaviour change wheel: a new method for characterising and designing behaviour change interventions. Implement Sci 6:42. https://doi.org/10.1186/1748-5908-6-42

22. Collins LM, Murphy SA, Nair VN, Strecher VJ (2005) A strategy for optimizing and evaluating behavioral interventions. Ann Behav Med 30:65–73

23. Peterson JC, Czajkowski S, Charlson ME, Link AR, Wells MT, Isen AM, Mancuso CA, Allegrante JP, Boutin-Foster C, Ogedegbe G, Jobe JB (2013) Translating basic behavioral and social science research to clinical application: the EVOLVE mixed methods approach. J Consult Clin Psychol 81:217–230

24. Coller BS (2008) Translational research: forging a new cultural identity. Mt Sinai J Med 75:478–487

25. Popper KR (1959) The logic of scientific discovery. Basic Books, New York

26. Schulz KF, Altman DG, Moher D, and the CONSORT Group (2010) CONSORT 2010 statement. Updated guidelines for reporting parallel group randomized trials. Ann Intern Med 152:726–732

27. Deardorff J, King K (2014) Chicago doctor's research fails federal smell test: federal agency says his studies on Sensa weight-loss product have no merit. Chicago Tribune. http://articles.chicagotribune.com/2014-01-19/health/ct-met-sensa-weight-loss-hirsch-20140119_1_hirsch-journals-studies

28. Korownyk C, Kolber MR, McCormack J, Lam V, Overbo K, Cotton C, Finley C, Turgeon RD, Garrison S, Lindblad AJ, Banh HL, Campbell-Scherer D, Vandermeer B, Allan GM (2014) Televised medical talk shows – what they recommend and the evidence to support their recommendations: a prospective observational study. BMJ 349:g7346. https://doi.org/10.1136/bmj.g7346

29. Kaufman SB, Gregoire C (2015) Wired to create: unraveling the mysteries of the creative mind. Perigee/Penguin, New York

30. Lehrer J (2008) The eureka hunt. The New Yorker 28:40–45

31. Reynolds M (2017) Inspiration points: entrepreneurs reveal what sparks their creativity. Chicago Tribune July 31

32. Hess RB (2012) Innovation generation: how to produce creative and useful scientific ideas. Oxford University Press, New York

33. Eckel RH, Jakicic JM, Ard JD, de Jesus JM, Houston Miller N, Hubbard VS, Lee IM, Lichtenstein AH, Loria CM, Millen BE, Nonas CA, Sacks FM, Smith SC Jr, Svetkey LP, Wadden TA, Yanovski SZ, American College of Cardiology/American Heart Association Task Force on Practice Guidelines (2014) 2013 AHA/ACC guideline on lifestyle management to reduce cardiovascular risk: a report of the American College of Cardiology/American Heart Association Task Force on Practice Guidelines. Circulation 129:579–599

34. James PA, Oparil S, Carter BL, Cushman WC, Dennison-Himmelfarb C, Handler J, Lackland DT, LeFevre ML, MacKenzie TD, Ogedegbe O, Smith SC Jr, Svetkey LP, Taler SJ, Townsend RR, Wright JT Jr, Narva AS, Ortiz E (2014) 2014 evidence-based guideline for the management of high blood pressure in adults: report from the panel members appointed to the Eighth Joint National Committee (JNC 8). JAMA 311:507–520

35. Stone NJ, Robinson JG, Lichtenstein AH, Bairey Merz CN, Blum CB, Eckel RH, Goldberg AC, Gordon D, Levy D, Lloyd-Jones DM, McBride P, Schwartz JS, Shero ST, Smith SC Jr, Watson K, Wilson PW, Eddleman KM, Jarrett NM, LaBresh K, Nevo L, Wnek J, Anderson JL, Halperin JL, Albert NM, Bozkurt B, Brindis RG, Curtis LH, DeMets D, Hochman JS, Kovacs RJ, Ohman EM, Pressler SJ, Sellke FW, Shen WK, Smith SC Jr, Tomaselli GF, American College of Cardiology/American Heart Association Task Force on Practice Guidelines (2014) 2013 ACC/AHA guideline on the treatment of blood cholesterol to reduce atherosclerotic cardiovascular risk in adults. A report of the American College of Cardiology/American Heart Association Task Force on Practice Guidelines. Circulation 129:S1–S45

36. American Diabetes Association (2020) Standards of medical care in diabetes – 2020. Diabetes Care 43:Supplement 1. https://doi.org/10.2337/dc20-Sint
37. Choudhry NK, Avorn J, Glynn RJ, Antman EM, Schneeweiss S, Toscano M, Reisman L, Fernandes J, Spettell C, Lee JL, Levin R, Brennan T, Shrank WH, Post-Myocardial Infarction Free Rx Event and Economic Evaluation (MI FREEE) Trial (2011) Full coverage for preventive medications after myocardial infarction. N Engl J Med 365:2088–2097
38. De Geest S, Sabate E (2003) Adherence to long-term therapies: evidence for action. Europ J Cardiovasc Nursing 2:323. https://doi.org/10.1016/S1474-5151(03)00091-4
39. Calvin JE, Shanbhag S, Avery E, Kane J, Richardson D, Powell LH (2012) Adherence to evidence-based guidelines for heart failure in physicians and their patients. Lessons from the Heart Failure Adherence Retention Trial (HART). Congest Heart Fail 18:73–78
40. Watts DJ (2017) Should social science be more solution-oriented? Nat Hum Behav 1:0015. https://doi.org/10.1038/s41562-016-0015
41. Davis R, Campbell R, Hildon Z, Hobbs L, Michie S (2015) Theories of behaviour change across the social and behavioral sciences: a scoping review. Health Psychol Rev 9:323–344
42. Ma J, Lewis MA, Smyth JM (2018) Translational behavioral medicine for population and individual health: gaps, opportunities, and vision for practice-based translational behavior change research. Transl Behav Med 8:753–760
43. Fagundo AB, de la Torre R, Jiménez-Murcia S, Agüera Z, Granero R, Tárrega S, Botella C, Baños R, Fernández-Real JM, Rodríguez R, Forcano L, Frühbeck G, Gómez-Ambrosi J, Tinahones FJ, Fernández-García JC, Casanueva FF, Fernández-Aranda F (2012) Executive functions profile in extreme eating/weight conditions: from anorexia nervosa to obesity. PLoS One 7:e43382. https://doi.org/10.1371/journal.pone.0043382
44. Bruch H (1978) The golden cage. The enigma of anorexia nervosa. Harvard University Press, Cambridge
45. Foerde K, Steinglass JE, Shohamy D, Walsh BT (2015) Neural mechanisms supporting maladaptive food choices in anorexia nervosa. Nat Neurosci 18:1571–1573
46. Guo J, Simmons WK, Herscovitch P, Martin A, Hall KD (2014) Striatal dopamine D2-like receptor correlation patterns with human obesity and opportunistic eating behavior. Mol Psychiatry 19:1078–1084
47. Gardner B (2013) A review and analysis of the use of 'habit' in understanding, predicting and influencing health-related behaviour. Health Psychol Rev 21:1–19
48. Lally P, Gardner B (2013) Promoting habit formation. Health Psychol Rev 7:S137–S158
49. Roberto CA, Kawachi I (2016) Behavioral economics and public health. Oxford University Press, New York
50. Wu R, Rebok GW, Lin FV (2016) A novel theoretical life course framework for triggering cognitive development across the lifespan. Human Dev 59:342–365
51. Ennett ST, Tobler NS, Ringwalt CL, Flewelling RL (1994) How effective is drug abuse resistance education? A meta-analysis of project DARE outcome evaluations. Am J Pub Health 84:1394–1401
52. Cima R (2016) DARE: the anti-drug program that never actually worked. https://priceonomics.com/dare-the-anti-drug-program-that-never-actually/
53. Hecht ML, Graham JW, Eiek E (2006) The drug resistance strategies intervention: program effects on substance use. Health Comm 20:267–276
54. Covey SR (1989) The 7 habits of highly effective people. Free Press, New York
55. Knowler WC, Barrett-Connor E, Fowler SE, Hamman RF, Lachin JM, Walker EA, Nathan DM, Diabetes Prevention Program Research Group (2002) Reduction in the incidence of type 2 diabetes with lifestyle intervention or metformin. N Engl J Med 346:393–403
56. Diabetes Prevention Program (DPP) Research Group (2002) The Diabetes Prevention Program (DPP): description of lifestyle intervention. Diabetes Care 25:2165–2171
57. Wansink B (2007) Mindless eating: why we eat more than we think. Bantam, New York
58. Seemann J (2012) Hybrid insights: where the quantitative meets the qualitative. Rotman Magazine, fall, pp 57–61

59. Antonucci M (2011) Sparks fly. Stanford Magazine https://alumni.stanford.edu/get/page/magazine/article/?article_id=28380
60. Dallery J, Cassidy RN, Raiff BR (2013) Single-case experimental designs to evaluate novel technology-based health interventions. J Med Internet Res 15:e22. https://doi.org/10.2196/jmir.2227
61. Dallery J, Raiff BR (2014) Optimizing behavioral health interventions with single-case designs: from development to dissemination. Transl Behav Med 4:290–303
62. Ridenour TA, Pineo TZ, Molina MMM, Lich KH (2013) Toward rigorous idiographic research in prevention science: comparison between three analytic strategies for testing preventive intervention in very small samples. Prev Sci 14:267–278
63. Shadish WR, Kyse EN, Rindskopf DM (2013) Analyzing data from single-case designs using multilevel models: new applications and some agenda items for future research. Psychol Methods 18:385–405
64. Zucker DR, Ruthazer R, Schmid CH (2010) Individual (N-of-1) trials can be combined to give population comparative treatment effect estimates: methodologic considerations. J Clin Epidemiol 63:1312–1323
65. Ridenour TA, Wittenborn AK, Raiff BR, Benedict N, Kane-Gill S (2016) Illustrating idiographic methods for translation research: moderation effects, natural clinical experiments, and complex treatment-by-subgroup interactions. Transl Behav Med 6:125–134
66. Jensen MD, Ryan DH, Apovian CM, Ard JD, Comuzzie AG, Donato KA, Hu FB, Hubbard VS, Jakicic JM, Kushner RF, Loria CM, Millen BE, Nonas CA, Pi-Sunyer FX, Stevens J, Stevens VJ, Wadden TA, Wolfe BM, Yanovski SZ, American College of Cardiology/American Heart Association Task Force on Practice Guidelines, Obesity Society (2014) 2013 AHA/ACC/TOS guideline for the management of overweight and obesity in adults: a report of the American College of Cardiology/American Heart Association Task Force on Practice Guidelines and the Obesity Society. Circulation 129:S102–S138
67. Brown T (2008) Design thinking. Harvard Business Review, Boston
68. Prahalad CK, Ramaswamy V (2004) Co-creation experiences: the next practice in value creation. J Interact Market 18:5–14
69. Strolla LO, Gans KM, Risica PM (2006) Using qualitative and quantitative formative research to develop tailored nutrition intervention materials for a diverse low-income audience. Health Educ Res 21:465–476
70. Shiffman S, Stone AA, Hufford MR (2008) Ecological momentary assessment. Ann Rev Clin Psychol 4:1–32
71. Nahum-Shani I, Smith SN, Spring BJ, Collins LM, Witkiewitz K, Tewari A, Murphy SA (2016) Just-in-Time Adaptive Interventions (JITAIs) in mobile health: key components and design principles for ongoing health behavior support. Ann Behav Med 52:446–462
72. Almirall D, Nahum-Shani I, Sherwood NE, Murphy SA (2014) Introduction to SMART designs for the development of adaptive interventions: with application to weight loss research. Transl Behav Med 4:260–274
73. Voils C, King HA, Maciejewski ML, Allen KD, Yancy WS, Shaffer JA (2014) Approaches for informing optimal dose of behavioral interventions. Ann Behav Med 48:392–401
74. Collins LM, Dziak JJ, Kugler KC, Trail JB (2014) Factorial experiments: efficient tools for evaluation of intervention components. Am J Prev Med 47:498–504
75. Dziak JJ, Nahum-Shani I, Collins LM (2012) Multilevel factorial experiments for developing behavioral interventions: power, sample size, and resource considerations. Psychol Methods 17:153–175
76. Spring B, Schneider K, McFadden HG, Vaughn J, Kozak AT, Smith M, Moller AC, Epstein LH, Demott A, Hedeker D, Siddique J, Lloyd-Jones DM (2012) Multiple behavior changes in diet and activity: a randomized controlled trial using mobile technology. Arch Intern Med 172:789–796
77. Ji Y, Wang SJ (2013) Modified toxicity probability interval design: a safer and more reliable method than the 3 + 3 design for practical phase I trials. J Clin Oncol 31:1785–1791

78. Ji Y, Liu P, Li Y, Bekele BN (2010) A modified toxicity probability interval method for dose-finding trials. Clin Trials 7:653–663

79. Pace NL, Stylianou MP (2007) Advances in and limitations of up-and-down methodology: a précis of clinical use, study design, and dose estimation in anesthesia research. Anesthesiology 107:144–152

80. Gustafson DH, McTavish FM, Chih MY, Atwood AK, Johnson RA, Boyle MG, Levy MS, Driscoll H, Chisholm SM, Dillenburg L, Isham A, Shah D (2014) A smartphone application to support recovery from alcoholism: a randomized clinical trial. JAMA Psychiat 71:566–572

81. Matthews M, Abdullah S, Gay G, Choudhury T (2014) Tracking mental well-being: balancing rich sensing and patient needs. Computer 474:36–43

82. Klasnja P, Hekler EB, Shiffman S, Boruvka A, Almirall D, Tewari A, Murphy SA (2015) Microrandomized trials: an experimental design for developing just-in-time adaptive interventions. Health Psychol 34:1220–1228

83. Brockwell PJ, Davis RA (2016) Introduction to time series and forecasting, 3rd edn. Springer, AG Switzerland

84. Spring B, Duncan JM, Janke EA, Kozak AT, McFadden HG, DeMott A, Pictor A, Epstein LH, Siddique J, Pellegrini CA, Buscemi J, Hedeker D (2013) Integrating technology into standard weight loss treatment: a randomized controlled trial. JAMA Intern Med 173:105–111

85. Tolley EE, Ulin PR, Mack N, Robinson ET, Succop SM (2016) Qualitative methods in public health: a field guide for applied research, 2nd edn. Jossey Bass, San Francisco

86. Weston AD, Hood L (2004) System biology, proteomics, and the future of health care: toward predictive, preventative, and personalized medicine. J Proteome Res 3:179–196

87. Mimezami R, Nicholoson J, Darzi A (2012) Preparing for precision medicine. N Engl J Med 366:489–491

88. Ma J, Rosas LG, Lv N (2016) Precision lifestyle medicine: a new frontier in the science of behavior change and population health. Am J Prev Med 50:395–397

89. Lei H, Nahum-Shani I, Lynch K, Oslin D, Murphy SA (2012) A "SMART" design for building individualized treatment sequences. Ann Rev Clin Psychol 8:21–48

90. Nahum-Shani I, Qian M, Almirall D, Pelham WE, Gnagy B, Fabiano GA, Waxmonsky JG, Yu J, Murphy SA (2012) Experimental design and primary data analysis methods for comparing adaptive interventions. Psychol Methods 17:457–477

91. Nahum-Shani I, Qian M, Almirall D, Pelham WE, Gnagy B, Fabiano GA, Waxmonsky JG, Yu J, Murphy SA (2012) Q-learning: a data analysis method for constructing adaptive interventions. Psychol Methods 17:478–494

92. Palmer CG, Hadley DW (2005) Evaluating the impact of genetic counseling and testing with signal detection methods. J Genet Couns 14:17–27

93. Eldridge S, Spencer A, Cryer C, Parsons S, Underwood M, Feder G (2005) Why modelling a complex intervention is an important precursor to trial design: lessons from studying an intervention to reduce falls-related injuries in older people. J Health Serv Res Policy 10:133–142

94. Hammond RA (2009) Complex systems modeling for obesity research. Prev Chronic Dis 6:1–10

95. Hammond RA, Dubé L (2012) A systems science perspective and transdisciplinary models for food and nutrition security. Proc Natl Acad Sci 109:12356–12363

96. Navarro-Barrientos J-E, Rivera DE, Collins LM (2011) A dynamical model for describing behavioural interventions for weight loss and body composition change. Math Comput Model Dyn Syst 17:183–203

97. Powell LH, Appelhans BM, Ventrelle J, Karavolos K, March ML, Ong JC, Fitzpatrick SL, Normand P, Dawar R, Kazalauskaite R (2018) Development of a lifestyle intervention for the metabolic syndrome: discovery through proof-of-concept. Health Psychol 37:929–939

98. Ridenour TA, Szu-Han K, Liu HY, Bobashev GV, Hill K, Cooper R (2017) The clinical trials mosaic: toward a range of clinical trials designs to optimize evidence-based treatment. J Person-Oriented Res 3:28–48

99. Mosnaim GS, Cohen MS, Rhoads CH, Rittner SS, Powell LH (2008) Use of MP3 players to increase asthma knowledge in inner-city African-American adolescents. Int J Behav Med 15:341–346

100. Friedman LM, Furberg CD, DeMets D, Reboussin DM, Granger CB (2015) Fundamentals of clinical trials, 5th edn. Springer Cham, Heidelberg

101. Freedland KE (2017) A new era for Health Psychology. Health Psychol 36:1–4

102. Colditz GA, Willett WC, Rotnitzky A, Manson JE (1995) Weight gain as a risk factor for clinical diabetes mellitus in women. Ann Intern Med 122:481–486

103. Stuart RB (1996) Behavioral control of overeating. Obes Res 4:411–417

104. Penick SB, Filion R, Fox S, Stunkard AJ (1971) Behavior modification in the treatment of obesity. Psychosom Med 33:49–55

105. Colditz GA, Willett WC, Stampfer MJ, Manson JE, Hennekens CH, Arky RA, Speizer FE (1990) Weight as a risk factor for clinical diabetes in women. Am J Epidemiol 132:501–513

106. Page RC, Harnden KE, Cook JT, Turner RC (1992) Can lifestyles of subjects with impaired glucose tolerance be changed? A feasibility study. Diabet Med 9:562–566

107. Bourn DM, Mann JI, McSkimming BJ, Waldron MA, Wishart JD (1994) Impaired glucose tolerance and NIDDM: does a lifestyle intervention program have an effect? Diabetes Care 17:1311–1319

108. Eriksson KF, Lindgärde F (1991) Prevention of type 2 (non-insulin-dependent) diabetes mellitus by diet and physical exercise. The 6-year Malmö feasibility study. Diabetologia 34:891–898

109. Wing RR, Koeske R, Epstein LH, Nowalk MP, Gooding W, Becker D (1987) Long-term effects of modest weight loss in type II diabetic patients. Arch Intern Med 147:1749–1753

110. Tuomilehto J, Knowler WC, Zimmet P (1992) Primary prevention of non-insulin-dependent diabetes mellitus. Diabetes Metab Rev 8:339–353

111. Wadden TA (1993) The treatment of obesity: an overview. In: Stunkard AJ, Wadden TA (eds) Obesity: theory and therapy. Raven, New York, pp 197–218

112. Wing RR (1993) Behavioral approaches to the treatment of obesity. In: Bray G, Gouchard C, James P (eds) Handbook of obesity. Marcel Dekker, New York, pp 855–873

113. Stamler R, Stamler J, Gosch FC, Civinelli J, Fishman J, McKeever P, McDonald A, Dyer AR (1989) Primary prevention of hypertension by nutritional-hygienic means: final report of a randomized, controlled trial. JAMA 262:1801–1807

114. Stevens VJ, Corrigan SA, Obarzanek E, Bernauer E, Cook NR, Hebert P, Mattfeldt-Beman M, Oberman A, Sugars C, Dalcin AT, Whelton PK (1993) Weight loss intervention in phase 1 of the Trials of Hypertension Prevention. The TOHP Collaborative Research Group. Arch Intern Med 153:849–858

115. Whelton PK, Appel LJ, Espeland MA, Applegate WB, Ettinger WH Jr, Kostis JB, Kumanyika S, Lacy CR, Johnson KC, Folmar S, Cutler JA (1998) Sodium reduction and weight loss in the treatment of hypertension in older persons: a randomized controlled trial of nonpharmacologic interventions in the elderly (TONE). TONE Collaborative Research Group. JAMA 279:839–846

116. Moore LL, Visioni AJ, Wilson PW, D'Agostino RB, Finkle WD, Ellison RC (2000) Can sustained weight loss in overweight individuals reduce the risk of diabetes mellitus? Epidemiology 11:269–273

117. U.S. Department of Health and Human Services (1996) Physical activity and health: a report of the Surgeon General. U.S. Department of Health and Human Services, Centers for Disease Control and Prevention, National Center for Chronic Disease Prevention and Health Promotion, President's Council on Physical Fitness and Sports. https://www.cdc.gov/nccdphp/sgr/pdf/sgrfull.pdf

118. Pate RR, Pratt M, Blair SN, Haskell WL, Macera CA, Bouchard C, Buchner D, Ettinger W, Heath GW, King AC, Kriska A, Leon AS, Marcus BH, Morris J, Paffenbarger RS, Patrick K, Pollock ML, Rippe JM, Sallis J, Wilmore JH (1995) Physical activity and public health. A recommendation from the Centers for Disease Control and Prevention and the American College of Sports Medicine. JAMA 273:402–407

119. Pereira MA, Kriska AM, Day RD, Cauley JA, LaPorte RE, Kuller LH (1998) A randomized walking trial in postmenopausal women: effects on physical activity and health 10 years later. Arch Intern Med 158:1695–1701

120. Wing R (2011) Development of a behavioral clinical trial: the road from discovery to action. Paper presented at the ORBIT NIH Workshop on innovative study designs and methods for developing, testing and implementing behavioral interventions to improve health, NIH, Bethesda. http://www.nihorbit.org/ORBIT%20Content/Workshops%20and%20 Conferences.aspx?PageView=Shared

121. Perri MG, McAllister DA, Gange JJ, Jordan RC, McAdoo G, Nezu AM (1988) Effects of four maintenance programs on the long-term management of obesity. J Consult Clin Psychol 56:529–534

122. Jeffery RW, Wing RR, Mayer RR (1998) Are smaller weight losses or more achievable weight loss goals better in the long term for obese patients? J Consult Clin Psychol 66:641–645

123. Joyner MJ, Paneth N, Ioannidis JP (2016) What happens when underperforming big ideas in research become entrenched? JAMA 316:1355–1356

124. Lee GC, Jonas S (2013) A proportional funding approach to understanding extramural behavioral and social sciences research and basic behavioral and social sciences research in the NIH's Research, Condition, and Disease Categorization (RCDC) System. Science and Technology Policy Institute, under contract to NIH, Bethesda

125. Naci H, Ioannidis JPA (2015) Comparative effectiveness of exercise and drug interventions on mortality outcomes: metaepidemiological study. Br J Sports Med 49:1414–1422

126. Tabak RG, Khoong EC, Chambers DA, Brownson RC (2012) Bridging research and practice: models for dissemination and implementation research. Am J Prev Med 43:337–350

Chapter 4
Hypothesized Pathway and Bias

"A proper theory sticks its neck out"

Lewens, 2016 [1].

> ## Fundamental Point
>
> *Articulation of a pathway by which a behavioral treatment is hypothesized to translate into a primary endpoint guides the design of a behavioral trial and maximizes an ability to interpret results and advance the science. This pathway should quantify targets for successful implementation of the behavioral treatment and for clinically significant levels of change in the behavioral risk factor and the primary clinical endpoint. A range of biases have been identified in medicine, epidemiology, biostatistics, and behavioral sciences that undercut the ability to test a scientific hypothesis and obtain a conclusive answer to the primary question of interest. Avoidance of these biases is a measure of the quality of a behavioral trial.*

Science proceeds by a progressive process of posing scientific hypotheses and conducting experiments to test them. When this process is directed toward a treatment to improve human health, it is called a clinical trial [2]. The great philosophers of science argued that a good scientific hypothesis "sticks its neck out" with a quantified prediction which can only be tested in an experiment that is free of bias. They further argued that failure should be welcomed as an opportunity to refine and progress, and replication is the best route available to obtain conclusive evidence that a treatment works. In behavioral clinical trials, the scientific hypothesis is translated as the hypothesized pathway. It is the quantified path by which a behavioral treatment is hypothesized to improve a behavioral, biomedical, or chronic disease endpoint. It guides the design of the trial, the interpretation of results, and the next step in a progressive, translational program of research. A trial is inconclusive when it falls prey to any of a number of known biases. Because a behavioral trial synthesizes a behavioral treatment with a health endpoint, biases identified in behavioral sci-

© Springer Nature Switzerland AG 2021
L. H. Powell et al., *Behavioral Clinical Trials for Chronic Diseases*,
https://doi.org/10.1007/978-3-030-39330-4_4

ences, medicine, epidemiology, and biostatistics can all pose potential problems. Mastery of this complete range of potential biases will promote the rigor and conclusiveness of any single behavioral trial.

SCIENTIFIC PRINCIPLES

The Logic of Scientific Hypotheses

The great philosopher of science, Karl Popper, advanced our understanding of the logic of scientific hypotheses. His contribution can be summarized into two key principles: (1) science proceeds by progressive deductive hypothesis testing; and (2) scientific hypotheses must be vulnerable to falsification.

> ### Karl R. Popper (1902–1994)
>
> *"Popper is incomparably the greatest philosopher of science that has ever been."*
> Sir Peter Medawar
> Nobel Prize, Medicine [3]
>
> *"There is no more to science than its method, and there is no more to its method than Popper has said."*
> Sir Hermann Bondi,
> Mathematician [3]

Science Proceeds by Deductive Hypothesis Testing

Inductive reasoning uses evidence from a specific observation to make a generalization about the universal. Inductive inferences guide everyday living. Observing that the sun rises every morning leads to the inductive inference that the sun always rises. Inductive inferences also guide science. Observations from a specific experiment form the basis for the inference that the result applies to the general.

Although Popper believed that the sun will always rise because it has always done so, it was the logic of this reasoning that troubled him. His discomfort stemmed from what is now referred to as Hume's challenge, first articulated in 1739:

> *"What, if anything, makes it possible to extrapolate from a limited sample to a broader generalization?" [4]*

Popper arrived at an answer to this challenge by considering the logic behind inductive and deductive reasoning in his now famous swan example (Fig. 4.1) [5]. The top of this figure portrays inductive inference. It starts with observations, not a hypothesis. With each observation, a white swan is observed. But no matter how many instances of white swans have been observed, one cannot make the inductive leap that *all* swans are white. There can always be a new observation, at any point in the future, in which a black swan is observed. From the point of view of pure logic, inductive reasoning is inconclusive. Neither existing scientific dogma in which there is consensus that all swans are white nor a large number of "past successes" in observing white swans can get around this inferential problem.

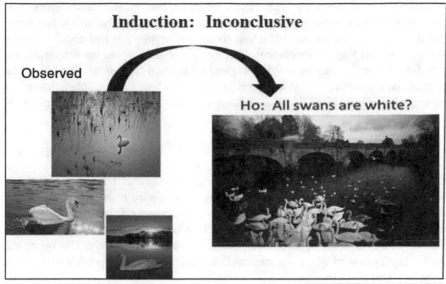

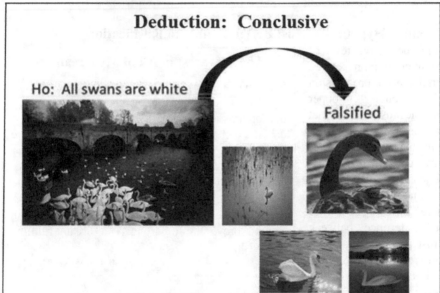

Fig. 4.1 Inductive and deductive logic using Popper's swan example

Deductive logic, portrayed on the bottom of the figure, infers from the general to the specific. It starts with a general hypothesis, makes a prediction that is an implication of that hypothesis, and conducts an experiment to determine whether or not the prediction is supported by empirical observation. In the swan example, if the hypothesis is that all swans are white and an experiment produces a white swan, then the hypothesis endures, waiting for a black swan to emerge. But if an experiment produces a black swan, the hypothesis that all swans are white is falsified conclusively. Although it is logically impossible to conclude with certainty that a hypothesis is true, we can conclude with certainty that it is false.

It is because of the certainty of deductive reasoning that the scientific method proceeds by repeatedly setting up hypotheses and conducting experiments to test them. But it is only with falsification of a hypothesis that certainty is realized. This is the rationale behind Popper's argument that negative results should be welcomed, not avoided. In Popper's mind, falsification and refinement were better for advancing science than maintaining existing beliefs while waiting for the "black swan" to appear. Falsification provides an opportunity, not a source of discouragement. In his own words,

> *"The wrong view of science betrays itself in the craving to be right" [5].*

This logic can be applied to behavioral clinical trials. When the hypothesis that a behavioral treatment will improve an outcome is supported in one clinical trial, the support is tentative, awaiting for a "black swan" to appear. If in a subsequent trial the treatment fails to show a benefit, the "black swan" has appeared, and the hypothesis that this treatment improves outcomes is falsified, conclusively. This opens the door to exploration of why the treatment failed in this trial, refinement, and, as such, progression of the science.

Scientific Hypotheses Must Be Vulnerable to Falsification

Since deductive tests of scientific hypotheses are crucial to the progression of science, Popper became interested in what constitutes a good scientific hypothesis. In the early days of his career, he compared science to what he called pseudoscience. He struggled with the difference between Einstein's theory of relativity, which he admired, and Freud's theory of psychoanalysis, of which

> ### The Cleverest of All of My Dreamers
>
> Freud had a patient he called "the cleverest of all of my dreamers." Freud's explained to her his theory that dreams are the fulfillment of wishes. The next day, the patient described to him a dream where she was traveling to spend a holiday with her mother-in-law, an idea she abhorred. She asked Freud whether or not this was a refutation of his theory. Freud countered that the theory was intact. Since her dream showed that Freud was wrong, her real wish was to prove Freud wrong. Her dream fulfilled that wish.
>
> Lewens, 2016 [1]

he was deeply suspicious. He concluded that the theory of relativity was heroically *vulnerable to destruction* if quantified predictions should show it false. In contrast, psychoanalytic theory was immune to destruction because it was couched in such elastic and noncommittal terms that it could easily stretch around whatever evidence it confronted (see box) [1].

Popper concluded that scientific hypotheses must be vulnerable to falsification. They must make specific predictions that are objective and quantified. A strong scientific hypothesis *"sticks its neck out."*

Tests of Scientific Hypotheses Should Be Free Of Bias

Popper was unwilling to hedge on his dichotomous view of falsification. If the results of an experiment disagree with the scientific hypothesis, then the hypothesis is wrong. But more recent philosophers of science, most notably Feyerabend [6], turned their attention to the quality of the experiment used to test a hypothesis. Could the experiment be a poor test because of some mistake in its design, operations, or interpretation? Scientific observations are value laden. Investigators see what they want to see. And what they see is influenced not only by their personal preferences but also by the reliability and validity of the measuring instruments they use. In Campbell's words:

> *"To the extent that experiments reveal nature to us,
> it is through a very clouded windowpane" [7].*

There is also bias in the larger research community. New hypotheses are often "born" into hostile contexts where there is wide investment in the status quo. This may be a particular problem for new behavioral treatments that are designed for use in established medical settings. Even if a test is unbiased, it can face criticism from a community invested in the status quo. Rather than abandoning a new treatment, it must be nurtured in its infancy [1] with what some have referred to as a "blind conviction" to persist by tinkering, refining, testing, and building resilience against skepticism [6]. Sometimes scientists, like horses, progress best when blinders are on [1].

Application of the Logic of Scientific Hypotheses

Popper and other philosophers of science operated in the world of abstract logic. But the world of medicine is urgent and messy. It is about saving lives, managing disease, and promoting health. Historically, medicine was an art, not easily captured by a set of rules but instead passed down from experienced clinician to student. But because this knowledge transfer was slow and inefficient, clinical research emerged as the partner of clinical medicine, and its "gold standard" became the rigorous clinical trial that guided action in the face of uncertainty [2]. Because of the importance of clinical trials, sophisticated methods in their design, conduct, analysis, and interpretation were developed by clinical researchers, statisticians, and epidemiologists and are now presented in an extensive number of books and papers. Several themes from this literature extend the logic of scientific hypotheses.

Statistical Hypothesis Testing

The inconclusive nature of inductive logic poses a problem for science which proceeds by inferring from specific observations to general applicability. This was the problem that gave rise to the field of inferential statistics which essentially applied deductive reasoning to practice. Statisticians writing in the early 1900s, most notably Fisher, Neyman, and Pearson, developed the basic concepts of statistical hypothesis testing. They did not reject the uncertainty of inductive logic but instead side-stepped around it by arriving at a method to use deductive logic to quantify the uncertainty of deductive inferences [8]. Using the vehicle of the null hypothesis, about which certain properties are known, statistical hypothesis testing aims to reject it with a known, and acceptable, probability of making an error. They never really solved the problem of induction posed by Hume. It remains a logical flaw to make the leap that rejection of the null hypothesis of no treatment benefit means that the hypothesis that a treatment has benefit should be accepted. (*See Chapter 5: Clinical Significance*.)

Statistical hypothesis testing drew on the strength of deductive inferences and quantified the probability of error in making them. It is the fundamental method of modern scientific inquiry. This is not to say that exploration, without pre-existing hypotheses, is inconsistent with scientific inquiry. But it is to say that exploration should be in the service of hypothesis generation. When it is not, it is based upon inconclusive inductive logic.

Quantification of Hypotheses

Falsification requires quantification. Predictive models in clinical trials quantify the level of improvement in a particular risk factor needed to produce a desired level of improvement on a particular outcome [9]. In drug trials, this quantification is developed in a series of *Phase I* and *II* studies aimed at isolating the dose of drug needed to affect the mechanism of action, within limits of safety, and achieve efficacy on surrogate targets. In behavioral trials, the existence of early treatment development studies makes it possible to articulate and refine a quantified hypothesized pathway for a *Phase II* or *Phase III* efficacy trial. (*See Chapter 3: Behavioral Treatment Development*.)

Quantification of the pathway by which a treatment is hypothesized to work results in a hypothesis that "sticks its neck out" for falsification. In Nobel Prize winner Sir Peter Medawar's words:

> *"No experiment should be undertaken without a clear preconception of the forms its results might take; for unless the hypothesis restricts the total number of possible happenings . . ., it will yield no information at all." [10]*

Biases That Render a Trial Inconclusive

Clinical research has gone well beyond philosophy by not only underscoring the importance of bias as an alternative explanation for why a scientific hypothesis was not supported but in providing detail about when and how these biases operate. The beauty of the randomized trial is the equivalence between arms created by random assignment. This fosters the inference that any results are due to treatment, since any pre-existing differences tend to be balanced across arms and thus unlikely to confound treatment effects. This is the reason that the key responsibility of a clinical trialist is to protect the random assignment. (*See Chapter 8: Protection of Random Assignment*.)

Biases can occur at all stages of a trial, including the process of randomization to treatment arms, the trial operations, and the analysis and interpretation of results. For this reason, a vast literature on bias in clinical trials has evolved. A fair estimate is that in excess of 30 different types of pre- and post-randomization biases have been identified [11–13]. The identification of clinical trial biases continues to evolve. New biases reveal themselves as the results of new trials with new designs are reported and critiqued.

Replications Determine the Worth of a Treatment

Medical practice needs answers that are both fast and conclusive. Statistical hypothesis testing provides answers that are fast but not necessarily conclusive. The need for fast tends to minimize the limitation of inconclusiveness. It has fostered the misinterpretation that rejection of the null hypothesis of no treatment benefit means that the treatment is beneficial. It is a logical error to infer that a low probability event under the null hypothesis is evidence that an alternative hypothesis is true. (*See Chapter 5: Clinical Significance.*)

Hume's challenge of what makes it possible to extrapolate from a limited sample to a broader generalization remains unanswered. Clinical research's best approach to solving this problem is through replication. Confidence that a treatment works is bolstered by replications of a trial result by the same or other groups and in the same or other populations. For example, meta-analyses have identified 147 clinical trials testing the benefit of beta blockers for managing blood pressure [14] and 92 clinical trials testing statins for the primary and secondary prevention of major coronary events and mortality [15]. The Diabetes Prevention Program [16] which showed the benefit of lifestyle change on preventing the conversion from insulin resistance to diabetes was replicated at least eight times in such diverse places as Japan, Scandinavia, China, Europe, India, and Finland [17–24].

Essentially, medicine's response to Hume's challenge can be illustrated by drawing on the example of the sun rising, presented earlier. If the sun rises consistently every day for many days, it is reasonable to make the inductive leap to the generalization that the sun always rises.

Summary

The philosophers of science advanced scientific inquiry by illustrating the strength of inferences that result when quantified scientific hypotheses are falsified in experiments that are free of bias. The statisticians extended this basic principle by developing methods to quantify the uncertainty with which inferences about falsification are made. Clinical research detailed the array of biases which could render any single test of a hypothesis inconclusive.

Science is an imperfect method. Belief that the sun always rises stems from the fact that it has done so every day in recorded history and the mechanism of the earth's rotation is understood. Belief that beta blockers are an effective treatment for high blood pressure is strong because 147 clinical trials have shown benefit and the mechanisms are understood. Replication bolsters belief but does not provide a guarantee. If only one trial is available, belief should be, but often is not, considerably weaker.

We must embrace uncertainty in science. In the face of an imperfect method, knowledge is transitory, and humility is appropriate. In Duchamp's words:

"Knowledge keeps like fish."
Marcel Duchamp, 1917

CHALLENGES FOR BEHAVIORAL TRIALS

A rigorous behavioral clinical trial is guided by a quantified hypothesis that is vulnerable to falsification and free of biases that would render results inconclusive. There are two practices common in the current behavioral trials culture that pose a challenge to this rigor.

Exploratory Aims in Confirmatory Trials

A translational science model for the progression of research on behavioral treatments for chronic diseases evolves from exploration and discovery in the early phases to confirmation in the later phases. As relevant questions progress, so too do the methods used to answer them. A challenge is posed for a behavioral trial when there is an attempt to mix these separate questions together into one single trial.

It is a common practice to guide a behavioral trial by an inclusive and explanatory conceptual model. These models represent a disease process by portraying a complex web of causal factors, including bidirectional and reciprocal causal associations and mediators and moderators of these associations. These models can be tested in experiments as well as observational studies using such methods as path analysis to determine strength, direction, and independence of various paths. An example of an explanatory conceptual model is portrayed in Fig. 4.2 at the top. It portrays the complex web of interacting factors that explain childhood obesity [25].

The conceptual model is inclusive, portraying the array of immutable, contextual, behavioral, and biological factors that together explain the problem of childhood obesity. Paths to obesity are bidirectional and reciprocal. Assessments of the strength

Conceptual Model

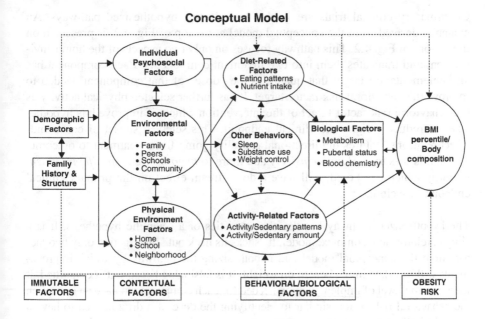

Hypothesized Pathway

Fig. 4.2 Conceptual model and hypothesized pathway for childhood obesity

and independence of specific paths are determined statistically. This model is likely to be a close approximation of the multitude of factors that influence the problem of childhood obesity.

When a behavioral trial is guided by a conceptual model, it is reasonable to explore a variety of outcomes in primary aims, including moderators and mediators of treatment benefit. These types of aims are consistent with the inclusive representation of reality portrayed in the conceptual model. Exploratory studies based upon conceptual models are important and necessary for behavioral treatment development. While they are highly informative in the early design phase, they are not well-suited to the later confirmatory phase.

Confirmatory clinical trials are guided by selective hypothesized pathways. An example, derived from the conceptual model at the top of Fig. 4.2, is presented on the bottom of Fig. 4.2. This pathway focuses on only two aspects of the home environment and translates them into two treatment components. Each component has an implementation target that quantifies the "dose" of that component needed to improve the behavioral risk factor target. It has further selected physical activity as the behavioral risk factor target of the intervention which, if improved, is hypothesized to reduce weight, the clinical endpoint. This selected subset of cause-and-effect relations features unidirectional causality going from treatment to outcome. The aim is less to *explain inclusively* and more to *hypothesize a specific treatment pathway* which, if altered, will have a downstream effect on the primary clinical endpoint of weight.

The hypothesized pathway has the characteristics of a scientific hypothesis. It is a simple, relative to a complex, model. It "sticks its neck out" by targeting only two factors from the conceptual model and hypothesizing the pathway by which improvements will translate into a benefit on weight. It is falsifiable because it is quantified. It identifies the level of implementation needed for each component to have an impact on the behavioral risk factor, similar to identifying the dose of a drug needed to have a biological effect. It identifies a clinically significant milestone for the level of improvement needed on the behavioral risk factor (e.g., physical activity) to achieve improvement on the clinical risk factor (e.g., weight). This clinically significant milestone was derived from clinical guidelines, based upon meta-analyses that identify the level of improvement needed to achieve improvement in cardio-metabolic risk. Each step in the pathway serves as a judge for the success of the behavioral treatment. Each step guides the choice of essential measurements in the trial that will include measures for each step in the pathway using the best, most objective, state-of-the-art instruments available.

The key difference between a conceptual model and a hypothesized pathway is the difference between the aims of discovery and confirmation. Exploratory studies discover associations. Confirmatory trials test quantified models. Early in the process of behavioral intervention development, exploration and discovery are at a premium. Conceptual models can and should inform the design of a treatment. But as development progresses, exploration shifts to confirmation, and conceptual models evolve into refined hypothesized pathways. Confirmation is selective. It "sticks its neck out."

Inadequate attention to the early phases of treatment development can lead to the temptation to conduct behavioral trials which aim to simultaneously discover and confirm. A key symptom of this is when a confirmatory trial features a wide variety of primary outcomes, moderators, and mediators. This runs the risk of posing scientific hypotheses that are not falsifiable. Chance alone will account for some positive associations.

Some exploration in a confirmatory clinical trial is a good use of resources. But it should be articulated as such in exploratory aims. Combining discovery and confirmation into primary aims of a clinical trial is inconsistent with progressive translational science, inconsistent with the scientific method, risks undue participant burden, and opens the door to bias, inconclusive results, and inability to replicate.

Discipline-Specific Approach to Bias

Methods are specific to disciplines. Most applied behavioral scientists came of age learning how to design experiments in the tradition of Campbell and Stanley [12]. This tradition places an emphasis on understanding the dynamics of a behavioral treatment. When the primary aim of a behavioral trial is to understand treatment dynamics, mechanisms, or moderators, as is characteristic of early *Phase I* and some *Phase II* studies, a short-term follow-up is common, and the biases that endanger validity are well-established within the behavioral sciences [12].

But when the aim is to determine efficacy on a chronic disease outcome or a surrogate for it, as is characteristic of *Phase III* efficacy trials and some *Phase II* efficacy trials, unique biases emerge. When participants are followed over extended periods of time, there is less experimental control. Participants can undergo a variety of nontrial treatments and/or they can lose interest in continuing to participate. Biases in *Phase III* clinical trials have been identified in a wide variety of publications, primarily in medical and epidemiological journals.

When the treatment under investigation is behavioral in nature and the efficacy of that treatment is based upon improvement in a chronic disease outcome or surrogate, a cross-disciplinary understanding of bias is needed. Biases identified in *both* the traditions of experimental design and clinical trials must be avoided to promote rigor.

OVERCOMING THESE CHALLENGES IN A BEHAVIORAL TRIAL

Guide Trial Design with a Hypothesized Pathway

Figure 4.3 presents a template for a hypothesized pathway. The hypothesis to be tested in a *Phase III* behavioral trial is that treatment (**A**) will have a clinically significant (CS⚠) benefit on clinical outcome (**D**). Early phase studies of this treatment show that it can be implemented by participants as designed (**A→B**) and that this level of implementation can produce a clinically significant change in the behavioral or biomedical risk factor target of treatment (**B→C**). The link between **A** and **B** demonstrates that participants can and will enact the treatment according to pro-

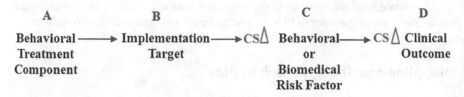

Fig. 4.3 Template for hypothesized pathway for a behavioral clinical trial

tocol. The link between **B** and **C** is that this level of implementation will produce a change in a behavioral risk factor that is strong enough to produce a change on a clinical endpoint. Note the emphasis on clinically significant (CS) change in both the behavioral risk factor (**C**) and the clinical endpoint (**D**). These are categorical milestones which, if achieved, will be linked to clinically meaningful reduction of disease risk.

Figure 4.3 can be modified for a *Phase II* behavioral trial by eliminating (**D**). By so doing, the primary outcome becomes the behavioral or biomedical risk factor in (**C**).

A hypothesized pathway, such as that shown in Fig. 4.3, should be articulated early in a program of research to guide progress at all subsequent stages. Feasibility studies can determine whether or not a treatment component can be implemented as designed. Refinement studies can determine whether a specific level of implementation is sufficient to improve a behavioral risk factor at a clinically significant level. Answers to these questions at early developmental phases provide the opportunity to refine the behavioral treatment, as well as the hypothesized pathway, before moving to a confirmatory *Phase II* or *Phase III* behavioral trial.

The structure of a hypothesized pathway can be extended to explore mediators (**C**) and biomedical mechanisms (**E**), as presented in Fig. 4.4. When mediators and mechanisms are included in a hypothesized pathway, they are confirmatory, not exploratory. Inclusion means that they *must* be improved for a treatment to have benefit on a clinical outcome. They become, in essence, a way to judge the success of a treatment. Although an understanding of mediators and mechanisms increases confidence in a behavioral treatment, without certainty that they are part of the pathway, it is risky to judge treatment success by change in them. Mechanisms of action in drugs are often elusive, and their immense biological subtlety often presents itself long after a drug has been on the market. Similarly, behavioral mediators and mechanisms are often elusive. Many behavioral treatments have produced clinically significant benefit without a clear understanding of the psychological or biomedical mechanisms of action [26].

When there is uncertainty, mediators and mechanisms are better included as secondary or exploratory aims rather than part of a hypothesized pathway. Inclusion of a mediator that is hypothesized *not* to change with treatment can be a powerful way to support the discriminant validity of that treatment. In a progressive, translational science model, mediators and mechanisms explored in the early phases of treatment

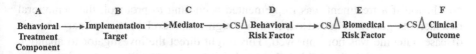

A		B		C		D		E		F
Behavioral	→	Implementation	→	Mediator	→	CS△ Behavioral	→	CS △ Biomedical	→	CS△ Clinical
Treatment		Target				Risk Factor		Risk Factor		Outcome
Component										

Fig. 4.4 Expanded template for hypothesized pathway for a behavioral clinical trial

development could promote more certainty about their role in producing a benefit from a treatment, thereby justifying their incorporation into the hypothesized pathway in a confirmatory *Phase II* or *Phase III* trial, as shown in Fig. 4.4.

Interpret Trial Results with a Hypothesized Pathway

A major benefit of having a simple, quantified, a priori hypothesized pathway is that it aids in the interpretation of results of a trial and decisions about appropriate next steps. It is obvious when the result of a trial is positive or null. But without a hypothesized pathway, it is less obvious why.

In a *Phase III* trial where the hypothesis is that a behavioral treatment will improve a disease outcome, it is a failure of the treatment if milestones were not achieved in the first step (A to B in Fig. 4.3) or in the second step (B to C in Fig. 4.3). It is a failure of the hypothesis when milestones were achieved in these first and second steps but they did not translate into achievement of the milestone in the third step (A to D in Fig. 4.3).

In a *Phase II* trial where the hypothesis is that a behavioral treatment will improve a behavioral or biomedical risk factor, it is a failure of the treatment if milestones were not achieved in the first step (A to B in Fig. 4.3) and a failure of the hypothesis if milestones were achieved in the first step, but they did not translate into benefit on the behavioral or biomedical risk factor at the second step (B to C in Fig. 4.3).

In the event of a positive trial where benefit on the primary outcome was achieved, generalizability depends upon an ability to determine if it was by a known or unknown pathway. If targets for every link in the hypothesized pathway were achieved, the pathway of benefit is known, and it would encourage replication by the same or another group, an effectiveness trial in a real-world setting, and/or a dismantling study to determine if the same effect could be produced more efficiently. Alternatively, if targets were not achieved on one or more steps of the hypothesized pathway, the interpretation would be that a positive effect was achieved by an unknown pathway. In this situation, it would be of interest to refine the pathway, based perhaps on qualitative studies in the participants, and determine if the same effect could be produced in a new trial using a refined hypothesized pathway.

In the event of a null trial, it is incumbent on the investigator to determine why the trial failed. In a *Phase III* trial, a failure of the hypothesis would be the right conclusion if a treatment was implemented according to protocol, the behavioral risk factor target was reduced to a clinically significant level, but the primary chronic disease outcome was not improved. This might direct the investigator to abandon this treatment approach, or this behavioral risk factor target, as a way to improve a chronic disease. Alternatively, a failure of the treatment would be the right conclusion if one or more links in the hypothesized pathway were not improved. Either the treatment could not be implemented as designed or it was not strong enough to achieve a clinically significant improvement on the behavioral risk factor. A failure of the treatment might direct the investigator to go back to the treatment development phase to refine and optimize in places where weakness occurred. In past behavioral clinical trials which produced null results, it is common to mistake a failure to deliver the treatment as a failure of the trial hypothesis [27–29].

When the hypothesized pathway is evaluated against results for a comparator group, it can provide insight into potential biases in the trial design or implementation. Unexpected improvement in a comparator condition, particularly to levels that are clinically significant, could be a sign of treatment crossover or the choice of a control that was more active than intended.

Following are concrete examples of the usefulness of a hypothesized pathway to the interpretation of results and decisions about next steps.

- In a null trial, the hypothesized pathway revealed that participants in the comparator arm underwent clinically significant improvement on the behavioral risk factor. This may suggest that the comparator was an active treatment. If the sample size in the trial was based upon the assumption that the comparator group would not change from their baseline level, the hypothesized effect size would be smaller than assumed, and the trial will be underpowered to detect it. A future direction could be to conduct a pilot study of several choices for comparators and determine empirically the best one. Significant change in the comparator group could also suggest treatment contamination where participants sought trial treatment on their own. Another future direction could be to repeat the trial, keep track of all treatments participants received, and improve the rigor of the trial operations by developing a culture characterized by equipoise, the honest belief that the answer to the question of which arm is better is unknown.

- In a null trial, the hypothesized pathway revealed that attendance at the treatment sessions was only 30% when the goal was 80%. This was a failure to implement the treatment. It would encourage qualitative analyses to obtain the perspective of the participants on what could help to improve engagement. If refinement of the protocol bolstered attendance and a small proof-of-concept study showed it produced clinically significant benefit, it would justify replication of the trial rather than abandonment of the treatment.

- In a positive trial, the hypothesized pathway revealed that attendance at the treatment sessions was only 30% when the goal was 80%. This could suggest that the implementation target was unnecessarily stringent and only 30% of the treatment "dose" is needed. It could also suggest that an alternative pathway may have produced benefit. A replication of the same trial but with a lower required dose of treatment in a small proof-of-concept study could help to disentangle these possible explanations.

Develop Cross-Disciplinary Sophistication in Common Trial Biases

Before making the judgment that a hypothesis has been tested and a conclusive result obtained, it is essential to rule out potential biases that may provide alternative explanations for results and thus compromise the trial. While it is clearly preferable to anticipate and minimize bias before undertaking a trial, identification of unexpected biases that may be emerging during the course of a trial, or have occurred in a completed trial, aids in its its interpretation. There are five general categories of bias.

1. *The Passage of Time.* Participants would have improved or worsened due to the passage of time, without any treatment. These biases provide the essential justification for use of a randomized design since participants in all arms will experience these extraneous factors similarly.

2. *Errors in Statistical Inference.* Violations of assumptions underlying statistical procedures can spuriously enhance or undercut an inference of covariation between a treatment and an outcome.

3. *Preferences.* When participants, staff, providers, and/or investigators view treatment arms as "favored" and "unfavored," reactivity to that value-laden label influences behavior. These biases provide the justification for extending the blind in as many ways, and to as many people, as possible.

4. *Unintended Treatments.* Part of active treatment could include other, unintended factors that covary with a defined treatment. This could spuriously potentiate the treatment effect but undercut the ability to replicate it. It is important to distinguish treatment effects from nuisance variables and clarify this before beginning a trial.

5. *Dissimilar Treatments.* Treatments that look different and have different operational demands can inadvertently promote differential trial procedures that affect the quality of data collection.

Table 4.1 presents a list of specific biases that have been identified within each of these five categories. All have presented problems for *Phase II* or *Phase III* behavioral clinical trials in the past. It is a synthesis of biases identified in experimental research in the behavioral and social sciences [12], clinical trials in medicine [30], and epidemiologic methods [11]. It includes a column labeled "Prevention" which presents a general suggestion for how to minimize the risk of the particular bias in trial design, implementation, or interpretation. Suggestions in bold apply to all biases in the category; other suggestions are type-specific.

SOURCE OF BIAS	SPECIFIC BIAS	EXPLANATION	PREVENTION
Passage of time		**Since the outcome could have occurred over time without treatment, it is a mistake to infer treatment caused it**	– Randomized design
	Spontaneous remission/ Maturation	Natural changes occurring in absence of treatment (e.g., older, sicker, spontaneous remission of disease)	
	Historical events/ Secular trends	Events occurring during follow-up that affect outcome (e.g., policy changes, advertising campaigns, secular trends in disease)	– Parallel cohort designs
	Regression	Participants selected because of extremeness tend to be less extreme upon retest (e.g., high blood pressure, elevated stress, overweight)	– Repeated baseline eligibility assessments
	Testing	Familiarity with a test due to repeated testing over time is confounded with treatment effects (e.g., cognitive function)	– Statistical adjustment for testing effects – Parallel forms of tests
	Instrumentation	Change in measuring instrument over time is confounded with treatment effects (e.g., adjudicators become more proficient)	– Ongoing calibration of measuring instruments and outcomes assessors
Statistical inference		**The inference of covariation between a treatment and outcome is weakened by violation of statistical assumptions**	
	Low power	Low probability of rejecting the null hypothesis when the alternative hypothesis is true and thus a high probability of Type II error	– Increase sample size – Increase strength of treatment – Decrease diversity of participants/settings – Less stringent comparator
	Violation of statistical assumptions	Data may not meet the parametric statistical test assumptions of normality of distribution or independence of observations	– Non-parametric tests for non- normal distributions – Cluster randomized designs for correlated observations

Table 4.1 Selected biases common in behavioral clinical trials

(continued)

Table 4.1 (continued)

SOURCE OF BIAS	SPECIFIC BIAS	EXPLANATION	PREVENTION
	Fishing/Data snooping/"*Cherry picking*"	Multiple statistical tests conducted on multiple outcomes increase the probability of a Type I false positive error	– Single primary outcome – Single behavioral risk factor target – Statistical adjustment of alpha
	Unreliable measures	Low reliability biases toward the null hypothesis	– Identify valid and reliable outcome measures before starting a trial
	Spectrum bias/ Restriction of range/Ceiling effect	Restricted range of disease outcome or behavioral risk factor promotes floor/ceiling effects and biases toward the null hypothesis	– Include diverse populations and tailor treatment to enhance efficacy within subgroups
Preferences		**Differential expectations of benefit undercut equivalence created by randomization**	**– Foster a culture of equipoise throughout trial** **– Extend the blind to as many players as possible** **– Blind to hypotheses but not to trial aims**
	Co-interventions/ Compensatory treatment	Providers, families offer more/ less non-trial treatment based upon expectations of benefit from the trial arm to which participant was randomized	– Assess all non-trial treatments undergone by participants
	Treatment contamination/ Underdog/John Henry	Participants randomized to comparator seek trial treatment on their own because they failed to get the desired treatment	– Assess all non-trial treatments undergone by participants
	Demoralization	Participants randomized to comparator lose interest, compromising adherence, outcomes assessment, and running the risk of differential dropout	– Monitor attendance and drop-out rates closely in both arms – Provide attractive compensation for completing the primary outcome at the end of the trial
	Ascertainment bias	Outcomes assessors become aware of the arm to which the participant is randomized and judge outcomes differentially based upon their arm-specific expectations of benefit	– Blind outcomes assessors to the treatment arm to which participant is randomized – Instruct participants not to engage in discussions with staff about treatment activities

(continued)

Table 4.1 (continued)

SOURCE OF BIAS	SPECIFIC BIAS	EXPLANATION	PREVENTION
	Pygmalion effect/ Rosenthal effect	When the same interventionists are used for different arms, their higher expectations for one arm positively influence the outcome of that arm	– Use different interventionists for different arms but insure similar levels of expertise
	Expectancy bias/ Optimistic bias/"True believer"	Principal investigator's strength of commitment to a specific outcome or treatment arm promotes preferences in staff and participants	– Investigator adopts a scientific mindset of equipoise throughout all aspects of trial – Investigator limits trial involvement to supervising the intervention
	Early unblinding to results	Knowledge of outcome before completion of follow-up changes expectations for remaining treatment and outcome assessment	– Protocols for unblinding to various outcomes are pre-specified and approved by a Data and Safety Monitoring Board – Interim results evaluated by Data and Safety Monitoring Board only, presented to them by an unblinded biostatistician
Unintended treatments		**Inadvertent and differential non-trial treatments**	
	Non-specific attention/ Hawthorne effect	Differential attention of any type improves outcomes	– Use attention control comparator – Include attention as a component of treatment
	Placebo response	Differential beliefs about efficacy and/or contextual factors in the treatment setting promote placebo response	– Use placebo control – Include contextual factors as components of treatment
	Interventionist expertise	Differential expertise of interventionists across arms	– Use highly experienced interventionists for all arms – Manualize treatment protocols – Ongoing supervision and fidelity checks of interventionists

(continued)

Table 4.1 (continued)

SOURCE OF BIAS	SPECIFIC BIAS	EXPLANATION	PREVENTION
	Implementation/ Adherence	Different demands in trial arms promote differential ability to implement them and/or willingness to adhere to them	– Feasibility pilot studies to assess and improve adherence to respective protocols
Dissimilar treatments		**Because treatments are not identical, they trigger differential reactivity to them**	
	Ascertainment bias	Differences in patient contact by trial arm influence staff awareness of events and outcomes and participant ability to recall them	– Use one standardized approach for outcome assessment in all participants – Separate reports of outcomes obtained during the course of intervening from those obtained using the standardized trial protocol
	"Faking good"/ Reactive self-reports/ Social desirability	Differential desire to please, by arm, promotes spurious self-reports	– Objective measures, rather than self-reports, whenever possible, especially for the primary outcome
	Post-randomization selection bias	Differential dropout results in post-randomization non-equivalence between arms	– Encourage dropouts to drop the intervention but stay in the trial – Minimize burden for dropouts by obtaining permission to assess primary outcome only – Budget travel to participant location for outcome assessment – Provide generous participant incentives to complete final outcome assessment – Intent-to-treat analyses with conservative assumptions for missing data on the primary endpoint

SELECTED EXPERIENCE FROM BEHAVIORAL TRIALS

The Hypothesized Pathway in a Successful Behavioral Trial

The Diabetes Prevention Program was among the greatest successes reported to date for a lifestyle program's ability to improve a chronic disease outcome [16, 31, 32]. The aim was to compare the benefits of lifestyle, metformin, and placebo on preventing the development of diabetes in patients who were insulin resistant. Results showed that lifestyle was 30% better than the best drug available and 60% better than a placebo pill.

This lifestyle treatment was developed progressively and systematically over approximately 40 years in an array to studies done by a variety of investigators. *(See Chapter 3: Behavioral Treatment Development, Table 3.9.)* This extensive development resulted in the ability to articulate a quantified hypothesized pathway by which the treatment

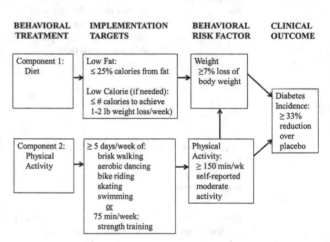

Fig. 4.5 Hypothesized pathway in the Diabetes Prevention Program

would translate into a reduction in diabetes incidence (Fig. 4.5) [32]. It can be seen that this pathway "sticks its neck out." It portrays two components, each of which is linked to a quantified implementation target and behavioral risk factor target. Physical activity has a direct path to the primary outcome and an indirect path to it through its ability to sustain weight loss over and above changes in dietary intake.

Results of the trial supported the hypothesis that this was the pathway by which the treatment reduced the incidence of diabetes. At the conclusion of the 6-month lifestyle treatment, 50% of participants met the goal of ≥7% loss of body weight, and 74% met the goal of ≥150 minutes of physical activity/week [16]. By the end of the average of 3.2 years of follow-up, 38% continued to meet the body weight goal, and 58% continued to meet the physical activity goal [16]. Although the percentages of people expected to meet the behavioral risk factor targets were not specified a priori, the success of the trial suggests that the percentage of participants who achieved each target was sufficient to reduce diabetes incidence. These percentages of success can be embedded into future hypothesized pathways as clinically significant targets. Further support for the validity of the hypothesized model is provided by the 10-year follow-up of the program [33]. There were no differences in diabetes incidence among the three randomized arms in the interval between the 3.2-year end of treatment and the 10-year follow-up. This is tracked with posttreatment weight regain over the same interval.

The Hypothesized Pathway Explains a Null Trial

The aim of the Women's Health Initiative Dietary Modification Trial was to determine if a low-fat eating pattern would reduce risk of cardiovascular disease, colorectal cancer, and breast cancer. A total of 48,385 women were randomized to a diet intervention or a usual care comparison in a 40:60 ratio, respectively. This was a null trial in which there was no benefit of the dietary intervention on any of the three primary clinical outcomes. This null result, in combination with the extraordinary expenditure of resources expended in this trial, justified working back through the hypothesized pathway to determine what happened.

The behavioral target of the intervention was a low-fat eating pattern, operationalized as ≤20% of intake from fat, 5 servings/day of vegetables and fruits, and 6 servings/day of grains. The results for the cardiovascular disease outcome are presented in Table 4.2 [34]. It can be seen that the diet improved but dietary goals were not met at the end of the 6-year follow-up period.

A post hoc, per-protocol investigation was aimed at determining benefit if participants had achieved dietary goals. The treated group was broken down into quartiles based upon the dietary changes achieved by 1 year. Rates of cardiovascular disease at 6 years were compared in those who were in the lowest quartile in the treated arm relative to those in the usual care comparator. Those who had an average intake of saturated fat <6.1%, had an average intake of trans fat <1.1%, or ate ≥6.5 servings of vegetables and fruits/day had a lower incidence of cardiovascular events than those randomized to usual care (HR = 0.81–0.88).

Table 4.2 Expected vs. observed dietary changes in the Women's Health Initiative Dietary Modification Trial

	Goal	Baseline	1 year	6 years
Percent energy from fat	≤20%	37.8%	24.3%	28.8%
Vegetable/fruit servings/day	5	3.6	5.1	4.9
Grains servings/day	6	4.7	5.1	4.3

Although post hoc findings are suggestive but not conclusive, they provide a valuable opportunity to consider reasonable next steps in a program of research after a null trial. Because a priori goals specified in the hypothesized pathway were not met, this was a failure of the treatment, not the hypothesis. Post hoc analyses suggested that the specific target for vegetable intake should be increased from 5 to 6.5 servings/day. They also suggested that the treatment be refined to target saturated and trans fat rather than total fat. A refined hypothesized pathway, and a more targeted intervention, may provide a conclusive test of the impact of diet on cardiovascular disease. But before such a rigorous replication is undertaken, it would be wise to conduct a small proof-of-concept study to determine if a refined and more targeted intervention is strong enough to achieve the revised clinically significant targets on vegetable, saturated fat, and trans fat intake.

Consequences of Mistaking a Failed Treatment for a Failed Hypothesis

The Trials of Hypertension Prevention (TOHP) Collaborative Research Group trials aimed to determine the best approach for preventing the development of hypertension in persons with high normal diastolic blood pressure. In the first of two trials, the Phase I TOHP-I trial tested the feasibility and efficacy of seven nonpharmacologic interventions on the primary endpoint of diastolic blood pressure [29]. These interventions included three lifestyle treatments (weight reduction, sodium restriction, stress management) and four dietary supplements. All were compared against a usual care control. The importance of TOHP-I was that only those interventions that were efficacious would go on to be tested in the larger Phase II TOHP-II trial which examined the impact of the interventions on the incidence of hypertension [35].

TOHP-I results indicated that only the weight loss and sodium restriction groups were effective at lowering diastolic blood pressure. Stress management was ineffective at both 6 and 18 months suggesting a *failure of the hypothesis* that reduction in stress was associated with a reduction in blood pressure. From the Abstract:

> *"Despite good compliance, stress management did not reduce diastolic blood pressure significantly (P>.05)."*

However, a closer look raises the possibility that this was instead a *failure of the intervention* aimed at managing stress. Although attendance at stress sessions was 86%, Table 4.3 shows that at the 18-month end of treatment, the stress management group experienced a significant *increase*, and the usual care group a *decrease*, in the frequency of hassles, the primary measure of stress (+1.9 vs. −0.5, respectively, $p < 0.05$). This translated into no difference between arms on diastolic blood pressure at 18 months, although both were below the clinically significant cutpoint for hypertension of 80 mmHg.

Table 4.3 Comparison of treatment effects in TOHP-I and TOHP-II at the 18-month follow-up

			TOHP- I			TOHP-II	
		N	Behavioral target: Δ 0–18 months	Diastolic blood pressure target: $\bar{X}$ 18 months	N	Behavioral target: Δ 0–18 months	Diastolic blood pressure target: $\bar{X}$ 18 months
Stress management	Treated	242	+1.9[*a]	78.4 mmHg[ns]	—	—	—
	Usual care	589	−0.5	78.9 mmHg	—	—	—
Weight reduction	Treated	308	−3.8 kg**	77.5 mmHg**	595	−2.0 kg***	81.5 mmHg***
	Usual care	589	+0.1 kg	80.1 mmHg	596	+0.7 kg	82.6 mmHg

[a]Frequency of Daily Hassles Scale
ns not significant
*$p < 0.05$
**$p < 0.01$
***$p < 0.001$

In contrast, Table 4.3 shows that the weight outcome in TOHP-I followed the expected pattern. Participants in the weight reduction intervention lost weight, and the usual care controls gained weight (−3.8 kg vs. +0.1 kg, respectively, $p < 0.01$). This translated into a statistically significant 2.6 mmHg difference between arms on diastolic blood pressure at 18 months ($p < 0.01$). Only the treated group achieved the clinically significant cutpoint for hypertension of <80 mmHg.

Because the stress management intervention did not produce a statistically significant reduction in blood pressure in TOHP-I, it did not move forward to be evaluated for its impact on incidence of hypertension in TOHP-II. However, the weight reduction treatment was evaluated in TOHP-II. It produced an average of 2.0 kg of weight loss and achieved a mean blood pressure of 81.5 mmHg at 18 months, both of which were statistically different from usual care ($p < 0.001$) due, to a certain extent, to the large sample size. The primary endpoint, incidence of hypertension, was reduced by 22% at 18 months ($p = 0.05$) and by 13% at 48 months ($p = 0.06$). This finding resulted in the recommendation to include weight reduction in clinical practice guidelines for patients with high normal blood pressure.

The failure to test the stress management intervention in TOHP-II was a missed opportunity. This decision was made based upon the inability to distinguish between a failure of the stress intervention and a failure of the hypothesis that reduction in stress improves diastolic blood pressure. The "red flags" were the increase in stress in the treated group and the decrease in stress in the usual care group. Whatever was going on in these two arms, both arms decreased diastolic blood pressure from a baseline of 82 mmHg (above the cutpoint for hypertension of 80 mmHg) to below this cutpoint.

This is an excellent example of how critical it is to make the distinction between a failure of the hypothesis and a failure of the treatment. The existence of a quantified hypothesized pathway would have helped make this distinction. In the face of a failed stress intervention, a reasonable next step would have been to increase its strength in a refinement study and replicate for the purpose of determining whether or not it should be a candidate for further evaluation in TOHP-II. Because the stress intervention was not evaluated in TOHP-II, it is unclear how it would have fared alone, or in combination with the other lifestyle factors. Another trial is needed. The clinical implication of this mistake is that experts in hypertension prevention interpret the TOHP results to mean that preventive efforts should focus on weight, but not on stress.

RECOMMENDATIONS

It is tempting to take the easy road in an academic career. It is, for example, comparatively easy to conduct a randomized trial guided by a complex conceptual model, compare treated to controls on a wide variety of outcomes, show a statistically significant difference on one or more of these outcomes, judge the treatment to be successful, get a publication needed to advance an academic career, and decide the job is done. This is a reasonable strategy, supported by a culture that includes not only investigators but also funders, institutions, and reviewers.

The problem with this "easy road" is that this is not good science. The result could have little to do with improving a chronic disease. It could be statistically, but not clinically, significant. It could be explained by simple design decisions such as the choice of the control, the size of the sample, or the number of comparisons conducted.

The "road not taken" is the harder road. It is the one that aims to identify behavioral treatments that improve chronic disease endpoints for the purpose of maximizing effective management. Should this road be taken, the roadmap for the trip is progressive treatment development guided by a hypothesized

> **The Road Not Taken**
>
> "... *Two roads diverged in the wood and I –*
> *I took the one less traveled by,*
> *And that has made all the difference.*"
>   Robert Frost
>   (1874–1963)

pathway. The pathway is created in the earliest stages of development and guides the studies, designs, and milestones evaluated at each subsequent stage. As an understanding of the treatment grows, the hypothesized pathway becomes simpler, more targeted, and more precise, and treatment evaluation progresses toward bigger, more rigorous, and more ambitious trials. The end game is an evidence-based behavioral treatment that meets the rigorous standards of evidence established in medical research.

For those who choose "the road not taken," several recommendations are offered.

Stick Your Neck Out

Karl Popper, the great philosopher of science, has provided behavioral trialists with two gifts that should be considered seriously. First, he encourages us to *welcome failure* as an opportunity to refine, simplify, and progress. This mindset is consistent with one of the key mantras of Silicon Valley: "*Failure provides the seedbed for innovation.*" Second, Popper encourages *humility*. Any claims about the benefits of a treatment can be overturned in the next trial. Embracing failure and humility in one's science and career encourages the freedom to have intellectual curiosity.

"Stick your neck out" means guiding your research program with a quantified hypothesized pathway. It means making bold hypotheses, seeing failure as an opportunity for refinement, persisting in the effort to understand, and progressing toward simplification. In behavioral treatments for chronic diseases, the web of causal factors is complex and progress can be slow. Those who are willing to "stick your neck out" will be aligning the method to the complexity of the problem.

Advance Academically as a Behavioral Trialist

Aspiring behavioral trialists may believe they are faced with a dilemma. Either advance one's academic career or do good science. Academic advancement is based upon products which most often take the form of external grants and publications. Doing good science as a trialist is characterized by a process that features treatments that fail and papers that have difficulties getting published.

The contradictory goals of academic advancement and good science are beginning to dissolve in the field of behavioral treatments for chronic diseases with recent evolutions in funding and publication practices. The National Institutes of Health now offer a variety of funding mechanisms for early treatment development studies and funding mechanisms that combine early feasibility studies with confirmatory trials but make success in the former contingent for continued funding for the latter. On the publication side, there has been an emergence of journals directed toward early phase studies. Publishing potential is maximized if early studies are positioned within the context of a progressive program of research, rather than an end unto themselves. Failures, guided by a priori hypothesized pathways, become important topics for papers if they not only document the failure but articulate why it is likely to have occurred and how it is a springboard to the next study guided by a refined hypothesized pathway. Guidelines now exist for the publication of intervention development studies [36].

Because behavioral treatment development is a slow process, it is wise to have other lines of research with shorter timelines for publications. Fruitful second lines of research can be developed through collaborations with investigators who are leading ongoing epidemiological studies or clinical trials. These investigators have a responsibility to their funding agency to show productivity in exchange for the large amount of resources they have been given to conduct such investigations. Affiliating with these investigators, learning how to work with their datasets, and writing papers from them is mutually beneficial. Beyond this, there are now many public use datasets that exist for completed studies. These datasets can be accessed without requiring collaboration with the principal investigator.

Become an Expert in Behavioral Clinical Trial Biases

Rigorous behavioral clinical trials require bridging disciplines and synthesizing insights. The challenge in a behavioral trial is to preserve the randomization over long periods of time, in the presence of treatment arms that often "look and feel" very different from one another, and under conditions where investigators often have a long-standing commitment to the treatment under investigation. Since the treatment is behavioral, mastery of biases in experimental design is needed. Since the outcome is a chronic disease or surrogate, mastery of biases in clinical trials is needed.

Interdisciplinary sophistication in the range of potential biases that could occur in a behavioral trial makes it clear that it is a mistake to assume that once randomization is accomplished, the problems with bias are over. In fact, new challenges are now beginning.

REFERENCES

1. Lewens T (2016) The meaning of science: an introduction to the philosophy of science. Basic Books, New York
2. Piantadosi S (2017) Clinical trials: a methodologic perspective, 3rd edn. Wiley, Hoboken
3. Magee B (1973) Karl Popper. Viking, New York
4. Hume D (1739-1740) A treatise of human nature. Edited by DF Norton, MJ Norton (2000). Oxford University Press, Oxford
5. Popper KR (1959) The logic of scientific discovery. Basic Books, New York
6. Feyerabend P (1975) Against method: outline of an anarchist theory of knowledge. Verso, New York
7. Campbell DT (1988) Methodology and epistemology for social science: selected papers. University of Chicago Press, Chicago
8. Fisher RA (1935) The design of experiments. Oliver and Boyd, Edinburgh
9. Susser M (1973) Causal thinking in the health sciences. Concepts and strategies of epidemiology. Oxford University Press, New York
10. Medawar PB (1979) Advice to a young scientist. Harper & Row, New York
11. Sackett DL (1979) Bias in analytic research. J Chron Dis 32:51–63
12. Shadish WR, Cook TD, Campbell DT (2002) Experimental and quasi-experimental designs for generalized causal inference. Houghton Mifflin, Boston
13. Shapiro SH, Louis TA (1983) Clinical trials: issues and approaches. Marcel Dekker, New York
14. Law MR, Morris JK, Wald NJ (2009) Use of blood pressure lowering drugs in the prevention of cardiovascular disease: meta-analysis of 147 randomised trials in the context of expectations from prospective epidemiological studies. BMJ 338:b1665. https://doi.org/10.1136/bmj.b1665
15. Naci H, Brugts JJ, Fleurence R, Tsoi B, Toor H, Ades AE (2013) Comparative benefits of statins in the primary and secondary prevention of major coronary events and all-cause mortality: a network meta-analysis of placebo-controlled and active-comparator trials. Eur J Prev Cardiol 20:641–657
16. Knowler WC, Barrett-Connor E, Fowler SE, Hamman RF, Lachin JM, Walker EA, Nathan DM, Diabetes Prevention Program Research Group (2002) Reduction in the incidence of type 2 diabetes with lifestyle intervention or metformin. New Engl J Med 346:393–403
17. Kosaka K, Noda M, Kuzuya T (2005) Prevention of type 2 diabetes by lifestyle intervention: a Japanese trial in IGT males. Diab Res Clin Pract 67:152–162
18. Saito T, Watanabe M, Nishida J, Izumi T, Omura M, Takagi T, Fukunaga R, Bandai Y, Tajima N, Nakamura Y, Ito M, Zensharen Study for Prevention of Lifestyle Diseases Group (2011) Lifestyle modification and prevention of type 2 diabetes in overweight Japanese with impaired fasting glucose levels. Arch Intern Med 171:1352–1360
19. Sakane N, Sato J, Tsushita K, Tsujii S, Kotani K, Tsuzaki K, Tominaga M, Kawazu S, Sato Y, Usui T, Kamae I, Yoshida T, Kiyohara Y, Sato S, Kuzuya H, Japan Diabetes Prevention Program (JDPP) Research Group (2011) Prevention of type 2 diabetes in a primary healthcare setting: three-year results of lifestyle intervention in Japanese subjects with impaired glucose tolerance. BMC Public Health 11:40. https://doi.org/10.1186/1471-2458-11-40
20. Lindahl B, Nilsson TK, Borch-Johnsen K, Oder ME, Soderberg S, Widman L, Johnson O, Hallmans G, Jansson J (2009) A randomized lifestyle intervention with 5-year follow-up in subjects with impaired glucose tolerance: pronounced short-term impact but long-term adherence problems. Scand J Pub Health 37:434–442
21. Pan XR, Li GW, Hu YH, Wang JX, Yang WY, An ZX, Hu ZX, Lin J, Xiao JZ, Cao HB, Liu PA, Jiang XG, Jiang YY, Wang JP, Zheng H, Zhang H, Bennett PH, Howard BV (1997) Effects of diet and exercise in preventing NIDDM in people with impaired glucose tolerance. Diabetes Care 20:537–544

22. Penn L, White M, Lindstrom J, den Boer AT, Blaak E, Eriksson JG, Feskens E, Ilanne-Parikka P, Keinanen-Kiukaanniemi SM, Walker M, Mathers JC, Uusitupa M, Tuomilehto J (2013) Importance of weight loss maintenance and risk prediction in the prevention of type 2 diabetes: analysis of European Diabetes Prevention Study RCT. PLoS ONE 8:e57143. https://doi.org/10.1371/journal.pone.0057143
23. Ramachandran A, Snehalatha C, Ram J, Selvam S, Simon M, Nanditha A, Shetty AS, Godsland IF, Chaturvedi N, Majeed A, Oliver N, Toumazou C, Alberti KG, Johnston DG (2013) Effectiveness of mobile phone messaging in prevention of type 2 diabetes by lifestyle modification in men in India: a prospective, parallel-group, randomized controlled trial. Lancet 1:191–198
24. Tuomilehto J, Lindström J, Eriksson JG, Valle TT, Hämäläinen H, Ilanne-Parikka P, Keinänen-Kiukaanniemi S, Laakso M, Louheranta A, Rastas M, Salminen V, Uusitupa M, Finnish Diabetes Prevention Study Group (2001) Prevention of type 2 diabetes mellitus by changes in lifestyle among subjects with impaired glucose tolerance. New Engl J Med 344:1343–1350
25. Lytle LA (2009) Examining the etiology of childhood obesity: the IDEA study. Am J Community Psychol 44:338–349
26. Mendes de Leon C, Powell LH, Kaplan BH (1991) Change in coronary-prone behaviors in the Recurrent Coronary Prevention Project. Psychosom Med 53:407–419
27. Jones DA, West RR (1996) Psychological rehabilitation after myocardial infarction: multicentre randomised controlled trial. BMJ 313:1517–1521
28. Robinson TN, Matheson DM, Kraemer HC, Wilson DM, Obarzanek E, Thompson NS, Alhassan S, Spencer TR, Haydel KF, Fujimoto M, Varady A, Killen JD (2010) A randomized controlled trial of culturally tailored dance and reducing screen time to prevent weight gain in low-income African American girls: Stanford GEMS. Arch Pediatr Adolesc Med 164:995–1004
29. The Trials of Hypertension Prevention Collaborative Research Group (1992) The effects of nonpharmacologic interventions on blood pressure of persons with high normal levels. Results of the Trials of Hypertension Prevention, Phase I. JAMA 267:1213–1220
30. Hulley SB, Cummings SR, Browner WS, Grady DG, Newman TB (2013) Designing clinical research, 4th edn. Lippincott Williams & Wilkins, Philadelphia
31. The Diabetes Prevention Program (DPP) Research Group (1999) The Diabetes Prevention Program. Design and methods for a clinical trial in the prevention of type 2 diabetes. Diabetes Care 22:623–634
32. The, Diabetes Prevention Program (DPP) Research Group (2002) The Diabetes Prevention Program (DPP): description of lifestyle intervention. Diabetes Care 25:2165–2171
33. Diabetes Prevention Program Research Group (2009) 10-year follow-up of diabetes incidence and weight loss in the Diabetes Prevention Program Outcomes Study. Lancet 374:1677–1686
34. Howard BV, Van Horn L, Hsia J, Manson JE, Stefanick ML, Wassertheil-Smoller S, Kuller LH, LaCroix AZ, Langer RD, Lasser NL, Lewis CE, Limacher MC, Margolis KL, Mysiw WJ, Ockene JK, Parker LM, Perri MG, Phillips L, Prentice RL, Robbins J, Rossouw JE, Sarto GE, Schatz IJ, Snetselaar LG, Stevens VJ, Tinker LF, Trevisan M, Vitolins MZ, Anderson GL, Assaf AR, Bassford T, Beresford SA, Black HR, Brunner RL, Brzyski RG, Caan B, Chlebowski RT, Gass M, Granek I, Greenland P, Hays J, Heber D, Heiss G, Hendrix SL, Hubbell FA, Johnson KC, Kotchen JM (2006) Low-fat dietary pattern and risk of cardiovascular disease: the Women's Health Initiative randomized controlled dietary modification trial. JAMA 295:655–666
35. The Trials of Hypertension Prevention Collaborative Research Group (1997) Effects of weight loss and sodium reduction intervention on blood pressure and hypertension incidence in overweight people with high-normal blood pressure. The Trials of Hypertension Prevention, Phase II. Arch Intern Med 157:657–667
36. Duncan E, O'Cathain AO, Rousseau N, Croot L, Sworn K, Turner K, Yardley L, Hoddinott P (2020) Guidance for reporting intervention development studies in health research (GUIDED): an evidence-based consensus study. BMJ Open 10:e033516. https://doi: 10.1136/bmjopen-2019-033516

Chapter 5
Clinical Significance

"To say that a great deal of mischief has been associated with the test of significance is hardly original. It is what 'everybody knows.'. . . . To say it 'out loud' is to assume the role of the child who pointed out that the emperor was really outfitted in his underwear."

Bakan 1966 [1]

"If this comment was hardly original in 1966, it can hardly be original now. Yet this naked emperor has been shamelessly running around for a long time."

Cohen, 1994 [2]

> ### *Fundamental Point*
>
> *In a behavioral clinical trial, change in the behavioral target of treatment must be strong enough to test the hypothesis that improving it produces a beneficial effect on a clinical outcome. Judgment of the strength of a behavioral treatment should be based more heavily on clinical, than statistical, significance. Clinical significance can be used to identify treatment targets, analyze trial results, and calculate sample size. By so doing, the strength of scientific conclusions that are possible from any single behavioral clinical trial can be enhanced.*

This chapter first considers the strengths and limitations of statistical inference. Its limitations are often overlooked relative to its convenience and immense popularity as a decision-making metric. This background provides the basis for the argument that statistical significance is not the only, or the best, judge for making the case that a behavioral treatment can move a chronic disease endpoint. More persuasive is a demonstration of clinical significance where a behavioral treatment is strong enough to neutralize the risk incurred by a behavioral risk factor. The second part of the chapter is directed toward how to identify clinically significant treatment targets, incorporate clinical significance into the analysis of trial results, and integrate clinical significance into the calculation of sample size. The contribution of any single behavioral trial is assessed by the

© Springer Nature Switzerland AG 2021
L. H. Powell et al., *Behavioral Clinical Trials for Chronic Diseases*,
https://doi.org/10.1007/978-3-030-39330-4_5

strength of the scientific conclusions drawn from it. This includes a clinically significant benefit of treatment, quantified certainty that this benefit is greater than a relevant comparator, biologic plausibility, and consistency with results from past studies. The conclusion that a behavioral treatment improves health is best answered progressively, through replication.

SCIENTIFIC PRINCIPLES

A "significant" result from a trial refers to an "important" result. A "statistically significant" result from a trial evaluates "importance" by determining the likelihood that an observed result would occur if the reality was that the treatment had no benefit. A "clinically significant" result from a trial evaluates "importance" by whether or not a result is large enough to be meaningful and useful to patients, providers, or other stakeholders.

Statistical significance is appealing because it is quantified, evaluated against a conventional standard in the form of the null hypothesis, and provides a simple, categorical answer. Clinical significance has less practical appeal because it is more subjective, context-specific, and multiply-determined. In a behavioral clinical trial aimed at improving a chronic disease endpoint, the value of the behavioral treatment is whether or not it is strong enough to reduce behavioral risk to a level sufficient to move this endpoint. Since this criterion is one of clinical significance, a "significant" result in a behavioral trial is a result that is clinically significant.

Inferential Statistics

The logic behind behavioral trials, drug trials, or any experiment is based upon inductive reasoning: an inference from an observation in a specific experiment to a general state of affairs. Although this logic is part of the fabric of science, it is fallible. Hume was the first to challenge inductive logic by questioning what makes it possible to extrapolate from a limited sample to a broader generalization [3]. Karl Popper, the great philosopher of science, devoted the early phase of his career to this challenge and concluded that it was logically impossible to generalize with certainty from an observation in a sample to a population [4].

This logical problem puts the foundation of science on shaky ground with no simple solution. It did, however, serve as a catalyst for innovation among statisticians of the 1920s and 1930s. These innovations provide the foundation of classical inferential statistics.

Statisticians, most notably Fisher, Neyman, and Pearson, accepted the philosophical argument that inductive inferences about a scientific hypothesis could never be made with certainty. So they proposed instead to use a statistical hypothesis that featured deductive inferences made from the general (i.e., the null hypothesis) to the specific (i.e., the experiment). Using this framework, they developed methods by which to quantify the risk of error in making such deductive inferences. Fisher articulated the approach in this way:

"Any inference must be attended with some degree of uncertainty. But this is not the same as to admit that such inference cannot be absolutely rigorous. For the nature and degree of uncertainty may itself be capable of rigorous expression." [5]

To quantify the risk of being wrong, the statisticians drew on two basic principles. The first is the *frequentist principle*. This assumes that characteristics of a population have an influence on a sample drawn from it. Therefore, dramatic departure from population characteristics makes it likely that a sample is from a different population [1]. The second principle is *once-ness*. This assumes that experiments are carried out with limited resources so methods need to offer a shortcut around the more time-intensive demands of science for repeated replication [1, 5].

The P-Value
Fisher's key contribution to modern statistical approaches was the "probability value" (p-value). Based upon the frequentist principle, the p-value, calculated after the experiment has been conducted, is the probability that the obtained result would occur if the null hypothesis of no-treatment effect was true. Convention has converged upon a p-value of ≤ 0.05, based upon the rationale that an event occurring only 5 times out of 100 is unlikely enough to be inconsistent with the null hypothesis of no treatment benefit. Since the p-value is calculated on the assumption that the null hypothesis is true, it does not provide a direct measure of the null hypothesis being false or that any alternative hypothesis is true [6]. Fisher argued that the p-value is just a simple tool, to be used only as one part of a fluid qualitative process of drawing a conclusion from observed data [7], consistent with the approach originally proposed by Bayes [8]. In Fisher's words:

". . . no scientific worker has a fixed level of significance at which from year to year, and in all circumstances, he rejects hypotheses; he rather gives his mind to each particular case in the light of his evidence and his ideas." [9]

The Hypothesis Test
The p-value provides the basis for an inference, not an action. If the null hypothesis is rejected, what is the correct course of action? This was the problem for which Neyman and Pearson developed a solution in the form of statistical hypothesis testing [10]. They applied the once-ness principle and found a shortcut around dependence on replication by developing a decision-making approach which produced a long-

term error rate that could be applied to statistical conclusions from any one experiment. Two hypotheses were posed: a null hypothesis of no effect and an alternative hypothesis of an effect. Accepting one required the rejection of the other. Two types of errors result: falsely concluding that the alternative hypothesis is true (Type I error) and falsely concluding that the null hypothesis is true (Type II error). It is critical to keep in mind that this error rate does not apply to a single experiment but to the error that would occur over many replications of the experiment. The acceptable error rate is built into the design of the trial before any result is obtained. In their own words:

> *"Without hoping to know whether each separate hypothesis is true or false, we may search for rules to govern our behavior with regard to them, in following which we insure that, in the long run, we shall not often be wrong." [10]*

These two approaches to statistical inference can be understood by borrowing an analogy from the legal system. P-values quantify the likelihood of making an error in convicting an innocent defendant. Hypothesis testing quantifies the overall rate of errors in convictions made by the court.

The Confidence Interval

Derived from the same frequentist mathematics as the p-value, the confidence interval represents the range of values that 95 times out of 100 would contain the true population parameter if an experiment were repeated many times. Because the emphasis is on the range of values possible for an observed effect, it provides more precise information about the degree of uncertainty and, as such, is gaining increasing acceptance in high-visibility journals. Although a step in the right direction, they are still used as surrogates for categorical p-values by looking to see if a null effect is contained within the interval. They do, however, provide an opportunity to determine a priori what a *clinically significant* effect would be and to reference the interval to see if it is contained within it. If it is, then a clinically significant benefit is a plausible result of the treatment [6].

Limitations of Inferential Statistics

Inferential statistics have become the preeminent criteria for decision-making in the scientific literature. But in such diverse disciplines as statistics, medicine, psychology, and business, and dating as far back as the time when these procedures were first introduced [11], criticisms abound. Most recently, the American Statistical Association (ASA) issued a statement on p-values and statistical significance. The rationale for this statement was that decades of saying what *not* do have gone mostly unheeded. In their words:

> *"It is as though statisticians were asking users of statistics to tear out the beams holding up the edifice of modern scientific research without offering solid materials to replace them. Pointing out old rotting timbers was a good start, but we now need more." [12]*

In their most recent statement, they have reiterated the "Don't's" articulated over the past decades. But now, in hopes of action, they have accompanied them with a list of "Do's" (see the box). The "Don't's" and "Do's" that are particularly pertinent for behavioral clinical trials can be summarized into the four key points presented in the box.

Misinterpretation

What we want to know is the probability that a scientific hypothesis is true. What we get from a p-value is the probability that the null hypothesis, created with some assumptions, is true. It is a logical error, referred to as proof by contradiction [2], to infer that a low probability event under the null hypothesis is evidence that the scientific hypothesis is true. To get the needed information, it is tempting to turn to hypothesis testing. But what we get is an alpha

American Statistical Association Statement On P-Values and Statistical Significance [12]	
DON'T	**DO**
Say "statistically significant"	Accept uncertainty: seek replication
Base conclusions on statistical significance	Be thoughtful: recognize difference between exploration and confirmation
Believe the p-value is the probability that a scientific hypothesis is true	Be open: judge value by a variety of criteria; one trial is rarely enough
Judge scientific value by statistical significance	Be modest: understand and express clearly the limitations of science and of one's own work

level, predetermined before any experiment is undertaken, that represents the level of error in accepting the scientific hypothesis that could be expected over many tests conducted over many repetitions. It says very little about error in any specific test.

It would be extremely convenient to have a single statistic that provides conclusive support for a scientific hypothesis. But since no single statistic can accomplish this, the interpretive error referred to as the *hybrid p-value* has arisen [2, 6]. Because the p-value and the alpha level look alike, both often being 0.05, it is easy to combine them into one hybrid statistic that quantifies error made in a single test when inferring that a research hypothesis is true. Making this error gives us what we want: the probability that a scientific hypothesis is true. Fisher, Neyman, and Pearson argued against this misinterpretation by saying that error cannot be quantified simultaneously as an event in the short run and a rate in the long run [6]. Beyond this interpretative error, categorization of a p-value into an acceptable error of ≤0.05 provides a convenient dichotomous decision rule: the treatment worked or it did not. But this rule is based upon flimsy and misleading evidence [13]. This misinterpretation has had a profound influence on the process of science by manufacturing convenient scientific conclusions that are not restricted by the limits imposed upon either p-values or hypothesis testing.

The ASA statisticians encouraged modesty in interpretations of results. This modesty is expressed by understanding the limitations of inferential statistics, retiring the term "statistical significance," reporting exact p-values, and replacing the term "confidence interval" with "compatibility interval" to show all the values that are reasonably compatible with the data [12, 13].

False Security

Basing scientific conclusions on statistical significance leads to a false sense of security about results from a single trial. Although a statistical verdict has legitimacy because it is quantitative and requires minimal interpretation, it promotes a tyranny of statistical evidence over such types of evidence as biologic plausibility and consistency with past research [6, 14]. Moreover, acceptance of the statistical verdict as definitive undercuts scientific progression, accumulation of knowledge, and replications that are central to the confidence that a treatment works [15]. The falseness of this security has been revealed by a high rate of non-replication of findings in clinical trials. This is likely due, in part, to claims of conclusive findings from a single trial evaluated using statistical significance criteria [16].

The ASA statisticians encouraged acceptance of uncertainty in making scientific conclusions. Uncertainty is reflected, in large part, in the drive to embrace variation in the effects of a treatment and to view statistical results as being much more incomplete and uncertain than is currently the norm [12].

Ease of Manipulation

One needs only to do the "sample size samba" several times to understand how easy it is to manipulate statistical significance by manipulating assumptions in the design of a trial [17]. The dance is set in motion as investigators and biostatisticians go back and forth varying design assumptions to get to a sample size that is within resources to implement. When the sample size comes out to be too high, assumptions about the treatment effect, the choice of a primary outcome, the dropout rate, and/or the stringency of the comparator are relaxed. This ease of manipulation opens the door to a potentially dangerous state of affairs where the design of the trial is informed by maximizing statistical significance rather than answering a key scientific question. This practice is reinforced by academic pressures for publications, combined with publication practices that seek papers with positive results.

The ASA statisticians encouraged thoughtfulness in the use of statistical procedures. "Statistical thoughtfulness" is reflected in sensitivity to the different objectives of exploratory and confirmatory studies and finding the right method for a question, rather than finding the right question for a method [12].

Statistical Significance Is Not Clinical Significance

It has long been recognized that a result can be statistically, but not clinically, significant. That is, it can be statistically significant but not very important to patients, providers, or other stakeholders. Alternatively, a result can be clinically, but not statistically, significant because of such design manipulations as a small sample size. *(See Chapter 3: Behavioral Treatment Development, Figure 3.3*, for an example.) While statistical significance shows the probability that an observed result is from a null distribution, clinical significance focuses on the potency of treatment, whether it is large enough to move the chronic disease needle and whether it will make a difference in patient's lives [18]. The problem is that statistical significance has become a proxy for clinical significance. In a systematic sampling of 869 journals in general medicine, clinical specialties, epidemiology, and public health, 81% equated statistical significance with clinical significance [19]. This is likely due, in part, to the fact that it is generally easier to get a statistically significant result than one that is clinically significant [20].

Prioritizing statistical over clinical significance in a *Phase III* behavioral trial is a Pyrrhic victory. When nature is the final arbiter, a short-term win from statistics sets the stage from a longer-term defeat from nature. It would be a mistake to assume that statistical significance has no role in scientific investigation. Indeed, it serves as a handrail that guides decisions and prevents researchers from getting carried away by hasty, impressionistic generalizations [21]. But the balance between statistical and clinical significance needs to be shifted so that quantitative methods are better integrated into the more general picture of clinical benefit.

The AHA statisticians encouraged openness in making scientific conclusions. This openness is expressed by judging conclusions in a particular trial not simply by a p-value but by relevant prior evidence, plausibility of the mechanism, study design, data quality, and the cost vs. benefit ratio [12].

CHALLENGES FOR BEHAVIORAL TRIALS

The ultimate rationale for conducting a *Phase III* behavioral efficacy trial is the strength of the hypothesis that a behavioral treatment can produce a clinically significant benefit on an important chronic disease outcome. The rationale for conducting a *Phase II* behavioral efficacy trial is the strength of the hypothesis that a behavioral treatment can produce a clinically significant reduction in behavioral risk and thereby neutralize the risk on the chronic disease endpoint which would be otherwise incurred. This chain of reasoning is straightforward, but progress in developing this rationale can be undercut in several ways.

"One-Size-Fits-All" Methods

Many applied behavioral scientists who develop interests in conducting behavioral clinical trials were trained in the tradition of experimental psychology. This is a tradition of discovery of mechanisms and how a treatment works. Experiments are designed to test hypotheses about mechanisms, mediators, moderators, and components. To make use of all of the data, predictors and outcomes tend to be continuous. They are analyzed for statistical significance using such procedures as correlations, regressions, and path analyses [22].

But when the focus progresses to testing the efficacy of behavioral treatments on chronic disease outcomes, the aim is to confirm and make decisions and the tradition shifts to clinical trial methodology. Hypotheses tend to compare a new treatment to existing care. Predictor and outcome data tend to be categorical, featuring clinically significant benchmarks for judging both the success of a treatment and the reduction in disease risk. Statistics of choice include rates, relative risks, and risk differences. Analytic procedures are often time-to-event.

Clinical trial methodology, a synthesis of clinical research, biostatistics and epidemiology, is part of the culture of medicine and the fabric of medical training, but it is not a part of traditional training in the behavioral sciences. By the same token, design of experiments, aimed at understanding the dynamics of behavioral treatments, is a part of the culture of behavioral sciences but is not part of traditional training in medicine or epidemiology. These training gaps come to a head when conducting behavioral clinical trials. Behavioral treatments which have not been optimized are tested by medical scientists with ripe and expensive clinical trial methods. Optimized behavioral treatments are tested by behavioral scientists using the experimental psychology methods of discovery and experimentation rather than methods aimed at confirmation, decision-making, and efficacy. A translational science model draws on methods from both of these traditions to link maturing questions about a behavioral treatment to an evolving, transdisciplinary set of methods.

Significance Tests Are the Status Quo

Significance testing is woven into the fabric of most scientific investigation. But psychology was one of the first disciplines to embrace it with enthusiasm, shortly after it was introduced by Fisher [15]. Use of significance testing was reported in 10% of the empirical papers in psychology published in the early part of 1900 but jumped to 90% of the papers published in the 1970s [23]. Significance testing is far more common in the social sciences than it is in such physical sciences as physics and chemistry where many scientists regard it as unscientific [24]. Some have referred to the extensive use of significance testing as a ritual, similar to compulsive hand washing [25]. In Bakan's words:

"Statistical hypothesis testing is profoundly woven into the psychological research enterprise, constituting a critical part of the total cultural-scientific tapestry. To pull out the strand of the test of significance would seem to make the whole tapestry fall apart." [1]

Despite Fisher's emphasis on the primitive nature of the p-value and the importance of restricting its use to problems about which we know very little [26], significance testing is used to test all types of interventions, at all phases of development, ignoring the mathematical and philosophical framework from which the test emerged.

While it is appealing to have one standard answer to all types of questions, it runs the risk of providing a conclusive answer to the wrong question. If, for example, interest is in whether or not a behavioral treatment is strong enough to improve a clinical outcome, statistical significance will provide a conclusive answer but not to that question. It is this very problem that has

Retire statistical significance [13]

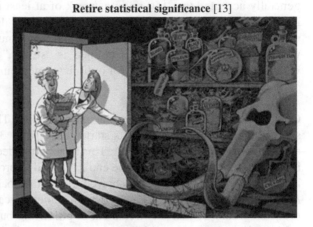

directed statisticians and clinical researchers toward Bayesian analyses which aim to enhance the quality of scientific conclusions through the use of a methodology that incorporates other ways of knowing beyond statistical significance including clinical significance, biologic plausibility based upon potential biological mechanisms, and past research [27, 28]. In the eyes of statisticians, significance testing is the bottom rung on a ladder of increasingly more informative hypothesis testing methods progressing to empirical Bayes methodology [29].

OVERCOMING THESE CHALLENGES IN A BEHAVIORAL TRIAL

A key question in developing and evaluating a behavioral treatment for a chronic disease is whether the treatment is strong enough to reduce risk incurred by a behavioral risk factor and, by so doing, improve a disease endpoint. This is a question of clinical significance. It is a categorical, yes/no decision. It requires a milestone for making a decision about readiness to move to a *Phase III* efficacy trial [30].

Clinically Significant Treatment Target

A "strong" behavioral treatment is one that can achieve a clinically significant improvement in a behavioral risk factor. This means finding a cutpoint on the scale of that behavioral risk factor at which risk for a chronic disease endpoint is decreased.

With established behavioral risk factors, the easiest way to find a cutpoint is to draw upon clinical practice guidelines and/or meta-analyses. For example, it is generally accepted that 150 minutes/week of at least moderate physical activity is needed to reduce cardiovascular risk factors and diseases [31]. Thus a treatment that was successful in achieving only 100 minutes/week of activity/week would be promising but not yet defined as "strong." This promising treatment would, however, be a candidate for optimization in pursuit of achieving the clinically significant target.

One could argue, instead, the continuous perspective. This treatment could be considered to be strong if participants started out at only 30 minutes/week of activity and improved to 100 minutes/week. This treatment indeed improved physical activity. If a *Phase II* efficacy trial is the end game and improvement in physical activity is the goal, it would have been achieved. But if the goal is to push toward a *Phase III* efficacy trial with the end game of improvement in cardiovascular risk, the interpretation would be that this treatment is promising but not yet strong enough to achieve clinical practice guidelines for level of physical activity needed to improve cardiovascular risk.

If clinical practice guidelines do not exist and the behavioral target of treatment is a novel risk factor, the epidemiologic literature can be helpful in identifying a milestone for success. Risk factor status is conferred upon factors that have been shown to be linked to disease incidence, most often in longitudinal epidemiologic studies. A variety of measures of risk potency, such as relative risks, odds ratios, risk ratios, and risk reduction, portray the strength of the risk factor by categorizing it into deciles, tertiles, or more fine-grained categories of equal sample size [18]. This categorization is generally done on large studies which provide sufficient numbers to calculate within-category disease rates. Often, relative risks reveal a natural break in categories where disease risk is increased. But when an association is graded, such a natural cutpoint will not exist, and judgment will be required.

Figure 5.1 portrays a hypothetical epidemiologic study of 300 participants aimed at determining the relationship between a behavioral risk factor (i.e., anger) and the incidence of coronary heart disease (CHD). To facilitate calculation of meaningful CHD rates, needed for a *Phase III* efficacy trial, the continuous anger scale has been categorized into tertiles of 100 participants each, based upon anger score. Figure 5.1a shows a natural break in disease risk. An anger score of <3 cuts disease risk by two-thirds or 67% (i.e., $(15–5)/15 = 0.67$). Thus, the clinically significant target for an anger treatment would be to reduce anger to a level of <3 on this scale.

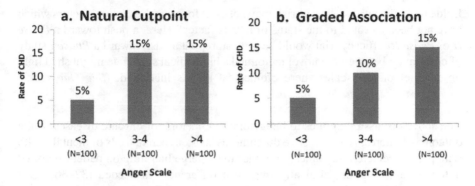

Fig. 5.1 Identification of a clinically significant target on an anger scale for an anger treatment to reduce CHD. Figure 5.1a shows a natural cutpoint at which CHD is increased. Figure 5.1b shows a graded association between anger and CHD where judgment is needed.

Figure 5.1b shows that there is a graded relationship between anger and disease. Since each progressive tertile is associated with an increase of 5% in CHD risk, the cutpoint for determining a clinically significant target for the anger intervention requires consideration of the trade-off: the stronger the treatment effect, the smaller the disease effect that can be detected. One approach would be to prioritize the ability to detect the disease effect by putting the demand on the treatment. Here the target of treatment would be a score of <3 on anger, the expected disease risks would be 5% (tertile 1) vs. 12.5% (mean of tertiles 2 + 3), and the CHD risk reduction that could be expected from this treatment would be 60% (i.e., (12.5–5)/12.5 = 0.6). An alternative approach would be to place less demand on treatment but design the trial to be able to detect a smaller benefit on disease. Here the target of treatment would be a score of ≤4, the disease risks would be 7.5% (mean of tertiles 1 + 2) vs. 15% (tertile 3), and the CHD risk reduction that could be expected from this treatment would be 50% (i.e., (15–7.5)/15 = 0.5). An aid to making the decision about which approach to pursue would be to consider the disease reduction achieved by the best treatments currently available. This level of improvement reflects the clinically significant standard of care. This also shows how important it is to optimize the strength of a behavioral treatment in early treatment development studies. Designing a trial to detect small improvements in a disease outcome usually translates into a huge sample size and a multi-site trial.

The search for cutpoints by which to judge behavioral treatment strength is not without its limitations. Reliance on cutpoints minimizes the clinical relevance of differences that are just above and just below the cutpoint. Alternative measures of risk potency, such as area under the curve, could serve as alternatives [18]. Cutpoints are more tentative when they are determined from only one epidemiologic study compared to cutpoints derived from clinical guidelines and/or meta-analyses. Thus, a range around the point estimate for judging treatment success may be in order.

Epidemiologic data for disease risk may not exist for novel behavioral factors which have not been elevated to the status of a "risk factor." Here, a push toward a *Phase II* or *Phase III* efficacy trial would be premature, but a push toward a *Phase I* study of covariation between the novel factor and a biomedical surrogate might shed light on a target on the scale where biomedical risk is increased. *(See Chapter 3: Behavioral Treatment Development.)*

The above discussion applies to behavioral risk factors for chronic diseases. If the outcome of interest is a subjective outcome, as is often seen in trials of mental health with patient-centered outcomes, reference to the large literature on patient-reported outcomes and minimal clinically important differences is needed [32–36]. *(See Chapter 9: Outcomes.)*

Clinically Significant Treatment Effect

Once a clinically significant benchmark for judging the ability of a behavioral treatment to reduce behavioral risk and thus move a clinical endpoint has been identified, it is a comparatively simple task to determine the clinical significance of a behavioral treatment effect. Simply add that benchmark to the figure that portrays the results from a *Phase II* trial.

Figure 5.2 portrays three sets of results from a hypothetical *Phase II* trial examining the strength of an anger management treatment on an anger scale. The only thing that is different between these three figures and the large number of similar figures common in the applied behavioral treatment literature is that the clinically significant goal needed to reduce risk of disease (i.e., anger ≤ 3) is portrayed. The addition of this goal essentially brings clinically meaningful reduction of risk of disease into the picture of results.

In Fig. 5.2a, there was a statistically significant difference in anger between treated and comparator arms, but only treated subjects achieved a clinically significant reduction in anger. This suggests that the treatment may be ready for testing in a *Phase III* behavioral trial examining the impact of treatment on disease, and the comparator arm is appropriate because it reduces anger but not to a clinically significant level. In Fig. 5.2b, there was a statistically significant difference between arms but neither achieved a clinically significant benefit. In this situation it would be appropriate to strengthen the treatment to achieve a clinically significant reduction in anger. In Fig. 5.2c, there was a statistically significant difference between arms, but both achieved clinically significant reductions in anger. If the purpose of the comparator was simply to control factors that jeopardize internal validity, the appropriate course of action would be to find a more inert comparator. In all three figures, the effect size of two points on the anger scale was the same.

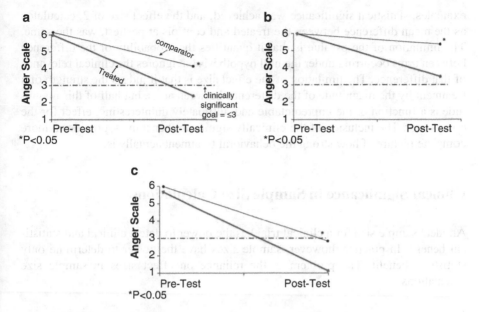

Fig. 5.2 Determination of the success of a behavioral treatment when (a) only the treated arm is clinically significant, (b) neither arm is clinically significant, and (c) both arms are clinically significant. In a, b, and c, the effect size and significance level are the same.

This example can be extended to the case where the clinically significant target is not a group mean (i.e., the average anger score achieved by the group), but instead the percent of participants in the treatment who achieved the clinically significant benchmark (i.e., the percent of participants who were able to get to an anger score of ≤3). In this case, the y-axis would be a percent rather than a mean. To judge success based upon the percent who achieve a clinically significant target, it is helpful to reference the success rates of other existing treatments. For example, on average, adherence to drug therapy is less than 50%, regardless of the drug class [37]. Thus, a new behavioral treatment that achieves success in ≥50% of those treated would have a reach that is comparable to drug approaches to anger management. Another example is provided by the Food and Drug Administration which has judged the success of weight loss interventions by whether or not ≥35% of treated participants achieve goal [38]. Thus, a new behavioral weight loss treatment that achieved success in ≥35% of those treated would provide a standard comparable to federal guidelines for successful weight loss programs. In both these cases, treatment response to the new treatment is judged by the standard for treatment response in other existing treatments.

Figure 5.2 illustrates an important limitation of sole reliance on statistical significance and effect sizes. When the figure includes the target needed to reduce disease, it brings disease into the picture even though disease is not measured. When the ultimate aim is to reduce disease, this addition is more useful for judging the worth of a treatment than either statistical significance or effect sizes. In all three of these examples, statistical significance was achieved, and the effect size of 2, calculated as the mean difference between the treated and controls at posttest, was the same. The limitation of the p-value is that it quantifies the probability of the difference between arms occurring under the null hypothesis but ignores the clinical relevance of that difference. The limitation of the effect size is that it judges the strength of a treatment by the magnitude of the difference between arms, but half of this magnitude is a function of the unpredictable and, ultimately uninteresting, effect for the comparator. The inclusion of the clinically significant benchmark provides a more complete picture of how strong the behavioral treatment actually is.

Clinical Significance in Sample Size Calculations

An ideal sample size for a clinical trial has the power to detect clinical and statistical benefit. In practice, however, sample sizes have the power to determine only statistical benefit. The problem is the reliance on effect sizes in sample size calculations.

Disaggregate the Effect Size

The use of an effect size in sample size calculations considers only the difference between treated and comparator arms and ignores the clinical significance of the treatment effect. There are at least two problems with this. First, the basis for estimating an effect size is often flimsy. Effect sizes estimated from small pilot studies tend to be overestimates [39]. Estimated treatment effects from past studies are often poor approximations because of different populations, treatments, settings, and time frames. Estimated comparator effects are even more unpredictable because they are generally not studied in any preliminary studies. When two flimsy estimates are combined into a single number, the result is an even flimsier estimate.

Second, effect sizes confound the question of *whether* a treatment works with questions about *why* or *compared to what*. The question of whether a treatment works is answered by whether or not a treatment can achieve a clinically significant benchmark. The question of why or compared to what is the rationale for a comparator group: does the treatment do better than the simple passage of time, non-specific attention, or a current treatment? If a treatment cannot reduce risk, the questions about *why* or *compared to what* are meaningless. A single number that confounds the questions of *whether* and *why* gives the comparator condition more importance than it deserves in designing a trial to determine the worth of a new behavioral treatment.

To include clinical significance in the determination of sample size, it is necessary to disaggregate an effect size into its two separate components (Table 5.1). Disaggregation preserves the ability to answer the question of whether a new treatment achieves clinically significant benefit because the estimate for the treated group is fixed at the clinically significant treatment target. Disaggregation also

Table 5.1 Parameters in a sample size calculation

PARAMETER	DESCRIPTION	SOURCE
Alpha	Probability of incorrectly rejecting the null hypothesis (false-positive error rate)	Convention
Power	Probability of correctly rejecting the null hypothesis (1-false-negative error rate)	Convention
Direction of H_o	One-tailed or two-tailed test	Convention
Variability	Standard error (continuous primary outcome)	Observed
	Shape of distribution (categorical primary outcome)	Observed
Treatment effect	Clinically significant effect of treatment on the primary outcome	Estimated from practice guidelines or epidemiologic studies
Comparator effect	Range of possible effects of comparator on primary outcome	Estimated from past studies using similar comparator

makes it possible to translate the uncertainty of the estimate for the comparator group into a range of possible responses that could be achieved, based upon similar comparator groups in the literature. Disaggregation simplifies the investigator's job who is now only responsible for determining the clinically significant treatment target and the range of possible responses in the comparator group. Variability in response, commonly assessed as the standard deviation or standard error, can be reliably obtained from pilot data [39]. Disaggregation of the effect size simplifies sample size calculations and makes them less open to manipulation. It identifies the sample size needed to achieve *both* clinical and statistical significance. Two examples follow.

Sample Size for a *Phase II* Efficacy Trial
Figure 5.3a presents the sample size calculations for a hypothetical *Phase II* trial of a treatment for anger management. This trial aims to determine if a new treatment for anger is strong enough to achieve a clinically significant reduction in anger. This is a preliminary study for a *Phase III* efficacy trial testing the value of this anger management treatment on reducing recurrent cardiac events.

The anger scale ranges from 1 to 6, with a higher value associated with greater anger. The baseline average on anger in both groups is a score of 6. From Fig. 5.1a (above), the clinically significant target needed to reduce cardiovascular disease is <3 on the anger scale. This fixes the clinically significant treatment effect, portrayed by the green line. Other parameters are fixed by convention or observation

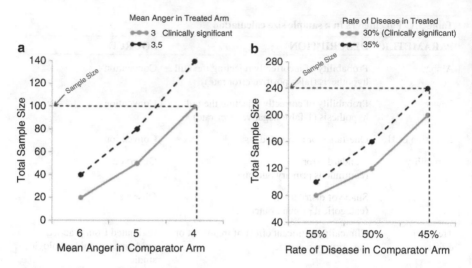

Fig. 5.3 **Sample size calculation for (a) a *Phase II* efficacy trial with a behavioral risk factor outcome (i.e., anger) and (b) a *Phase III* clinical trial with a disease outcome. All calculations fix the following parameters: alpha =0.05; power = 0.80; two-tailed test; variability estimated from pilot studies.**

(alpha = 0.05; power = 0.80; two-sided test; standard error taken from a pilot study). This leaves only one parameter that is free to vary: the range of possible responses in the comparator group. From past research with a similar comparator, the level of anger could be uninfluenced (i.e., an anger score of 6) or could be altered considerably (i.e., an anger score of 4). Thus, the horizontal x-axis portrays estimates for comparator response ranging from 6 to 4 on the anger scale. This range does not extend to less than 4 as this would suggest clinical benefit from the comparator condition, and a statistical difference between the two arms would be meaningless. Sample size is on the vertical y-axis. Using the parameters in Table 5.1, a sample size curve is plotted for the clinically significant result of 3 in the treated group and anything between 6 and 4 in the comparator group (green line). A similar curve is calculated for a treatment benefit of only 3.5 on anger (dotted black line) to provide a more complete picture of sample size needed to detect a statistical difference if treatment approached, but did not achieve, clinical significance.

The choice of a sample size of 100 makes it possible to detect both a clinical and statistical benefit of treatment when the range of response in the comparator group goes from no response, all of the way through a response as large as a 4 on the anger scale. The dotted black line shows that when treatment approaches, but does not achieve, a clinically significant target on anger (i.e., a score of 3.5), and the comparator has a strong benefit on anger (i.e., a score of 4), a statistical difference will not be detected. Failure to achieve statistical significance in this state of affairs is an appropriate result as it would direct the investigator to optimize the treatment to achieve the clinically significant target and/or reconsider the choice of a comparator before moving to a *Phase III* efficacy trial.

Sample Size for a *Phase III* Efficacy Trial

Figure 5.3b shows that the same approach is used for sample size calculations when the primary outcome is a rate of disease, rather than a behavioral risk factor. The challenge here is how to determine a clinically significant threshold for benefit on a disease outcome. This is a clinical question that bears on the significance of the trial. A new behavioral treatment may offer clinically significant benefit, compared to a state-of-the-art standard treatment, when it is superior on a primary outcome, no different on the primary outcome but has fewer side effects, is less costly in time, money, or resources, or is preferred by all or a subgroup of patients [40, 41]. A determination of a threshold for clinical significance for a new behavioral treatment on a disease outcome is the work of early treatment development that guides decision-making throughout the progressive program of research. *(See Chapter 3: Behavioral Treatment Development.)*

SELECTED EXPERIENCE FROM BEHAVIORAL TRIALS

Clinically Significant Treatment Target from Epidemiology

The field of psychosocial epidemiology aims to identify psychosocial risk factors for disease. The strongest studies are prospective designs where subjects free of the disease are assessed on the predictor of interest at baseline and then followed over time to determine disease status in those who did and did not have that predictor.

The Kuopio Ischemic Heart Disease Risk Factor Study enrolled 2682 participants from Eastern Finland between March 1984 and December 1989 and followed them over time to identify prospective links between baseline psychosocial risk factors and incidence of disease. Of considerable interest was to determine if stress was linked to cardiovascular outcomes. Two studies are relevant for present purposes.

The first study examined baseline anger and incident hypertension [42]. Eligible for study were 537 men who were free of hypertension at baseline. They were assessed on level of expressed (anger-out) and suppressed (anger-in) anger at baseline and then followed for an average of 4.2 years. Associations between anger expression and incidence of hypertension were assessed using age-adjusted logistic regression models with anger scores modeled both continuously and categorically. Categories were tertiles based upon anger scores that included equal numbers of subjects within the low, medium, and high anger tertiles.

Both continuous and categorical measures of anger were significantly associated with incident hypertension, after adjusting for known cardiovascular risk factors. The categorical results are presented in Fig. 5.4. It can be seen that there is a threshold effect for both the measures of anger-out and anger-in. The cutpoint on the anger scale that marked the end of the second tertile is an estimate of a clinically significant cutpoint on anger. That is, a clinically significant target for an anger management treatment that aims to reduce hypertension would be to get to a score below the beginning of the third tertile. Although the authors did not report the value on the scale associated with the end of the second tertile, it may be possible to obtain it by communicating with them.

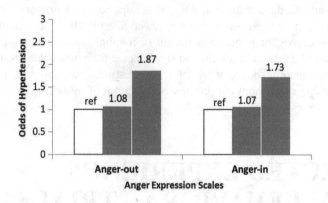

Fig. 5.4 Identification of a clinically significant cutpoint on two anger scales [42]

The same epidemiologic study was used to study the relationship between systolic blood pressure reactivity (i.e., being a "hot reactor") and incidence of stroke [43]. In this report, 2303 men, who were free of stroke at baseline, were followed for an average of 11.2 years to determine the relationship between baseline systolic blood pressure reactivity and incidence of stroke.

Reactivity was modeled both continuously, and categorically using a median split. The categorical analyses are portrayed in Fig. 5.5. In the median split, "hot reactors" were defined as men whose systolic blood pressure rose ≥ 19 mmHg in anticipation of exercise. They had a 72% greater risk of stroke over the subsequent 11.2 years than men who were less reactive ($p < 0.006$). Thus a clinically significant cutpoint for the

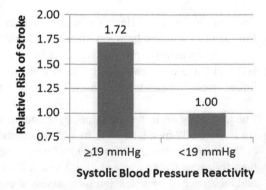

Fig. 5.5 Identification of a clinically significant cutpoint on blood pressure reactivity [43]

variable of cardiovascular reactivity could be estimated as ≥19 mmHg increase. A promising stress management treatment would have as its target <19 mmHg increase in systolic blood pressure in anticipation of exercise.

Clinically Significant Sample Size Calculation for a *Phase II* Efficacy Trial

A junior investigator was interested in obtaining support for a program of research aimed at promoting adherence to asthma controller medications in teenagers from the inner city [44, 45]. She worked with a technology firm to develop a device that provided culturally sensitive cues to remind participants to adhere and culturally sensitive feedback when controller medication was taken as prescribed. With this treatment, she aimed for a clinically significant target of 70% adherence, consistent with clinical guidelines from the Allergy and Immunology Society. To argue for funding, she conducted a proof-of-concept study in four subjects and showed that adherence increased from 40% to over the clinically significant threshold of 70% with the onset of the intervention.

Since the proof-of-concept study suggested that it was plausible that the intervention could produce a benefit on adherence, she was now ready to design a *Phase II* randomized efficacy trial to provide a more rigorous evaluation. Figure 5.6 presents the sample size calculation for the trial. The effect size was disaggregated into its

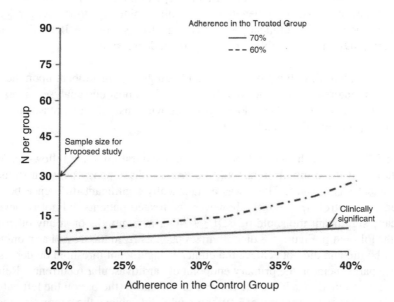

Fig. 5.6 Sample size calculation for a *Phase II* efficacy trial

component parts: the clinically significant rate of adherence in the treated and the expected range of adherence in the controls. The clinically significant rate of adherence in the treated was fixed at the guideline goal of 70% (the green line). The expected rate of adherence in the controls was estimated, from the literature, to range between 20% and 40% (the x-axis horizontal line). Included in this calculation was a curve for a treatment effect of 60% adherence (blue hashed line). This inclusion was based upon the argument that if treatment improved adherence, but not to a clinically significant level, an ability to detect this statistically would encourage further optimization of the treatment to achieve a clinically significant benefit. The resulting choice of sample size (30 per group) made it possible to insure both clinical and statistical significance if the treatment effect was as low as 60% and the control effect was as high as 40%.

Clinical Versus Statistical Significance in *Phase III* Efficacy Trials

ENRICHD was a multi-site behavioral trial aimed at, among other things, reducing depression after a myocardial infarction (MI) for the purpose of reducing cardiovascular recurrence (death or recurrent MI) [46]. The trial compared a treated arm that received cognitive behavior therapy for depression, to an arm receiving usual care, in 2481 post-MI patients. This sample size was based upon a two-sided test, alpha = 0.05, power = 80%, and a 3-year estimated MI event rate of 18% in the treated and 23% in usual care. Treatment for depression continued for 6 months, after which patients were followed for an average of 23 additional months to accumulate MI events. To achieve benefit on the primary outcome, the target for depression remission was the clinically significant goal of ≤ 7 on the Beck Depression Inventory (BDI), a goal established by experts in depression.

This was a null trial. In the presence of null findings, it is incumbent upon the principal investigators to determine what happened. Such post hoc analyses are exploratory and not conclusive. They do, however, provide insight into a reasonable next step in the program of research.

Figure 5.7 examines change in depression over the duration of the follow-up. At the conclusion of the 6-month treatment, there was a discrepancy between statistical and clinical significance. There was a statistically significant difference between treated and controls ($p < 0.001$); however, the treated patients did not achieve the clinically significant threshold of BDI ≤ 7 either at 6 months or at any other time over the follow-up. Figure 5.8 dichotomizes patients from the treated arm only into those who did and did not achieve the clinically significant threshold on depression and compares them on the primary endpoint of cardiovascular recurrence. Relative to those who failed to achieve the depression threshold (the bar on the left with the hazard ratio set as the referent at 1.0), those who did achieve the depression thresh-

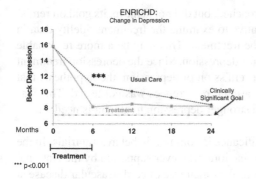

*** p<0.001

Fig. 5.7 Clinically vs. statistically significant change in depression in ENRICHD

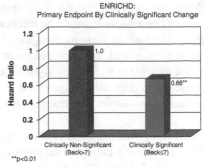

Fig. 5.8 Primary endpoint in the treated arm by clinically significant change in depression in ENRICHD

old had a 33% lower chance of cardiovascular recurrence (the bar on the right, hazard ratio = 0.66), after adjusting for factors that differed between these groups at baseline ($p < 0.01$).

The ENRICHD investigators interpreted their results based upon statistical significance:

> *"ENRICHD achieved significant improvements in depression . . . yet did not demonstrate a parallel benefit on mortality and recurrent infarction." [46]*

An accompanying editorial placed greater emphasis on the discrepancy between the statistical and clinical findings:

> *"The impact on depression scores, although statistically significant (p<.001) was only between 1.5 and 2.8 points, depending upon the scale used. . . . A statistically significant difference with a small effect size has unclear clinical importance . . . Depression remains a CAD risk factor in search of a successful intervention." [47]*

But despite this discrepancy, the title of the editorial "Depression—A Cardiac Risk Factor in Search of a Treatment" suggests that cognitive behavior therapy was not the right treatment, and the editorial goes on to suggest that exercise, SSRI's, or omega-3 supplementation might be more promising [47].

This is an excellent example of the importance of clinical significance relative to statistical significance. Since the sample size of the trial was based upon an ability to detect a difference on the primary outcome of cardiovascular recurrence, it was considerably overpowered to detect a statistical difference between arms on depression. The resulting direction of the bias is that very small differences can turn out to be highly statistically significant. In contrast, clinical significance is independent of sample size. When clinical significance is considered, the picture changes and it is clear that the cognitive behavior therapy approached, but did not achieve, its goal on remission of depression. It would be informative to examine the treatment fidelity data in pursuit of finding ways to strengthen the treatment. This may be a more reasonable next step than seeking a new treatment for depression. Since the depression treatment failed to achieve a clinically significant remission of depression, the hypothesis that reduction in depression reduces cardiovascular recurrences was not tested. This was an inconclusive trial. Replication with a stronger depression treatment is needed.

Prioritizing statistical over clinical significance is common in behavioral trials. In the Women's Health Initiative, the largest behavioral trial ever supported by the National Institutes of Health, 48,835 postmenopausal women free of cardiovascular disease at baseline were randomized to a dietary intervention or an education comparison group and followed for an average of 8.1 years for a primary endpoint of cardiovascular events [48]. The clinically significant dietary target was ≤20% of energy intake from fat and ≤ 7% energy intake from saturated fat. This was a null trial. With such a large sample, statistical significance was easily achieved at year 6 on fat intake between the treated and comparator arms ($p < 0.001$), but the treated arm fell short of the clinically significant goal and achieved 28.8% energy intake from fat and 9.5% energy intake from saturated fat. Unplanned post hoc analyses showed that those who achieved the lowest intake of saturated fat had a significant benefit on cardiovascular disease ($p = 0.001$). Nonetheless, the conclusion in the Abstract of the trial suggested that statistical significance was prioritized over clinical significance:

"Over a mean of 8.1 years, a dietary intervention that reduced total fat intake . . . did not significantly reduce the risk of CHD, stroke, or CVD in postmenopausal women . . ."

The intervention did not reduce total fat intake to clinically significant levels. This was a failure of the intervention to hit its goal on fat intake, not a failure of the hypothesis that reduced fat intake and reduced risk of cardiovascular events. But if the intervention had hit the clinically significant target, it may very well have translated into reduced risk on cardiovascular events. The only way to know is to do the trial again with a stronger intervention.

RECOMMENDATIONS

The essential question of interest to a behavioral trialist is:

"Does this behavioral treatment improve a chronic disease outcome?"

Statistical significance alone will not provide an answer. When nature is the disinterested final arbiter, as it is with a chronic disease outcome, it is clear that this *"emperor is not wearing much."* To answer this essential question, recommendations include interpreting results from behavioral trials with a progressive set of questions.

Does the Treatment Achieve a Clinically Significant Benefit?

The first question in evaluating the results of a behavioral trial is *whether* the treatment achieved a clinically significant benefit. Prioritization of clinical significance insures that improving health is the end game. Early identification of how strong a behavioral treatment needs to be in order for it to reduce the risk of chronic disease, and judging the strength of the behavioral treatment against this criterion, applies to all stages of behavioral treatment development and all outcomes used at these various stages.

A subtle way that clinical significance is undervalued in clinical trial design is the pervasive use of an effect size to estimate a treatment's efficacy on a primary endpoint. This ignores the important question of whether or not the treatment was strong enough to move a clinical endpoint and judges a treatment's strength instead by how it stacks up against the unpredictable response of a comparator group. Effect sizes should be disaggregated, and separate estimates for treated and comparator groups should be built into the design, analyses, and interpretation of behavioral trials.

Does the Treatment Achieve a Better Response than a Comparator?

If the treatment has achieved a clinically significant benchmark, this justifies going to a second question of *Why?* or *Compared to what?* The answer to this second question is meaningless when the first question is answered in the negative. If a treatment does not improve health, a reasonable direction would be to strengthen the treatment rather than studying its comparative advantage.

An answer to this second question draws on statistical analyses to quantify what "better" means. Statisticians are intensifying their arguments against statistical significance being a substitute for scientific importance. They are in active rebellion against what they believe has become a tyrant. This is shown in the strength of their words [12, 13].

> *"Never use 'no difference' or 'no association' based upon a p-value.*
> *Statistically significant—don't say it and don't use it."*

Nowhere is it more important to reduce reliance on statistical significance than in the field of applied behavioral clinical trials. Overreliance on statistical significance has impeded progress by creating false security about the conclusiveness of findings, providing a convenient substitute for scientific conclusions, a lack of interest in replication, and, if a replication is conducted, an inability to reproduce the finding.

A statistical comparison between a treatment and a comparator provides a useful metric for quantifying the certainty that exists, contingent upon assumptions, that there is a true difference between them. To answer the question of the comparative advantage of the treated relative to the comparator, the actual p-value and confidence interval should be reported along with a thoughtful discussion of the uncertainty they imply. This is in keeping with best practices in statistics and is consistent with the uncertainty that is implicit in the use of these statistical tools. Reporting actual p-values and confidence intervals is far superior to the false security implied by the dichotomous decision that the finding is "statistically significant" because the p-value is less than 0.05 or the confidence interval does not include 1.

What Is the Scientific Conclusion from This Trial?

The word "significance" is confusing. It applies to both the description of the importance of a scientific conclusion (e.g., a *"significant"* finding) and to the statistical results (e.g., a *"significant"* result). A significant scientific conclusion from a behavioral trial emerges from the integration of a variety of types of evidence, of which clinical significance (i.e., strength of a treatment to move a clinical endpoint) is at the top of the ladder and statistical significance (i.e., probability of a result under the null hypothesis) is closer to the bottom [29].

Because of the confusion surrounding the word "significant," and the judgment it implies, it may be wise to stop using it altogether and replace with the specific scientific conclusion drawn from a trial. The criteria for making a scientific conclusion in a behavioral trial are presented in the box. To arrive at a rigorous and thoughtful scientific conclusion from a single behavioral trial, spend less time with statistical software and more time thinking [13].

> **Basis for Scientific Conclusions**
>
> QUALITY OF THE TRIAL
>
> - Accuracy of assumptions in sample size calculations made for:
>   - Treatment effect
>   - Comparator effect
>   - Estimate of variability
>   - Drop-out rate
>   - Non-adherence rate.
>
> - Protection of randomization
> - Freedom from bias
>
> SCIENTIFIC CONTRIBUTION
>
> - Treatment produces a clinically significant benefit on the primary outcome
> - The certainty of the difference between the treated and comparator is quantified
> - Consistency with results from similar trials
> - Biological plausibility
> - Cost relative to benefit

How Conclusive Is the Evidence That This Treatment Improves Health?

> **Be open.**
> **One study is rarely enough.**
>
> *"The words 'groundbreaking new study' might be loved by news writers but must be resisted by researchers. Breaking ground is only the first step in building a house. It will be suitable for habitation only after much more hard work." [12]*

One trial alone is suggestive, but not conclusive, evidence for the hypothesis that a behavioral treatment can improve health. Although there is an extensive literature aimed at correcting the misinterpretation that a statistically significant result provides conclusive evidence that a treatment works, the misinterpretation is nonetheless sustained for many reasons. Among them are the seductive thrill of victory, the frustration with getting replications funded because they are not that innovative, and the fear that any victory is short-lived in the face of the high risk of inability to replicate.

Replications of results in new trials may not be "innovative," but they are essential to the progression of science. Although it is often assumed that the Diabetes Prevention Project [49] was, unto itself, a definitive test of lifestyle treatment to prevent the development of diabetes, it was not alone. Replications were conducted in Japan [50–52], Scandinavia [53], China [54], Europe [55], India [56], and Finland [57].

The best way for science to approach a conclusive determination of whether or not a treatment actually works is through replication. In the context of behavioral trials, reviews of grant proposals and papers should eliminate the criterion of innovation to judge the scientific contribution. This could make investigators less concerned about innovation and more concerned about getting to the essential goal of finding behavioral treatments that actually work.

It is also helpful to have patience and a healthy dose of humility. Elizabeth Barrett-Connor, the prolific and inspirational epidemiologist and clinical researcher, was a believer in the scientific method. She reminded her mentees repeatedly of it with her words (see box).

> *"The only reason to have a hypothesis is to try to disprove it. If you can't, you might be right—not guaranteed to be right, but you might be right."*
> Elizabeth Barrett-Connor
> (1935-2019)

REFERENCES

1. Bakan D (1966) The test of significance in psychological research. Psych Bulletin 66:423–437
2. Cohen J (1994) The earth is round (p < .05). Am Psych 49:997–1003
3. Hume D (1739-1740) A treatise of human nature, V1, Norton DF, Norton MJ (eds) (2000), Oxford University Press, Oxford
4. Popper KR (1959) The logic of scientific discovery. Basic Books, New York
5. Fisher RA (1935) The design of experiments. Oliver and Boyd, Edinburgh
6. Goodman SN (1999) Toward evidence-based medical statistics. 1: The P-value fallacy. Ann Intern Med 130:995–1004
7. Fisher RA (1973) Statistical methods and scientific inference, 3rd edn. Macmillan, New York
8. Bayes T (1763) Essay towards solving a problem in the doctrine of chances. Phil Trans Roy Soc 53:370–418. (Reprinted: Biometrika 1958:45:293–315)
9. Fisher RA (1956) Statistical methods and scientific inference, 1st edn. Oliver & Boyd, Edinburg
10. Neyman J, Pearson E (1933) On the problem of the most efficient tests of statistical hypotheses. Phil Trans Roy Soc 231:289–337
11. Tyler RW (1931) What is statistical significance? Ed Res Bull 10:115–118
12. Wasserstein RL, Schirm AL, Lazar NA (2019) Moving to a world beyond "p<0.05". Am Stat 73:1–19
13. Amrhein V, Greenland S, McShane B (2019) Retire statistical significance. Nature 567:305–307
14. Skeelam J (1969) Models, inference, and strategy. Biometrics 25:457–475
15. Armstrong JS (2007) Significance tests harm progress in forecasting. Intl J Forecasting 23:321–327
16. Ioannidis JPA (2005) Why most published research findings are false. PLoS Med 2:e124. https://doi.org/10.1371/journal.pmed.0020124
17. Bacchetti P (2010) Current sample size conventions: flaws, harms, and alternatives. BMC Med 8:17. https://doi.org/10.1186/1741-7015-8-17
18. Kraemer HC, Morgan GA, Leech NL, Gliner JA, Vaske JJ, Harmon RJ (2003) Measures of clinical significance. J Am Acad Child Adolesc Psychiat 42:1524–1529
19. Silva-Aycaguer LC, Suarez-Gil P, Fernandez-Somoano A (2010) The null hypothesis significance test in health sciences research (1995–2006): statistical analysis and interpretation. BMC Med Res Meth 10:44. https://doi.org/10.1186/1471-2288-10-44
20. Jacobson NS (1991) Clinical significance: a statistical approach to defining meaningful change in psychotherapy research. J Consul Clin Psych 59:12–19
21. Lecoutre B, Lecoutre MP, Poiteveneau J (2001) Uses, abuses, and misuses of significance tests in the scientific community: Won't the Bayesian choice be unavoidable? Intl Stat Rev 69:399–417
22. Rutledge T, Loh C (2004) Effect sizes and statistical testing in the determination of clinical significance in behavioral medicine research. Ann Behav Med 27:138–145
23. Hubbard R, Ryan PA (2000) The historical growth of statistical significance testing in psychology — and its future prospects. Educ Psych Meas 60:661–681
24. Schmidt FL, Hunter JE (1997) Eight common but false objections to the discontinuation of significance testing in analysis of research data. In: Harlow LL, Mulnik SA, Steiger JH (eds) What if there were no significance tests? Erlbaum, London, pp 35–60
25. Gigerenzer G (2004) Mindless statistics. J Socio-Econ 33:587–606
26. Gigerenzer G, Swijtink Z, Porter T, Daston L, Beatty J, Kruger L (1989) The empire of chance. How probability changed science and everyday life. Cambridge University Press, Cambridge
27. Efron B, Hastie T (2016) Computer age statistical inference. Algorithms, evidence, and data science. Cambridge University Press, New York

28. Goodman SN (1999) Toward evidence-based medical statistics. 2: The Bayes factor. Ann Intern Med 130:1005–1013
29. Efron B (August 2018) Personal communication
30. Czajkowski SM, Powell LH, Adler N, Naar-King S, Reynolds KD, Hunter CM, Laraia B, Olster DH, Perna FM, Peterson JC, Epel E, Charlson M (2015) From ideas to efficacy: the ORBIT model for developing behavioral treatments for chronic diseases. Health Psychol 34:971–982
31. 2018 Physical Activity Guidelines Advisory Committee (2018) 2018 Physical Activity Guidelines Advisory Committee Scientific Report. US Department of Health and Human Services, Washington DC
32. McGlothlin AE, Lewis RJ (2014) Minimal clinically important difference defining what really matters to patients. JAMA 312:1342–1343
33. Nezu AM, Nezu CM (2008) Evidence-based outcome research: a practical guide to conducting randomized controlled trials for psychosocial interventions. Oxford University Press, New York
34. Lambert MJ, Hansen NB, Bauer S (2008) Assessing the clinical significance of outcome results. In: Nezu AM, Nezu CM (eds) Evidence-based outcome research: a practical guide to conducting randomized controlled trials for psychosocial interventions. Oxford University Press, New York, pp 359–378
35. Gitlin LN, Czaja SJ (2016) Behavioral intervention research. Designing, evaluating, and implementing. Springer, New York
36. Calvert M, Kyte D, Mercieca-Bebber R, Slade A, Chan AW, King MT, SPIRIT-PRO Group (2018) Guidelines for inclusion of patient-reported outcomes in clinical trial protocols: the SPIRIT-PRO Extension. JAMA 319:483–494
37. De Geest S, Sabate E (2003) Adherence to long-term therapies: evidence for action. Europ J Cardiovasc Nursing 2:323. https://doi.org/10.1016/S1474-5151(03)00091-4
38. Colman E (2012) Food and Drug Administration's obesity drug guidance document. A short history. Circulation 125:2156–2164
39. Kraemer HC, Mintz J, Tinklenberg J, Yesavage JA (2006) Caution regarding the use of pilot studies to guide power calculations for study proposals. Arch Gen Psychiat 63:484–489
40. Bacchetti P, McCulloch CE, Segal MR (2008) Simple, defensible sample sizes based on cost efficiency. Biometrics 64:577–594
41. Willan AR (2008) Optimal sample size determinations from an industry perspective based on the expected value of information. Clin Trials 5:587–594
42. Everson SA, Goldberg DE, Kaplan GA, Julkunen J, Salonen JT (1998) Anger expression and incident hypertension. Psychosom Med 60:730–735
43. Everson SA, Lynch JW, Kaplan GA, Lakka TA, Sivenius J, Salonen JT (2001) Stress-induced blood pressure reactivity and incident stroke in middle-aged men. Stroke 32:1263–1270
44. Mosnaim G, Li H, Martin M, Richardson D, Belice PJ, Avery E, Silberstein A, Leigh J, Kenyon R, Jones S, Bender B, Powell LH (2015) A tailored mobile health intervention to improve adherence and asthma control in minority adolescents. J Allergy Clin Immunol Pract 3:288–290
45. Mosnaim G, Li H, Martin M, Richardson D, Belice PJ, Avery E, Ryan N, Bender B, Powell LH (2013) The impact of peer support and mp3 messaging on adherence to inhaled corticosteroids in minority adolescents with asthma: a randomized, controlled trial. J Allergy Clin Immunol Pract 1:485–493
46. Berkman LF, Blumenthal J, Burg M, Carney RM, Catellier D, Cowan MJ, Czajkowski SM, DeBusk R, Hosking J, Jaffe A, Kaufmann PG, Mitchell P, Norman J, Powell LH, Raczynski JM, Schneiderman N, Enhancing Recovery in Coronary Heart Disease Patients Investigators (ENRICHD) (2003) Effects of treating depression and low perceived social support on clinical events after myocardial infarction: the Enhancing Recovery in Coronary Heart Disease Patients (ENRICHD) Randomized Trial. JAMA 289:3106–3116

47. Frasure-Smith N, Lesperance F (2003) Depression – A cardiac risk factor in search of a treatment. JAMA 289:3171–3173
48. Howard BV, Van Horn L, Hsia J, Manson JE, Stefanick ML, Wassertheil-Smoller S, Kuller LH, LaCroix AZ, Langer RD, Lasser NL, Lewis CE, Limacher MC, Margolis KL, Mysiw WJ, Ockene JK, Parker LM, Perri MG, Phillips L, Prentice RL, Robbins J, Rossouw JE, Sarto GE, Schatz IJ, Snetselaar LG, Stevens VJ, Tinker LF, Trevisan M, Vitolins MZ, Anderson GL, Assaf AR, Bassford T, Beresford SA, Black HR, Brunner RL, Brzyski RG, Caan B, Chlebowski RT, Gass M, Granek I, Greenland P, Hays J, Heber D, Heiss G, Hendrix SL, Hubbell FA, Johnson KC, Kotchen JM (2006) Low-fat dietary pattern and risk of cardiovascular disease: the Women's Health Initiative Randomized Controlled Dietary Modification Trial. JAMA 295:655–666
49. Knowler WC, Barrett-Connor E, Fowler SE, Hamman RF, Lachin JM, Walker EA, Nathan DM, Diabetes Prevention Program Research Group (2002) Reduction in the incidence of type 2 diabetes with lifestyle intervention or metformin. New Engl J Med 346:393–403
50. Kosaka K, Noda M, Kuzuya T (2005) Prevention of type 2 diabetes by lifestyle intervention: a Japanese trial in IGT males. Diab Res Clin Pract 67:152–162
51. Saito T, Watanabe M, Nishida J, Izumi T, Omura M, Takagi T, Fukunaga R, Bandai Y, Tajima N, Nakamura Y, Ito M, Zensharen Study for Prevention of Lifestyle Diseases Group (2011) Lifestyle modification and prevention of type 2 diabetes in overweight Japanese with impaired fasting glucose levels. Arch Intern Med 171:1352–1360
52. Sakane N, Sato J, Tsushita K, Tsujii S, Kotani K, Tsuzaki K, Tominaga M, Kawazu S, Sato Y, Usui T, Kamae I, Yoshida T, Kiyohara Y, Sato S, Kuzuya H, Japan Diabetes Prevention Program (JDPP) Research Group (2011) Prevention of type 2 diabetes in a primary healthcare setting: three-year results of lifestyle intervention in Japanese subjects with impaired glucose tolerance. BMC Public Health 11:40. https://doi.org/10.1186/1471-2458-11-40
53. Lindahl B, Nilsson TK, Borch-Johnsen K, Oder ME, Soderberg S, Widman L, Johnson O, Hallmans G, Jansson J (2009) A randomized lifestyle intervention with 5-year follow-up in subjects with impaired glucose tolerance: pronounced short-term impact but long-term adherence problems. Scand J Pub Health 37:434–442
54. Pan XR, Li GW, Hu YH, Wang JX, Yang WY, An ZX, Hu ZX, Lin J, Xiao JZ, Cao HB, Liu PA, Jiang XG, Jiang YY, Wang JP, Zheng H, Zhang H, Bennett PH, Howard BV (1997) Effects of diet and exercise in preventing NIDDM in people with impaired glucose tolerance. Diabetes Care 20:537–544
55. Penn L, White M, Lindstrom J, den Boer AT, Blaak E, Eriksson JG, Feskens E, Ilanne-Parikka P, Keinanen-Kiukaanniemi SM, Walker M, Mathers JC, Uusitupa M, Tuomilehto J (2013) Importance of weight loss maintenance and risk prediction in the prevention of type 2 diabetes: analysis of European Diabetes Prevention Study RCT. PLoS ONE 8:e57143. https://doi.org/10.1371/journal.pone.0057143
56. Ramachandran A, Snehalatha C, Ram J, Selvam S, Simon M, Nanditha A, Shetty AS, Godsland IF, Chaturvedi N, Majeed A, Oliver N, Toumazou C, Alberti KG, Johnston DG (2013) Effectiveness of mobile phone messaging in prevention of type 2 diabetes by lifestyle modification in men in India: a prospective, parallel-group, randomized controlled trial. Lancet 1:191–198
57. Tuomilehto J, Lindström J, Eriksson JG, Valle TT, Hämäläinen H, Ilanne-Parikka P, Keinänen-Kiukaanniemi S, Laakso M, Louheranta A, Rastas M, Salminen V, Uusitupa M, Finnish Diabetes Prevention Study Group (2001) Prevention of type 2 diabetes mellitus by changes in lifestyle among subjects with impaired glucose tolerance. New Engl J Med 344:1343–1350

Chapter 6
The Choice of a Comparator

"I would rather have questions that can't be answered than answers that can't be questioned."

Richard Feynman
Nobel Prize in Physics, 1965

Fundamental Point

The choice of a comparator is one of the most important decisions in the design of a behavioral trial. It should be driven by the primary research question that the trial is intended to answer. A comparator that is chosen on any other basis may leave that question unanswered.

The choice of a comparator in a behavioral trial is often based upon implicit rules that sustain the status quo. In many cases, this status quo is a "one-size-fits-all" comparator that controls for non-specific treatment factors. The recent emergence of frameworks for comparator choice aims to create explicit rules which place a priority on the primary purpose of the trial within its developmental context. This chapter reviews implicit and explicit criteria for making decisions about an optimum comparator and presents two new frameworks that facilitate decision-making: the Pragmatic Model for Comparator Selection in Health-Related Behavioral Trials; and the Purpose-Guided Trial Design Framework. Both encourage an evolution of a trial's purpose as understanding of a behavioral treatment progresses, prioritize purpose over logistic and scientific limitations of any particular comparator, and raise caution about the danger of choosing a comparator that inadvertently changes the purpose of the trial.

© Springer Nature Switzerland AG 2021
L. H. Powell et al., *Behavioral Clinical Trials for Chronic Diseases*,
https://doi.org/10.1007/978-3-030-39330-4_6

SCIENTIFIC PRINCIPLES

Researchers have a wide variety of comparators from which to choose when designing randomized trials of behavioral interventions [1]. The choice is an easy one in some cases. In a comparative effectiveness trial, for instance, the research goal is to compare two or more existing interventions or strategies. Here, the groups essentially choose themselves. In other cases, however, the choice can be quite difficult due to long-standing uncertainties and disagreements about whether, when, and how to use certain comparators.

These disputes are manifestations of a deeper controversy about decision-making frameworks. There are multiple frameworks for choosing comparators. There is, to date, no firm consensus on which one(s) to use.

Decision-Making Frameworks

Table 6.1 summarizes seven common frameworks that are explicitly or implicitly used to guide decisions about the appropriate comparator in a behavioral trial. Each of these frameworks is described below.

Implicit Rules
Comparator choices in behavioral intervention research are often determined by implicit rules. Among these rules are the following.

Maintain the Status Quo. If a particular comparator has been used in similar studies, then it must be the (safe, smart, or right) choice for (my or your) study too. This rule assumes that the comparator in question was the best choice for the previous studies even though it might not have been, and it privileges conformity over logic.

Table 6.1 Decision-making frameworks

Source of Guidance	Key Attributes
Implicit rules	Offers tacit guidance, absorbed from and reinforced by cultural environment
Explicit rules	Offers more transparent guidance, but may be excessively rigid
Quality-guided decisions	Aims to ensure that the trial's methodology will be judged favorably
Phase-guided decisions	Recommends different comparators for different phases of intervention research
Purpose-guided decisions	Asserts that the trial's primary purpose outweighs other considerations
Context-guided decisions	Recognizes constraints on comparator choices imposed by contextual factors
Evidence-based decisions	Provides empirical data that can either support or challenge any of the above

Tougher is Always Better. This rule implies that comparators that are relatively hard for interventions to outperform are inherently better than ones that are relatively easy to outperform. It derives from widespread dissatisfaction with the laxity of no-treatment and wait-list comparators [2, 3], a belief that placebo effects play problematic roles in psychotherapeutic and other behavioral interventions [4], and a desire to emulate the rigorous, double-blind, placebo-controlled designs that are used in drug research [5]. It would be easier to choose comparators for behavioral interventions if "tougher" *were* always better, but sometimes it is not, for reasons to be discussed later in this chapter.

Implicit rules can be learned without ever having been articulated overtly. One can follow them without having been told to do so and without being aware of doing so [6]. Implicit rules facilitate decision-making under uncertainty. To the extent that they seem self-evident, they relieve us from any burden of proof. Holding the same ones as our mentors and peers also gives us an entrée to a shared culture and a sense of belonging. These factors can make implicit rules easy to adopt, easy to follow, and hard to abandon even when confronted with evidence that contradicts them.

When different researchers inculcate different implicit rules, they tend to disagree about comparator choices even if their respective positions are not very well defined or supported. Such disputes can be difficult to resolve and slow the progress of behavioral intervention research when they adversely influence the fate of grants and papers.

Explicit Rules

Explicit rules for behavioral trials that would mandate or prohibit the use of various comparators could resolve disputes created by implicit rules but create other problems.

The most restrictive rule would mandate a single, one-size-fits-all comparator for behavioral trials. Drug research is one of the inspirations for this idea, as it is for the belief that *tougher is always better*. It posits that because most drug trials are placebo-controlled, the best comparator for behavioral research would be an all-purpose placebo condition. A less restrictive version recognizes that different circumstances may call for different comparators, but holds that explicit rules should determine the choice. Proponents of this position point to the fact that the Food and Drug Administration (FDA) regulates the design of pharmaceutical trials and that this helps to make drug research orderly and predictable.

In reality, the FDA regulations provide flexible *guidelines* for comparator choices rather than mandatory rules or standards. The "Adequate and Well-Controlled Studies" section of the Code of Federal Regulations (21CFR314.126) states that five different comparators are generally recognized in drug trials (see box). The FDA Drug Study Designs Information Sheet states that these comparators "can be useful in particular circumstances" and that "no general preference is expressed for any one type, but the study design chosen must be adequate to the task" [7]. It also discusses the advantages and disadvantages of these comparators and the usual circumstances in which each one may be used. In short, the FDA offers guidance instead of dictating comparator choices.

FDA's "Recognized" Comparators
Placebo concurrent comparator
Dose-comparison concurrent comparator
No treatment concurrent comparator
Active treatment concurrent comparator
Historical comparator

Nevertheless, the FDA is more likely to accept evidence from trials that are responsive to their guidelines than evidence from other trials.

Quality-Guided Decisions

The FDA is not in the business of approving behavioral interventions, so behavioral trials are not designed with FDA approval in mind. However, other kinds of approval may be sought for behavioral interventions, such as recommendations in evidence-based clinical practice guidelines. Whether trials are included in high-impact meta-analyses and clinical practice guidelines depends on whether they are methodologically rigorous according to research quality measures such as the Cochrane Collaboration's tool for assessing risk of bias in randomized controlled trials [8]. Consequently, researchers have incentives to design their trials in ways that merit high ratings on such measures.

The Cochrane risk of bias tool lists a number of specific methodological deficiencies that could cause a behavioral trial to be classified as having a high risk of bias, such as the use of an inadequate randomization procedure. However, it does not include any specific criteria for the choice of comparators. Neither does the Grading of Recommendations Assessment, Development, and Evaluation (GRADE) system of rating the quality of evidence [9]. Although quality of evidence rating measures may be useful guides for many different behavioral trial design decisions, they offer little guidance for choosing comparators.

Phase-Guided Decisions

A seminal paper by Mohr et al. [10] explains why different comparators may be needed in different phases of behavioral intervention development. Early trials of novel behavioral interventions tend to be small and to ask whether the treatment has any detectable effects. Type II errors (i.e., failing to find a true benefit) can have more serious consequences than Type I errors (i.e., finding a spurious benefit) in early-phase research because they can thwart continued development of promising interventions and/or promote premature abandonment of them. This favors the use of relatively lenient comparators such as wait-list or no-treatment conditions in early-phase trials. In contrast, later-phase trials tend to be larger and to ask whether the treatment has robust and clinically meaningful effects. The dominant concerns in this phase of research shift to avoiding Type I errors to maximize the clinical implications of the trial. These considerations favor more formidable and clinically relevant comparators.

Mohr et al. [10] argue that the comparators that best serve the needs of the ultimate stakeholders in an intervention (including patients and providers) also shift as individual research programs progress from *Phase I* studies through *Phase III* and *IV* trials. Different comparators may be needed for early investigations of an intervention than for trials conducted when understanding of the intervention is more mature. For example, Bower [11] recently suggested that research on mindfulness interventions for cancer survivors has advanced to a point at which wait-list comparators have outlived their usefulness and more formidable and clinically relevant comparators are needed.

Purpose-Guided Decisions

Purpose-Guided Trial Design (PGTD) [12] is a heuristic framework for choosing comparators for behavioral trials. Its fundamental principle is that the design of a behavioral trial should be guided by its primary purpose. A unique feature of PGTD is that it recognizes the existence of conflicting demands in the trial design process and asserts that compatibility of the design with the primary purpose of the trial outweighs any conflicting methodological considerations or secondary aims. The primary purpose is the main justification for conducting the trial. If it is sacrificed for the sake of less important considerations, the trial loses its *raison d'être*.

For example, the primary purpose of a trial may be to determine whether a behavioral intervention that requires multiple therapeutic contacts produces better outcomes than are typically obtained in routine clinical practice settings where such an intervention is not available. The comparator that would best serve the primary purpose of such a trial might be called usual care (UC), treatment as usual (TAU), or standard care, depending upon the area of research. For simplicity, it will be called usual care.

Although UC would fit the primary purpose of the trial, it would also have limitations. An obvious one is that the UC participants would not have any contacts with a trial therapist, whereas those in the intervention arm would have multiple contacts. Consequently, exposure to the intervention will be confounded with contact time. If the outcomes are significantly better in the intervention than the UC arm, it could be argued that this does not constitute evidence that the experimental intervention is efficacious. It is possible that simply spending the same amount of time with the participants, minus the elaborate intervention, might yield similar benefits.

This criticism focuses on a possible *rival explanation* for the apparent effects of the intervention. Comparators can be designed to rule out various rival explanations. In this example, the investigator could have chosen a comparator that provides the same amount of contact with a therapist that the intervention provides. In doing so, however, they would have created a comparator that is decidedly unlike routine clinical care. Hence the trial would not answer the key question of whether the intervention is superior to routine care.

PGTD acknowledges the importance of threats to internal validity and other rival explanations for treatment effects, but places highest priority on compatibility with the primary purpose of the trial, even if this makes it difficult to rule out certain rival explanations for the findings. This is not an excuse for methodological weaknesses or a way to downplay internal validity. It simply acknowledges that the trial design process often involves trade-offs, and, when it does, the primary purpose of the trial should take precedence over other concerns. If a trial does not serve its primary purpose, it is not worth conducting.

Context-Guided Decisions

The context within which a behavioral trial is conducted can impose constraints on comparator choices. For example, if a trial with a "no-treatment" comparator focuses on a disorder that is treated routinely in clinical practice, some of the participants may receive treatment for the disorder outside of the trial. This could occur even if the investigator were to urge the participants to refrain from seeking any non-trial care for the disorder during the course of the trial. Thus, even if the investigator were to call the comparator a "no-treatment" group, contamination by non-trial care would effectively turn it into a UC condition [1].

Evidence-Based Decisions

A small but growing empirical literature on comparators is challenging some long-held beliefs and may help to guide the selection, design, and implementation of comparators for future behavioral trials. For example, formidability (i.e., the expected amount of pre-post change on the primary outcome measure) is one of the most important considerations in choosing among comparators. Certain comparators are expected to be more formidable (i.e., more likely to produce change) than others. All else being equal, many investigators would expect to see more pre-post improvement in participants who are randomly assigned to TAU than to a wait-list condition.

However, Mohr et al. [13] performed a meta-analysis of a number of comparator features in trials of psychotherapy for depression. One of their analyses showed, contrary to expectation, that comparisons of depression interventions to wait-list control conditions yielded effect sizes that were not significantly larger than comparisons between depression interventions and TAU. This suggests that the formidability of TAU and wait-list comparators may be more similar in depression treatment trials than was previously believed. The formidability of the comparator is an important consideration in designing behavioral trials, and findings such as the ones reported by Mohr et al. are not only raising questions about reliance on traditional beliefs about comparator formidability but also fostering empirically informed design decisions. Feasibility pilot studies that test the formidability of a comparator on primary and secondary outcomes for a planned trial is an underutilized, but nonetheless extremely valuable, part of preparation for *Phase II* and *Phase III* efficacy trials.

CHALLENGES FOR BEHAVIORAL TRIALS

Historical Perspective

The pros and cons of various comparators have been debated ever since the dawn of psychotherapy research [14]. The discussion began in 1936 when the eminent psychologist, Saul Rosenzweig, argued that despite claims to the contrary by proponents of particular brands of therapy, all forms of psychotherapy have similar effects and common factors, such as clinical attention, which account for a substantial proportion of their efficacy [15]. He likened this to the scene in *Alice's Adventures in Wonderland* by Lewis

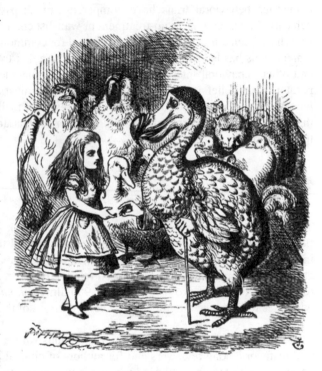

Carroll wherein a dodo bird organized a race in which everyone was allowed to start and stop whenever they liked. At the end of the race, the dodo bird declared, "Everybody has won, and all must have prizes."

Rosenzweig's proposition, which came to be known as the "Dodo Bird Conjecture," gained empirical support with the 1997 publication of an influential meta-analysis of research on "bona fide" psychotherapies [16]. The meta-analysis was limited to trials that had directly compared two (or more) different forms of psychotherapy. It was found that the effect sizes were homogeneously distributed around zero, consistent with the Dodo Bird Conjecture. There is evidence to the contrary, but it is equivocal. Even if some psychotherapeutic interventions are superior to others for certain disorders, common factors are important components of all of them.

Something resembling the dodo bird shows up in many other areas of behavioral intervention research, beyond the traditional terrain of psychotherapy. For example, a widely publicized meta-analysis found minimal differences in efficacy among a variety of popular weight loss diets, but all of them achieved a common factor of reduction in calories [17]. Novel interventions often generate a lot of enthusiasm, but the sobering reality is that dramatic breakthroughs are rare in behavioral intervention research. Incremental advances tend to be a more realistic goal.

Numerous behavioral trials have compared various psychotherapeutic or other behavioral interventions to no-treatment or wait-list comparator groups [18]. These trials have been criticized for failing to control for common factors and for being too lenient. This has led some researchers to conclude that trials of psychotherapeutic and other behavioral interventions should always include a common factor comparator. This belief is reinforced by the fact that most standard drug trials are placebo-controlled. Despite the appeal of this response to the Dodo Bird Conjecture, there are circumstances in which common factor comparators create more problems than they solve.

The Status Quo

There has never been a consensus about which framework(s) should guide the selection of comparators for behavioral trials. Starting from different premises and relying on different frameworks, different researchers often reach different conclusions about which comparator should be used in any given trial. The present situation is reminiscent of Akira Kurosawa's classic 1950 film *Rashomon*, in which a number of witnesses to a crime contradict each other's versions of the same incident.

This is problematic for individual grant applicants whose comparator choices may find disfavor among reviewers and for authors of clinical trial reports whose comparator choices may be criticized when it is far too late to do anything about them. It is also problematic for the entire field of behavioral clinical trials. Consequently, many researchers are looking for some sort of consensus to emerge and wondering whether a new framework will prevail.

OVERCOMING THESE CHALLENGES IN A BEHAVIORAL TRIAL

There are two emerging frameworks that provide guidance on the choice of an appropriate comparator in a behavioral trial. These frameworks release the investigator from implicit rules and facilitate reasoned decision-making.

The Pragmatic Model for Comparator Selection in Health-Related Behavioral Trials

The Office of Behavioral and Social Sciences Research (OBSSR) in the National Institutes of Health recently responded to the unsatisfactory state of affairs in choosing a comparator for a behavioral trial by convening an expert panel on the selection of comparators for trials of behavioral interventions. They asked the panel to develop a set of recommendations on how to decide on the optimal comparator and publish them in 2019. After reviewing existing frameworks (discussed above), the panel developed a decision-making approach called the Pragmatic Model for Comparator Selection in Health-Related Behavioral Trials [19]. This model advocates decision-making in six steps (Fig. 6.1).

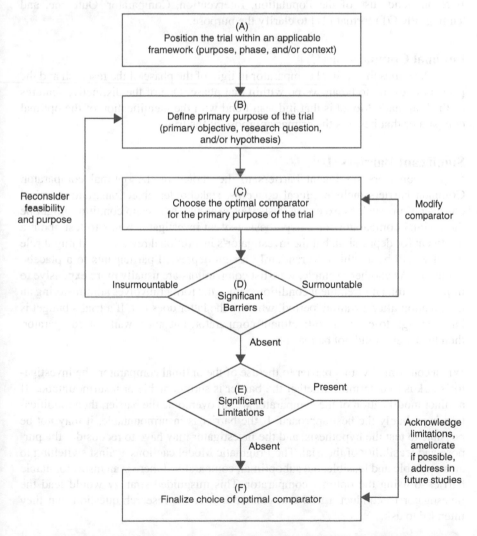

Fig. 6.1 The Pragmatic Model for Comparator Selection in Health-Related Behavioral Trials

Relevant Framework (A)

Step A positions the trial within an applicable translational research framework, such as the ORBIT model [20]. Showing how and where the trial fits into a sequence of studies or a program of translational research clarifies its purpose. It enables the investigator to differentiate between aims that will be addressed in the present trial and those that have already been addressed in previous studies or that will be addressed in studies planned for the future.

Primary Purpose of the Trial (B)

Step B defines the primary purpose of the trial. Like the Purpose-Guided Trial Design Framework (see below), the Pragmatic Model asserts that the optimal comparator for any behavioral trial is the one that best serves the trial's primary purpose. It recommends use of the Population, Intervention, Comparator, Outcome, and Timing (PICOT) format [21] to clarify the purpose.

Optimal Comparator (C)

Step C specifies the optimal comparator in light of the phase of the research and the primary question to be answered within that phase. One of the distinctive features of the Pragmatic Model is that it doesn't end with the identification of the optimal comparator that best fits the primary purpose of the trial.

Significant Barriers (D)

Step D considers significant barriers to the choice of the optimal comparator. Common barriers include ethical concerns, stakeholder objections, and practical considerations such as excessive costs. For example, a placebo condition might be the optimal comparator for a hypothesis that an investigator wants to test about a treatment for depression, but the investigator's institutional review board might rule that it would be unethical to randomly assign depressed participants to a placebo condition. As another example, wait-list comparators are usually more expensive to implement than no-treatment conditions, since the former involves administering an intervention after a waiting period, whereas the latter does not. If a trial's budget is large enough to cover a no-treatment comparator, but not a wait-list comparator, then the latter would not be feasible.

When confronted with a barrier to the use of the optimal comparator, the investigator's task is to determine whether the barrier is surmountable or insurmountable. If a minor modification of the comparator would overcome the barrier, then modification is probably the best approach. If the barrier is insurmountable, it may not be possible to test the hypothesis, and the investigator may have to reconsider the purpose and feasibility of the trial. The Pragmatic Model cautions against switching to an acceptable and feasible, but suboptimal, comparator if there is an insurmountable barrier to using the optimal comparator. This misguided strategy would lead the investigator to conduct a trial that cannot answer the research question that they intended to ask.

Significant Limitations (E)

Step E asks investigators to explicate the *limitations* of the optimal comparator. Unlike insurmountable barriers, limitations do not prevent an optimal comparator from being implemented, but they often do affect the validity of the conclusions that can be drawn from a trial. If, for example, a trial is designed to determine if the addition of a behavioral intervention to usual care improves the outcomes, the randomized arms would be usual care alone versus usual care plus the behavioral intervention. The groups will differ with respect to the amount of contact. This does not create a barrier to implementing the comparator, but it will make it difficult to draw any firm conclusions about the extent to which contact time per se explains the effects of the intervention.

Finalize Choice (F)

In Step F, the choice of the comparator is finalized. This choice places optimality *ahead* of barriers and limitations when decisions about comparators are being made. Many disagreements about comparators result from giving greater weight to barriers and limitations than to the optimality of a comparator for the purpose of the trial. One of the most important contributions of the Pragmatic Model is that it separates and sequences the establishment of the primary purpose of the trial, the identification of the comparator that best fits this purpose, the recognition of barriers to the use of the optimal comparator, and an explication of its limitations.

The Pragmatic Model will probably not answer every controversial question to the satisfaction of everyone who has a strong opinion about how behavioral trials should or should not be designed. However, it will help to resolve some of the most difficult questions. It will also provide clarity to the research community about the selection of comparators for behavioral trials. It can be cited by grant applicants and authors of papers reporting on behavioral trials. It is hoped that this enhanced clarity will have a significant positive influence on the selection and design of comparators in the years ahead and, more generally, on the entire culture of behavioral clinical trial design.

Purpose-Guided Comparator Choices

The principle that a comparator should fit the purpose of the trial is a central premise of the Purpose-Guided Trial Design (PGTD) Framework [12]. The main purpose of a trial should be obvious to an investigator, but it often becomes confused. Such confusion is exacerbated by the fact that comparator choices can change the primary purpose of the trial. The PGTD Comparator Grid aims to help investigators clarify the main purpose of the trial and then to align this purpose with the appropriate comparator (Table 6.2). The use of the grid illuminates the intimate relationship between comparator choice and the primary purpose of the trial.

Table 6.2 Purpose-Guided Trial Design comparator grid

Primary Purpose of the Comparator	Primary Purpose of the Behavioral Trial			
	Conduct Experiment	Investigate Intervention	Improve Outcomes	Increase Utility
Control				
Compare				

Purpose of the Trial

The grid's columns list the four primary reasons for conducting a behavioral trial.

Conduct Experiment. Experiments test causal hypotheses about the rela- tionship between a manipulable variable (e.g., a behavioral factor) and an outcome (e.g., a behavioral or biomedical factor).

Observational research can establish covariation between a behavioral factor and an outcome, but it has a limited ability to rule out confounding factors that could account for this covariation. Randomized designs provide a more powerful test of cause and effect by hypothesizing that change in one factor (e.g., the behavioral factor) will produce change in an outcome (e.g., a behavioral or biomedical factor). The design of these randomized experiments maximizes change in the treated arm, minimizes change in the comparator arm, and determines change on the outcome. Because these designs must maximize change in the treated arm, established treatments with known benefit on behavior are often used. The focus is not on the dimensions of the behavioral treatment but rather on the causal effects of a change in behavior. The comparator arm is chosen to minimize any change on the behavioral factor and thus maximize the ability to test the causal hypothesis.

An example of a randomized experiment was conducted by Sloan and colleagues [22]. Epidemiological studies have shown that anger and hostility predict cardiovascular disease, and laboratory studies have shown covariation between anger/hostility and autonomic dysfunction. Thus, autonomic dysfunction might be one of the mechanisms by which anger and hostility promote cardiovascular disease. The investigators randomized 158 adults, all of whom were elevated on anger and hostility, to an established cognitive behavioral therapy program for hostility reduction, or to a wait-list, and evaluated the effect on cardiac autonomic modulation. Although the results showed that the treatment was successful in reducing anger and hostility, and the wait-list controls did not change, autonomic modulation did not improve. The authors concluded that one of the possible explanations for this finding is that autonomic dysfunction is not a pathophysiological mechanism in the anger/hostility-cardiovascular disease pathway.

Investigate Intervention. The main purpose of an *intervention-oriented* trial is to answer a question about the intervention itself. These questions are commonly asked during the course of developing the intervention. They include questions about whether or not specific components of a multi-component intervention are active and questions about the optimum mode, dose, and duration of delivery of the intervention. *(See Chapter 3: Behavioral Treatment Development, Phase Ib.)* In these designs, the comparator tends to be self-evident, including various combinations of treatment components, alternative modes of delivery, dose, and duration, and comparators that control for alternative explanations for treatment efficacy such as non-specific attention.

Improve Outcomes. The main purpose of an *outcome-oriented* trial is to determine whether the intervention produces better outcomes than can be obtained through an alternative approach. This alternative is often the status quo. For example, a trial might be conducted to determine whether adding a behavioral adherence intervention to usual medical care for a particular chronic condition yields better medical outcomes than usual care alone. Similar to experiments, the focus is on the outcome. But unlike experiments, the test is whether or not the treatment can enhance outcomes over that which currently exists.

The Women's Health Initiative hormone trial is one of the best-known examples of an outcome-oriented trial. Decades of observational evidence had suggested that healthy postmenopausal women would be protected from the development of coronary disease by taking a combination of estrogen plus progestin. This hypothesis was tested by randomizing postmenopausal women to hormone therapy or placebo. Results of the trial showed that the risks of this hormone combination substantially exceeded the benefits. The increased risks of cardiovascular events and invasive breast cancer were so significant, in fact, that the trial was stopped by the Data and Safety Monitoring Board [23]. The randomized design made it possible to show that estrogen plus progestin therapy did not reduce coronary disease and should not be used for this purpose. The apparent benefits in observational studies were more likely due to confounding factors such as the younger age and higher socioeconomic status in women who opted to take this therapy on their own [23]. The placebo comparator created a double-blind design, thus minimizing any placebo effects and creating a formidable benchmark against which to compare the effects of hormone therapy.

Increase Utility. The main purpose of a *utility-oriented* trial is to determine whether it is possible to increase the reach, cost-effectiveness, or efficiency of an evidence-based intervention. For example, a trial might be conducted to determine whether an established behavioral intervention for individuals living with HIV can be effectively delivered by community health workers rather than by doctoral-level therapists.

The Diabetes Prevention Program community studies provide an excellent example of this type of study. A *Phase III* efficacy trial showed that this program exerted a powerful effect on preventing conversion of insulin resistance to incidence of diabetes [24]. This opened the door to implementation studies aimed at determining whether or not such a program could be delivered with similar efficacy in community settings, by lay people, or with reduced dose or duration [25–27].

Purpose of the Comparator

The Comparator Grid's rows differentiate between two different purposes of comparators.

Control.   One of the functions of a comparator in a randomized controlled trial is to make it possible to determine *why* a treatment works by ruling out an assortment of rival explanations for the apparent effects. This is the comparator's *control* function. Possible rival explanations include the classic threats to internal validity [28, 29] as well as others, such as differential expectancies [30, 31]. Most of the comparators in behavioral trials rule out the classic threats to internal validity, but they differ in their ability to rule out other rival explanations. For example, a behavioral trial comparing an intensive behavioral intervention for anxiety to a no-treatment control runs the risk of differential expectations of benefit across the arms. If the trial shows a benefit for the anxiety treatment, it will be difficult to disentangle the active treatment from expectations about that treatment.

Compare.   A comparator can also have a *comparison* function. This is the case when a behavioral trial is conducted to determine whether a behavioral treatment differs from some other treatment option. The principal question in this type of trial is not about *why* the outcomes differ, but *whether* they differ. For example, a superiority trial might be conducted to determine whether a recently developed behavioral treatment produces better outcomes than an older, established behavioral treatment. It could establish superiority by comparing the new treatment to usual care, the standard of care, or enhanced care. It could also establish superiority by comparing the standard of care potentiated by a behavioral treatment to the standard of care alone. The comparator can also serve a control function, but it is not the dominant function.

In some trials, the comparison function (i.e., whether the groups differ) is more important than the control function (i.e., why the groups differ). This is often the case in *Phase III* efficacy trials. In other trials, the comparison function is relatively (or completely) unimportant, and the control function dominates. This is often the case in experiments in which participants are either exposed or not exposed to an experimental manipulation and the research question is about the causal effects of exposure.

SELECTED EXPERIENCE FROM A BEHAVIORAL TRIAL

Rural Behavioral Health: Methodology Over Meaning

Divergent frameworks for choosing comparators can have profound effects on behavioral intervention research. An excellent example of this has been presented by Brenes and colleagues [32, 33]. The problem these investigators were trying to solve was significant. They observed that generalized anxiety disorder is prevalent among older adults in rural settings, but outpatient treatment services for this condition are difficult to access or unavailable. Consequently, they aimed to conduct a trial to determine whether telephone-delivered cognitive behavior therapy (CBT) was effective at treating older adults with generalized anxiety disorder living in rural settings. They chose CBT because prior evidence provided support for its value as the nonpharmacological treatment of choice for this condition. Like pharmacotherapy, it was evidence-based. But unlike pharmacotherapy, it could be delivered via telephone and thus had the potential for wide reach in a rural setting.

The choice of the comparator for this trial was telephone-delivered nondirective supportive therapy (NST). The rationale was that NST is structurally equivalent [34] to CBT and thus the two interventions would be comparable with respect to outcome expectations and credibility [33]. The co-primary outcomes were anxiety severity and worry severity. They randomly assigned 141 older adults with generalized anxiety disorder to telephone-delivered CBT or to telephone-delivered NST. The results showed that there was significantly greater improvement in worry severity at 4 months in the CBT than in the NST group, but no difference in anxiety severity. Some of the secondary outcomes were also significantly better in the CBT than in the NST group. The authors concluded that telephone-delivered CBT was superior to telephone-delivered NST in reducing worry, other anxiety symptoms, and depressive symptoms [32].

Implicit Decision-Making

The implicit rule that the investigators followed in choosing a comparator was to that the groups should be similar in terms of structure, outcome expectations, and credibility. Structural aspects of psychotherapy interventions include a variety of characteristics such as the number and length of the sessions and the modality of delivery [34]. Although the investigators did not explain why they held this implicit rule, it suggests that they were placing priority on internal validity, stringency, and formidability over other considerations.

The *implicit* decision-making rule for the comparator in this trial may have been used in the absence of any *explicit* rules or regulations for them to follow. Implicit, in this context, does not mean private or idiosyncratic. The fact that the trial was funded by a grant from the National Institute of Mental Health and published in a high-impact journal (*JAMA Psychiatry*) suggests that multiple reviewers probably held beliefs about comparator choices that resembled those of the investigators. In other words, the implicit rules that guided the investigators' comparator choice were compatible with, and probably influenced by, the cultural expectations of their research community.

Purpose-Guided Decision-Making

Despite the popularity and appeal of the implicit rules that appear to have guided the design of this trial, some of the other decision-making frameworks might have led the investigators to choose a different comparator. A purpose-guided perspective would encourage the choice of a comparator that best fit the primary purpose of the trial. The problem that the investigators set out to address was that there is a limited access to outpatient treatment services in rural areas and they hypothesized that telephone-delivered CBT might be a good way to overcome these access barriers and improve clinical outcomes. Thus, the primary purpose of their trial was to improve outcomes by improving access.

Unfortunately, the comparator that they chose had nothing whatsoever to do with the primary purpose of the trial. Neither face-to-face nor telephone-delivered NST are evidence-based treatments for generalized anxiety disorder. Thus, NST was a clinically irrelevant comparator. Furthermore, the question of whether telephone-delivered CBT is a viable solution to the problem of inadequate mental health care for rural participants cannot be answered by comparing two different telephone-delivered therapies.

Several different alternatives for a comparator might have emerged from the Purpose-Guided Comparator Choice framework. One would be to compare telephone-delivered CBT to face-to-face CBT at the urban clinics or academic medical centers where it is usually provided. This would be a difficult trial to conduct since the participants in the face-to-face arm would have to travel considerable distances for their weekly treatment sessions, running the risk of low adherence. Nevertheless, non-adherence to the status quo is part of the problem to be solved. A properly designed comparison of telephone-delivered vs. face-to-face CBT in the settings where it is currently available would have addressed the question of whether a more accessible, but possibly less powerful, treatment delivery modality improves outcomes over a less accessible, but possibly more powerful, alternative.

A second alternative for a comparator would be to compare telephone-delivered CBT to face-to-face CBT provided at more convenient rural locations. This would also be a difficult trial to conduct as the investigators would have to rent suitable spaces in multiple rural locations and send trained therapists out to these locations to conduct the face-to-face treatment sessions. If such a trial showed that face-to-face was superior to the telephone, the benefit compared to the increased cost would be a reasonable additional evaluation.

As difficult as either of these two trials might have been to conduct, both would have answered a potentially important question about telephone-delivered CBT for rural patients, i.e., how its outcomes compare to those of face-to-face CBT. Moreover, both of these comparators could have been designed to be structurally similar to telephone-delivered CBT, at least in most respects.

However, a purpose-guided framework would have led the investigators to a third alternative, which would be to compare telephone-delivered CBT to usual care for patients with generalized anxiety disorder living in rural settings. Given the problem the investigators wanted to address, this would probably be the best choice. It would have enabled the investigators to determine whether telephone-delivered CBT is superior to the meager care for generalized anxiety disorder that these participants would otherwise receive in the real world of rural mental health care.

The limitations of a usual care comparator are that it would not answer the question of whether telephone-delivered CBT is as effective as face-to-face CBT. Moreover, this comparator would be structurally dissimilar to telephone-delivered CBT, it may lack credibility as an intervention for generalized anxiety disorder, and it may run the risk of differential outcome expectations. It would also be the least formidable of all of the possibilities, thus maximizing the expected effect size. Purpose-guided decision-making suggests that these drawbacks are acceptable prices to pay for choosing a comparator that fits the primary purpose of the trial.

The use of telephone-delivered NST did not serve the primary purpose of the trial. It is easy to understand why this choice was made. It is difficult to design and implement a face-to-face comparator, and a usual care comparator has shortcomings in controlling for threats to internal validity. Although the choice of the comparator was well rationalized and the trial was well designed and conducted, it had limited applicability. When clinical administrators and policy-makers consider whether telephone-delivered CBT would be a suitable solution to the inadequate care that rural participants usually receive for generalized anxiety disorder, the results of this trial will not give them answers.

The Purpose-Guided Trial Design Comparator Grid (Table 6.3) could have helped clarify the primary question of interest and the optimum comparator. The investigators could consider the primary purpose of their trial in terms of: (1) investigating an intervention (i.e., telephone-delivered CBT); (2) improving outcomes (i.e., improving anxiety outcomes for elderly participants in rural areas); or (3) improving the utility of an established intervention. In their framing of the problem, they were less interested in learning something new about CBT and more interested in improving anxiety outcomes. By linking this problem to the purpose of the trial, they would have determined that their primary purpose was to improve outcomes.

If the aim is to improve outcomes, it is necessary to ask, *Compared to what?* The answer to this question is whether or not the intervention is superior to a clinically relevant alternative. This is only possible if the comparator actually *is* a clinically relevant alternative. They would have identified *comparison* as the primary purpose of the comparator and chosen one that was as clinically relevant as possible, which in this case would have been usual care. Identification of the primary purpose of the trial and its optimum comparator would lead the investigators to the **Intended** box below.

Table 6.3 **Application of Purpose-Guided Trial Design comparator grid to Brenes et al. [32, 33]**

Primary Purpose of the Comparator	Primary Purpose of Behavioral Trial			
	Conduct Experiment	Investigate Intervention	Improve Outcomes	Increase Utility
Control		Actual		
Comparison			Intended	

What actually happened is that their choice of a comparator *determined* the primary purpose of the trial. The implicit rules which the investigators seemed to have followed led them to decide that the appropriate comparator was a *control*. In making this choice, the purpose of the trial shifted to an investigation of the intervention, and the control aimed to rule out rival explanations for any apparent effects of CBT. This turned the trial into an investigation of the mechanisms of action of CBT rather than the original purpose which was to improve outcomes. On the grid, it moved the trial from the **Intended** box to the **Actual** box.

Phase-Guided Decision-Making

Phase-guided decision-making would also have pointed to a usual care comparator. This is not because of its clinical relevance, and not in spite of its low formidability, but instead *because* of its low formidability. Since this was the first trial to ask whether telephone-delivered CBT could be helpful for rural participants with general anxiety disorder, a non-formidable comparator would have minimized the risk of making the Type II error of failing to find a benefit that is truly there.

No single trial can answer every question that might be asked about an intervention. Both the Pragmatic and Phase-Guided frameworks advocate for placement of the trial within an appropriate developmental framework. This is consistent with progressive translational research and is an alternative to expecting any one trial to carry more weight than it can bear. A phase-guided framework might suggest, for example, conducting an initial trial of telephone-delivered CBT with a usual care comparator and then conducting a comparative effectiveness trial with a more formidable alternative such as a collaborative care intervention. If these studies demonstrated that the intervention was efficacious, one of the next questions to address would be whether even better outcomes could be achieved by refining the intervention. If the refinements do not make much difference, then the investigators might ask whether outcomes that are as good, or nearly as good, as those of telephone-delivered CBT could be achieved by less expensive interventionists. Each of these studies progresses from the one before it. Each would require different comparators to achieve the evolution of their purposes.

RECOMMENDATIONS

Stalking the Elusive Dodo Bird

The actual dodo bird (*Raphus cucullatus*) has been extinct since 1662. But the behavioral dodo bird is alive and well. Persistent demands to control for common factors reflect persistent concerns that even our best interventions may not be much better than non-specific therapies.

It is clear that common factors are both therapeutic and an integral part of most behavioral interventions, particularly those delivered by human therapists. For the past several decades, these common factors have proven to be fairly hard to surpass, despite many efforts to develop better interventions. However, that does not mean that common factors are satisfactory answers to difficult behavioral and psychosocial problems. Non-specific interventions that offer nothing more than common factors do not yield very high remission rates in conditions such as major depression or post-traumatic stress disorder or very high success rates for sustained improvement in maladaptive lifestyle behaviors such as smoking or physical inactivity. Indeed, even the most efficacious, evidence-based interventions that do better than non-specific comparators leave many participants behind. While some participants derive great benefits, others have an incomplete response, and some do not respond at all.

An endless cycle of repeatedly showing that behavioral interventions are only modestly better than non-specific common factors is impeding progress. Non-specific factors will always play an important role in behavioral interventions. But controlling for them is not where every effort should be directed. The overarching goal of behavioral intervention research should be to progress to significantly better outcomes in the future than were possible in the past. Non-specific factors will play a proportionately smaller role in highly effective interventions than they do in the current generation of modestly effective ones. Efforts should be directed toward development of increasingly powerful behavioral interventions, progressively testing them, and choosing comparators that evolve with aims and do not kill them off prematurely.

No matter which comparator one chooses, and no matter how one arrives at the decision, a dodo bird will be watching. Progressing toward stronger behavioral interventions will make our dodo a bird we can live with instead of one we wish were extinct.

What Should Investigators Do in the Meantime?

The publication of models for comparator selection in health-related trials [12, 19] will help to quell some long-standing controversies. But it will not eliminate them altogether. What should investigators do when planning their trials, when even well-chosen and well-designed comparators may be criticized or rejected?

Several of the existing frameworks suggest that one size does *not* fit all when it comes to comparators and that it is necessary to think carefully about the rationale for choosing the comparator for any given trial. If there are several different contenders, the trial proposal or grant application should discuss the pros and cons of each and the reasons why the chosen comparator is the best one for the proposed trial, even if it is imperfect in some ways. Support for or against various choices can now be found in the OBSSR expert panel's report [19]; published framework papers, such as the ORBIT model [20]; and the emerging empirical literature on comparators.

It is better to consider and cite these sources, despite whatever shortcomings they may present, than it is to simply follow one's own implicit rules and hope for the best. This is essential because reviewers and applicants can hold different implicit rules. Making implicit rules explicit may facilitate a consideration of the rule, rather than simply a critique of the choice. Reviewers may or may not agree with whichever framework might have guided the applicant's choice. But this is the luck of the draw. Despite the controversies and preferences that surround the choice of comparators, a clear explication of the rationale for the investigator's choice can be extremely persuasive.

REFERENCES

1. Freedland KE, Mohr DC, Davidson KW, Schwartz JE (2011) Usual and unusual care: existing practice control groups in randomized controlled trials of behavioral interventions. Psychosom Med 73:323–335
2. Schwartz CE, Chesney MA, Irvine MJ, Keefe FJ (1997) The control group dilemma in clinical research: applications for psychosocial and behavioral medicine trials. Psychosom Med 59:362–371
3. Rifkin A (2007) Randomized controlled trials and psychotherapy research. Am J Psychiatry 164:7–8
4. Wampold BE, Minami T, Tierney SC, Baskin TW, Bhati KS (2005) The placebo is powerful: estimating placebo effects in medicine and psychotherapy from randomized clinical trials. J Clin Psychol 61:835–854
5. Rains JC, Penzien DB (2005) Behavioral research and the double-blind placebo-controlled methodology: challenges in applying the biomedical standard to behavioral headache research. Headache 45:479–486
6. Reber AS (1993) Implicit learning and tacit knowledge: an essay on the cognitive unconscious. Oxford University Press, New York
7. Food and Drug Administration (1998) Drug study designs. Guidance for Institutional Review Boards and Clinical Investigators. Food and Drug Administration, Rockville
8. Sterne JAC, Savovic J, Page MJ, Elbers RG, Blencowe NS, Boutron I, Cates CJ, Chen H-Y, Corbett MS, Eldridge SM, Emberson JR, Hernan MA, Hopewell S, Hrobjartsson A, Junqueira DR, Juni P, Kirkham JJ, Lasserson T, Li T, McAleenan A, Reeves BC, Shepperd S, Shrier I, Stewart LA, Tilling K, White IR, Whiting PF, Higgins JPT (2019) RoB2: a revised tool for assessing risk of bias in randomised trials. BMJ 366:14898. https://doi.org/10.1136/bmj.14898
9. Guyatt G, Oxman AD, Akl EA, Kunz R, Vist G, Brozek J, Norris S, Falck-Ytter Y, Glasziou P, DeBeer H, Jaeschke R, Rind D, Meerpohl J, Dahm P, Schunemann HJ (2011) GRADE guidelines: 1. Introduction-GRADE evidence profiles and summary of findings tables. J Clin Epidemiol 64:383–394
10. Mohr DC, Spring B, Freedland KE, Beckner V, Arean P, Hollon SD, Ockene J, Kaplan R (2009) The selection and design of control conditions for randomized controlled trials of psychological interventions. Psychother Psychosom 78:275–284
11. Bower JE (2016) Mindfulness interventions for cancer survivors: moving beyond wait-list control groups. J Clin Oncol 34:3366–3368
12. Freedland KE (2020) Purpose-guided trial design in health-related behavioral intervention research. Health Psych 39:539–548
13. Mohr DC, Ho J, Hart TL, Baron KG, Berendsen M, Beckner V, Cai X, Cuijpers P, Spring B, Kinsinger SW, Schroder KE, Duffecy J (2014) Control condition design and implementation features in controlled trials: a meta-analysis of trials evaluating psychotherapy for depression. Transl Behav Med 4:407–423
14. American Psychological Association (1958) Research in psychotherapy. American Psychological Association, Washington DC
15. Rosenzweig S (1936) Some implicit common factors in diverse methods in psychotherapy. Am J Orthopsychiatry 6:412–415
16. Wampold BE, Mondin GW, Moody M, Stich F, Benson K, Ahn H-n (1997) A meta-analysis of outcome studies comparing bona fide psychotherapies: Empirically, "all must have prizes." Psychol Bull 122:203–215
17. Johnston BC, Kanters S, Bandayrel K, Wu P, Naji F, Siemieniuk RA, Ball GD, Busse JW, Thorlund K, Guyatt G, Jansen JP, Mills EJ (2014) Comparison of weight loss among named diet programs in overweight and obese adults: a meta-analysis. JAMA 312:923–933

18. Huhn M, Tardy M, Spineli LM, Kissling W, Forstl H, Pitschel-Walz G, Leucht C, Samara M, Dold M, Davis JM, Leucht S (2014) Efficacy of pharmacotherapy and psychotherapy for adult psychiatric disorders: a systematic overview of meta-analyses. JAMA Psychiat 71:706–715

19. Freedland KE, King AC, Ambrosius WT, Mayo-Wilson E, Mohr DC, Czajkowski SM, Thabane L, Collins LM, Rebok GW, Treweek SP, Cook TD, Edinger JD, Stoney CM, Campo RA, Young-Hyman D, Riley WT (2019) The selection of comparators for randomized controlled trials of health-related behavioral interventions: recommendatins of an NIH expert panel. J Clin Epidemiol 110:74–81

20. Czajkowski SM, Powell LH, Adler N, Naar-King S, Reynolds KD, Hunter CM, Laraia B, Olster DH, Perna FM, Peterson JC, Epel E, Boyington JE, Charlson ME (2015) From ideas to efficacy: the ORBIT model for developing behavioral treatments for chronic diseases. Health Psychol 34:971–982

21. Thabane L, Thomas T, Ye C, Paul J (2009) Posing the research question: not so simple. Can J Anaesth 56:71–79

22. Sloan RP, Shapiro PA, Gorenstein EE, Tager FA, Monk CE, McKinley PS, Myers MM, Bagiella E, Chen I, Steinman R, Bigger JT Jr (2010) Cardiac autonomic control and treatment of hostility: a randomized controlled trial. Psychosom Med 72:1–8

23. Manson JE, Hsia J, Johnson KC, Rossouw JE, Assaf AR, Lasser NL, Trevisan M, Black HR, Heckbert SR, Detrano R, Strickland OL, Wong ND, Crouse JR, Stein E, Cushman M, for the Women's Health Initiative Investigators (2003) Estrogen plus progestin and the risk of coronary heart disease. N Engl J Med 349:523–534

24. Knowler WC, Barrett-Connor E, Fowler SE, Hamman RF, Lachin JM, Walker EA, Nathan DM, Diabetes Prevention Program Research Group (2002) Reduction in the incidence of type 2 diabetes with lifestyle intervention or metformin. N Engl J Med 346:393–403

25. Aziz Z, Absetz P, Oldroyd J, Pronk NP, Oldenburg B (2015) A systematic review of real-world diabetes prevention programs: learnings from the last 15 years. Implement Sci 10:172. https://doi.org/10.1186/s13012-015-0354-6

26. Mudaliar U, Zabetian A, Goodman M, Echouffo-Tcheugui JB, Albright AL, Gregg EW, Ali MK (2016) Cardiometabolic risk factor changes observed in diabetes prevention programs in US settings: a systematic review and meta-analysis. PLoS Med 13:e1002095. https://doi.org/10.1371/journal.pmed.1002095

27. Haw JS, Galaviz K, Straus AN, Kowalski AJ, Magee MJ, Weber MB, Wei J, Narayan KMV, Ali MK (2017) Long-term sustainability of diabetes prevention approaches: a systematic review and meta-analysis of randomized clinical trials. JAMA Intern Med 177:1808–1817

28. Shadish WR, Cook TD, Campbell DT (2001) Experimental and quasi-experimental designs for generalized causal inference. Houghton Mifflin, Boston

29. Campbell DT, Stanley JC (1966) Experimental and quasi-experimental designs for research. Houghton Mifflin, Boston

30. Wilkins W (1973) Expectancy of therapeutic gain: an empirical and conceptual critique. J Consult Clin Psychol 40:69–77

31. Rutherford BR, Wager TD, Roose SP (2010) Expectancy and the treatment of depression: a review of experimental methodology and effects on patient outcome. Curr Psychiatr Rev 6:1–10

32. Brenes GA, Danhauer SC, Lyles MF, Hogan PE, Miller ME (2015) Telephone-delivered cognitive behavioral therapy and telephone-delivered nondirective supportive therapy for rural older adults with generalized anxiety disorder: a randomized clinical trial. JAMA Psychiat 72:1012–1020

33. Brenes GA, Danhauer SC, Lyles MF, Miller ME (2014) Telephone-delivered psychotherapy for rural-dwelling older adults with generalized anxiety disorder: study protocol of a randomized controlled trial. BMC Psychiatry. https://doi.org/10.1186/1471-244X-14-34

34. Baskin TW, Tierney SC, Minami T, Wampold BE (2003) Establishing specificity in psychotherapy: a meta-analysis of structural equivalence of placebo controls. J Consult Clin Psychol 71:973–979

Chapter 7
Feasibility and Pilot Studies

"It usually takes me two or three days to prepare for an impromptu speech"
Mark Twain

> ### *Fundamental Point*
>
> *Scientists usually collect data to discover new phenomena or to test hypotheses, predictions, or causal models with the goal of producing generalizable findings. Feasibility and pilot data have very different purposes. Scientists conduct them to pave the way for a proposed or planned project and to reassure themselves, other scientists, and funding agencies that it is possible to conduct the trial as planned.*

This chapter defines feasibility and pilot studies according to the 2010 CONSORT guidelines. Feasibility studies are always linked to a planned clinical trial. Pilot studies are a subset of feasibility studies that use an identical randomized design as the planned clinical trial but are conducted to answer questions about the feasibility of a protocol. Pilot studies are distinct from miniature efficacy trials. Although both are conducted on a small number of participants and use a randomized design, pilot studies focus on feasibility, but miniature efficacy trials claim to provide estimates of efficacy. The evolving literature on behavioral trial methodology has shown a variety of problems that result from estimating efficacy with underpowered miniature efficacy trials. Recommendations are to prepare for a definitive behavioral clinical trial by making a strong case for its credibility, plausibility, and feasibility and by estimating effect sizes using targets needed to achieve clinically significant benefit. The popular practice of conducting miniature efficacy trials which are loosely linked to a planned behavioral trial, calling them pilot studies, drawing conclusions about potential efficacy, and using results to estimate sample size should be discontinued.

© Springer Nature Switzerland AG 2021
L. H. Powell et al., *Behavioral Clinical Trials for Chronic Diseases*,
https://doi.org/10.1007/978-3-030-39330-4_7

SCIENTIFIC PRINCIPLES

Terminology

When a study is called a randomized controlled trial (RCT), there are general expectations. Participants will be randomly assigned to one condition or another, outcomes will be assessed, and the resulting data will be analyzed to determine whether the different conditions produce different results on the outcomes. Although the structure tends to be the same, there are many kinds of randomized controlled trials conducted for many different reasons.

When a study is called *feasibility*, *pilot*, or *preliminary*, it may have little in common with an RCT. Thus, it is not necessarily clear what to expect. Fortunately, consensus definitions for the first two terms have been provided in an extension to the Consolidated Standards of Reporting Trials (CONSORT) guidelines that addresses the purpose, structure, and reporting of feasibility and pilot studies [1].

The guidelines define a feasibility study as one that asks whether a proposed or planned RCT "can be done, should be done, and if so, how." A feasibility study may or may not resemble the future trial. For example, an investigator might convene a focus group of clinicians to find out whether or not they would be willing to refer potentially eligible patients to a study coordinator to assess their interest in participating in a trial. A focus group does not resemble a clinical trial in any way. Yet it might help to address a question about the feasibility of a recruitment approach for a planned clinical trial.

According to the guidelines, a pilot study is a special type of feasibility study. It also asks questions about feasibility, but it has a special design feature: it is a smaller version of the future definitive RCT. So, for example, if the planned RCT has three arms, the pilot study would have the same three arms. But the pilot study would have far fewer participants than the planned definitive trial. Thus, unlike other kinds of feasibility studies, pilot studies and the planned RCT to which it is linked have identical designs (Fig. 7.1).

These definitions help to clarify three long-standing points of confusion about feasibility and pilot studies:

1. Feasibility and pilot studies are not stand-alone endeavors. They must be explicitly tied to a proposed or planned RCT or at least to a concrete plan to propose an RCT. It is not sufficient to link a feasibility or pilot study to a vague call for future research. It should be designed to answer a specific question about the feasibility of a specific planned trial.

2. Pilot studies are a type of feasibility study. Whereas a feasibility study can use a variety of quantitative and qualitative designs, a pilot study is

designed as a smaller version of a planned or proposed RCT. If a study is not a smaller version of a planned RCT, it is not a pilot study. If a study is a smaller version of a planned RCT, but it is not aimed at determining feasibility, it is not a pilot study.

3. If this restricted definition of pilot studies is widely adopted, many studies that might have been called pilot studies in the past will have be called something else in the future. There are hundreds, if not thousands, of "pilot trials" or "pilot studies" published in recent decades that have *not* been designed to evaluate the feasibility of a planned or proposed RCT. The publication of the CONSORT extension pushes for an increase in conceptual precision and a decrease in confusion by calling these studies something other than pilots.

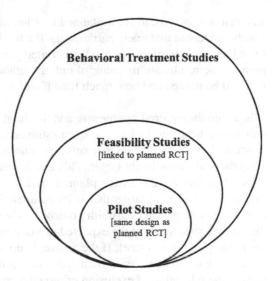

Fig. 7.1 Relationship among behavioral treatment studies using CONSORT guidelines

What Is Feasibility?

The feasibility of a trial refers to whether or not it can be successfully conducted. It does not refer to whether its outcomes are going to support the investigator's hopes or hypotheses. Many different questions about the feasibility of a planned or proposed trial can be raised, including questions about recruitment, processes, resources, management, and treatments [2]. All of these could be evaluated in one or more feasibility studies.

Recruitment
The ability to recruit adequate numbers of participants is one of the most important keys to the successful conduct of a clinical trial. Conversely, inability to enroll adequate numbers of participants is one of the most common reasons for the early termination of a clinical trial [3]. Consequently, recruitment rates are one of the most common foci of feasibility studies.

Recruitment provides a good example of why a feasibility study should be tied to a specific, planned, or proposed trial. It is necessary to have an estimate of the sample size that will be needed for a planned trial before one can determine whether it is feasible to recruit that many participants. If a feasibility study is conducted to determine how many participants can be recruited per unit of time (e.g., per week or per month), the results are meaningful only in relation to the numbers of participants that will be needed and how much time it will take to recruit them.

When both the required sample size and the duration of the recruitment phase for an anticipated behavioral trial have been estimated, then a feasibility study might be conducted to determine whether sufficient numbers of participants are available to meet the trial's enrollment target. This implies that (1) the feasibility study has the same eligibility criteria as the planned trial; (2) the feasibility study's objectives include an enrollment target that is based upon the expected needs of the planned trial; and (3) the primary feasibility outcome is binary (i.e., *Yes*, we are able to enroll the needed participants at the expected rate or higher, or *No*, we are unable to enroll the participants at that rate). If the answer is no, the feasibility study data can help the investigator to take corrective action, such as the identification of new recruiting sites or the relaxation of exclusion criteria that are causing too many otherwise eligible candidates to be ineligible. If either or both of these options are not possible, the question then becomes whether the behavioral trial will be feasible.

Trial Processes and Procedures
Beyond recruitment, the processes that are involved in a behavioral trial include assessment, treatment, and retention. Any processes that are necessary, but that cannot be implemented, can prevent a behavioral trial from being successfully conducted. For example, the plan for a trial involving medical patients might include assessment using a 6-minute walk test immediately before discharge. This assessment procedure might not be feasible if patients face too many competing demands when they are being discharged. The feasibility target would depend on the percentage of missing test data that would be acceptable in the trial. If that target were determined to be, for instance, <10%, the feasibility criterion would be ≥90% of participants completed walk tests before discharge. If a feasibility study were then conducted on 20 patients and only 12 (60%) of them completed the walk tests, the feasibility of this procedure would be called into question. The investigators either would have to find ways to improve upon this percentage, relax the criterion and assess the 6-minute walk either before or after discharge, or redesign the trial.

Resources
Resource constraints can make it difficult to conduct a behavioral trial. For example, the trial may require access to a specialized piece of equipment, such as a heavily used magnetic resonance imaging scanner. A feasibility study could be conducted, for example, to determine the percentage of participants who can be scheduled for their scans within one week of their target evaluation date.

Trial Management

The staff of a behavioral trial must be able to coordinate their efforts with each other and with service providers upon whom they depend. For example, the staff of a technology-intensive trial may need direct and timely access to technical support services for specialized software or devices. A feasibility study could be conducted to evaluate the team's access to support services and the ability of the service providers to resolve critical problems.

Interventions and Comparators

Many questions about the feasibility of interventions and comparators can arise when planning a behavioral trial. Treatment fidelity is a key question involving whether the interventionists are able to deliver the interventions as specified in the protocol and whether the participants will understand, accept, and implement actions required in the protocol. Another key question is dropout rates. Differential dropout is especially problematic because it adversely affects the equality created by the randomization. A feasibility study might be conducted to determine the percentages of participants who drop out of the intervention and comparator arms. If there are too many dropouts overall, the trial may not be feasible. If differential dropouts occur, the investigator could conduct qualitative studies to identify reasons for dropouts and refine the protocol to prevent this from occurring in the planned trial. Fortunately, similar levels of attrition have been observed in intervention and comparator arms in most trials [4, 5]. But this is not a guarantee that differential attrition will not happen in a proposed study with unique participants within unique contexts.

Inferences Based on Feasibility Data

Because feasibility studies concern a planned or proposed trial, inferences based on feasibility data are generalizable primarily to the conduct of that particular trial. This has two important implications:

First, the results of a feasibility study can rarely be generalized to anything *other* than that trial. Many feasibility studies are irrelevant to other investigators in other settings, even if they are planning to conduct similar trials. For example, a finding that one's own research team can recruit ample numbers of eligible cancer participants at the medical center with which they are affiliated suggests that they will be able to meet their recruitment targets for a planned behavioral trial. It does not imply that other research teams at other cancer centers will be able to do just as well, even if using the same recruitment approach. They will probably have to find out for themselves, in their own feasibility studies.

This is one of the reasons it is often difficult to publish feasibility studies. The main target audiences for the feasibility findings are the study section, the institutional review board, and the investigators themselves. When reviewers read a report of a feasibility study, they tend to ask why anyone other than those entities should be interested in the results. If the report includes some generalizable lessons learned, some creative or novel solution to a common feasibility problem, or preparatory work for a major, high-visibility multi-site trial, other researchers may have something to gain from reading it. But in general, the feasibility of a planned or proposed trial is of little interest to others, and the prospects for publication are quite uncertain. The main motive for conducting a feasibility study should be to pave the way for a planned behavioral trial. If anyone else is interested in the findings and the results do get published, this is icing on the cake.

The second implication of the pairing of feasibility studies with specific trials is that the main findings should be reported in the form of descriptive, rather than inferential, statistics. A foundation of any basic statistics course is that statistical tests enable us to use data from a limited sample of a population to make inferences about the entire population. Feasibility studies pertain to the work of particular investigators or research teams within particular settings. Extrapolation of feasibility findings to larger populations (i.e., to other investigators, settings, or participants) is not the goal. Thus, if a statistical test is applied to the enrollment data from a feasibility study and the result is $p < 0.05$, that is not very informative. In contrast, a simple descriptive finding that the recruitment rate was 40% *is* informative, especially if a feasibility target rate of $\geq 30\%$ was established in advance.

The Fallibility of Feasibility

Feasibility data promote confidence but not certainty. Even if the results of a feasibility study are encouraging, there is no guarantee that a planned behavioral trial will turn out to be feasible. For example, if the recruitment target is to enroll $\geq 30\%$ of screened participants, 50 are screened in a feasibility study, and 20 (40%) agree to participate, investigators will be reassured. But this is not a guarantee that 40% of screened participants will agree to be enrolled in the subsequent trial. The 40% rate might be excessively optimistic if, for example, the recruiter targeted the most accessible, cooperative, and enthusiastic participants. It is not uncommon for participants who are accessible, eligible, and enthusiastic about volunteering for research grow scarce over the course of a lengthy recruitment phase.

This is one of the reasons that some experts recommend calculating confidence intervals around feasibility data [2]. Unlike inferential statistical tests and *p*-values, confidence intervals can help to convey the uncertainty that surrounds the feasibility findings. For example, if the point estimate of the recruitment rate from a feasibility study is 40%, but the confidence interval ranges from 25% to 55%, this would serve as a warning that the actual recruitment rate in the planned behavioral trial could turn out to be well below 40%. If the recruitment rate turns out to be as low as 25%, the investigator would have to consider whether the trial is truly feasible or would have to develop a backup plan that can rely upon new recruiting sites in the event of such a turn of events.

There is a more basic reason that feasibility studies often reveal less about a planned behavioral trial than desired. This more basic reason is that some important feasibility questions will inevitably remain unasked and unanswered. Feasibility studies are typically funded by small grants and are thus limited in the questions that can be asked. But they are designed to lay the groundwork for much larger grants where a number of feasibility issues arise. If, for example, an early career investigator wins a $5000 grant from his or her own institution to evaluate the feasibility of a planned behavioral trial that will require hundreds of thousands of dollars per year, all of the important questions about recruitment rates, intervention fidelity, quality of assessment, and quality of data transmittal cannot be answered.

Therefore, to some extent one is always gambling on feasibility when embarking on a behavioral trial. It is the exception, rather than the norm, that a behavioral trial will run smoothly. Seasoned trialists learn to expect the unexpected and are usually not surprised when their behavioral trial requires ongoing troubleshooting. Moreover, they often have the advantage of being able to use their past experience in trials to encourage confidence in the feasibility of the next trial, thereby obviating at least some of the need for separate feasibility studies. Early career investigators seldom have this track record. Thus, it is a great advantage to be attuned to the feasibility questions that are likely to arise when their behavioral trial proposals are reviewed. Even more importantly, it is a great advantage for a new investigator to work as a member of a research network, research center, or institute. By so doing, they can use the experience of seasoned investigators to support the feasibility of their own trial.

The Purposes of Pilot Studies

A pilot study is a feasibility study with the special design feature of being a smaller version of a planned or proposed behavioral trial. In most cases this means that a pilot study will have a randomized design. Many feasibility questions can be, and have been, addressed in studies that do not fit this description. For instance, structured queries of electronic medical record systems are often used to estimate the numbers of potentially eligible participants. It is not necessary to conduct a small randomized pilot study to obtain this information.

Randomized pilot studies can provide certain types of feasibility data that cannot be obtained from other kinds of feasibility studies. For example, some potential participants may be willing to participate in a trial investigating a particular treatment but be unwilling to be randomized to a comparator condition in which they will not receive that treatment. Other potential participants may agree to randomization and play the odds that they will receive their desired treatment. If they lose, they may respond by being non-adherent to the protocol or dropping out of the trial completely. Randomized pilot studies can yield important insights into the impact of randomization on recruitment and dropout rates that could not be obtained from feasibility studies not using a randomized design.

Summary

In summary, there are a number of questions that are important in assessing the feasibility of a planned behavioral clinical trial. The need for answers to these questions provides the justification for feasibility and pilot studies. The most common questions and the optimum way to answer them are summarized in Table 7.1.

Table 7.1 Key feasibility questions and the optimum source for answering them

Source	Feasibility questions
Feasibility study	– Duration of recruitment period needed to recruit the desired number of participants
	– Number of recruitment sites needed
	– Accuracy of electronic medical record algorithms in identifying prospective participants
	– Percent of eligible prospective participants who agree to participate
	– Accuracy of data transmittal
	– Volume of participants who can be assessed by a high-usage piece of equipment per unit of time
	– Level of interest, support, and referrals from medical providers
Randomized pilot study	– Acceptability of random assignment
	– Estimate of differential dropout by arm
	– Estimate of variability in response to the primary outcome
	– Estimate of refusal rate
	– Ability to implement treatment according to protocol
	– Ability to implement comparator according to protocol
	– Participant preferences for specific treatment arm
	– Participant satisfaction with trial protocol
	– Participant satisfaction with treatment protocol
From the literature	– Estimate of expected effect size
	– Clinically significant target for improvement from the treatment

CHALLENGES FOR BEHAVIORAL TRIALS

Miniature Efficacy Trials

For many years, behavioral trialists have assumed that pilot studies were miniature efficacy trials (also called Preliminary Efficacy Trials (PETS)), not merely feasibility studies. These trials aimed to test efficacy hypotheses but on a smaller scale than a full-fledged *Phase II* or *Phase III* behavioral efficacy trial. It was also widely assumed that it was acceptable for these miniature efficacy trials to be less rigorous than full-fledged trials. For example, although rigorous behavioral trials typically include procedures for assessing treatment fidelity [6], many miniature efficacy trials were conducted without them.

Miniature efficacy trials were meant to serve several purposes:

- They were intended to find signals of efficacy in studies that were less expensive and time-consuming than full-fledged trials. Such a signal was interpreted as a sign that a full-fledged trial was warranted.

- They were included in the preliminary research sections of grant proposals to reassure reviewers that the intervention had a high probability of being efficacious and that the full-fledged behavioral trial now being proposed was therefore likely to produce positive results.

- They produced a between-group effect size that could be used as the estimate for the effect size in the sample size calculations for the planned behavioral trial proposal.

- They could make the case in a publication that they provided "preliminary evidence of efficacy" and that further research was needed.

All of this made perfectly good sense, or so we thought. Unfortunately, these ideas are misguided.

A Wake-Up Call

In 2006, a landmark paper was published by Kraemer and colleagues [7] raising concerns about the use of pilot studies to estimate effect sizes. They argued that this practice results both in the premature abandonment of promising treatments and in the testing of treatments that are underpowered to find hypothesized effects. While the details of their statistical reasoning are beyond the scope of this chapter, they demonstrated clearly that the standard errors of effect sizes estimated from miniature efficacy trials are extremely imprecise, tending to under- or overestimate true effect sizes. When these imprecise effect sizes turn out to be small, they discourage investigators from submitting grant proposals for larger trials. When they turn out to be large, they run the risk of inflating the actual effect size and, when used to estimate power in a planned behavioral trial, result in many trials that are underpowered and produce null results.[1]

Even if small pilot studies could produce highly precise effect size estimates, they would be estimating the *wrong* effect. The effect size that *should* be used in sample size calculations for a definitive behavioral trial is what Kraemer et al. call the *threshold of clinical significance*. This is the smallest effect that has the potential to affect clinical decision-making, health service policies, or participant preferences. The identification of the threshold of clinical significance for a given trial requires a judgment call that is based on multiple considerations [7, 8]. Pilot trials rarely yield much, if any, of the information needed to form this judgment. (*See Chapter 5: Clinical Significance.*)

Consider a hypothetical example in which a research team has developed a caregiver stress intervention for the partners of cancer patients. They conduct a small study and find that the intervention and control groups differ after treatment by an average of 3 points on a well-established measure of caregiver stress. This finding is not informative with respect to whether 3 points is a clinically meaningful difference on this measure. That sort of information typically must be found elsewhere, such as in observational, epidemiological, or clinical studies, and it may point to a very different value than the one that happened to emerge from the study.

Suppose that previous epidemiological studies showed that caregivers do not feel or function any better when their stress scores improve by only 3 points, but improvement of ≥6 points is enough to have a meaningful impact on a caregiver health and quality of life. These findings could be used to define the threshold of clinical significance as ≥6 points on the stress scale. If the investigator used the pilot study effect size of 3 instead of the threshold of clinical significance of ≥6 to determine the sample size for the definitive RCT, many more subjects would have to be enrolled because it takes a larger sample to detect a 3-point than a 6-point difference. However, the larger sample would be hard to justify because a difference as small as 3 points would be unlikely to provide any benefit on stress and the quality of life of the caregivers.

Kraemer et al. framed their concept of the threshold of clinical significance within the context of a *Phase III* efficacy trial where results influence clinical decision-making, healthcare services, public health policies, etc. However, clinical significance is relevant for behavioral interventions at all phases of their development, well before they can have an immediate, transformative impact on clinical care. (*See Chapter 4: Hypothesized Pathway and Bias.*)

---

[1] Although small pilot studies yield imprecise effect size estimates, they can produce useful estimates of the variability of the outcome measure(s). Estimates based on pilot study sample sizes as small as 20 or 30 participants are often sufficiently stable for use in calculations of sample size needed for planning definitive behavioral trials.

False Reassurance

We now know that pilot studies that claim to provide "preliminary signals of efficacy" are actually miniature efficacy trials that produce misleading estimates of effect sizes, are uninformative about clinical benefit, and result in an over- or underestimate of the power to detect benefit in a planned definitive behavioral trial. However, there is also another reason why investigators should not seek "preliminary signals of efficacy" in pilot studies and reviewers should not ask for them. The principle of equipoise is the ethical foundation of the clinical trial enterprise [9]. Equipoise means that clinical trials should only be conducted if there is genuine uncertainty about the results they will produce. *(See Chapter 10: Equipoise and Blinding.)*

If the answer to a clinical question is a foregone conclusion, the trial should not be conducted. Investigators and reviewers should not seek anything like a tacit guarantee that a proposed trial will turn out to support a hypothesis and prove that the intervention is efficacious. Instead, the decision to go forward with a definitive behavioral trial should be based upon whether the research question is an important one, and whether the trial is well-designed and has a good chance of providing a conclusive answer to that question, regardless of whether the answer is positive or negative.

OVERCOMING THESE CHALLENGES IN A BEHAVIORAL TRIAL

Investigators and reviewers must be able to make informed decisions about whether a behavioral intervention is worth testing in a *Phase II* or *Phase III* behavioral clinical trial. If they shouldn't base these decisions on the results of underpowered miniature efficacy trials, what *should* they base them on? A good alternative is to inform these decisions using the criteria of *credibility*, *plausibility*, and *feasibility*.

Credibility

The Old French Market in New Orleans opened in 1791. Given its age, it may seem surprising that it is still one of the best places in town to purchase the latest in pain control technology, namely, magnetized bracelets. These attractive, high-tech devices are guaranteed to eliminate hand, wrist, and arm pain. Larger sizes are available for ankle and foot pain.

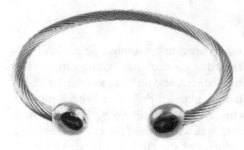

Despite the popularity and guaranteed benefits of these magical bracelets, few behavioral scientists would think it wise to apply for grant support to test their efficacy in an RCT, and few reviewers would respond favorably to such a proposal. Both the placebo effect [10] and the history of quackery, in which magnetic healing devices have played a prominent role [11], are too well known for that. In contrast, behavioral interventions that are grounded in the science of behavior change [12] and have been systematically developed and refined [13–15] are much more likely to be viewed as credible. However, perceived credibility is a necessary, but not sufficient, criterion to reassure reviewers that a behavioral intervention should be tested in a full-fledged behavioral efficacy trial.

Plausibility

Reviewers cannot rely upon effect sizes from miniature efficacy trials that determine the merit of conducting a full-fledged behavioral trial. What they can rely upon, however, is whether a positive outcome is *plausible*. Proof-of-concept studies are one of the best ways to support plausibility. In this context, *proof of concept* refers to evidence that an intervention *can* benefit a primary outcome. The essential elements of a proof-of-concept study are that attention is on the treatment and benefit is assessed using a predetermined, clinically significant target. The treatment can be tested in a small, unrepresentative, uncontrolled, quasi-experimental or time series design. The key question is whether or not, in this small, ideal situation, the treatment *can* achieve a clinically significant benefit. The focus is on whether; not why. The answer to the question of why a benefit might occur needs a randomized design. If the proof of concept achieves a clinically significant benefit, it is *plausible* that the treatment could produce a benefit using a more rigorous design and further investigation is warranted. If it does not achieve a clinically significant benefit, more refinement of the treatment is needed.

Consider, for example, a clinical population in which ≥80% adherence to a preventive medication regimen is necessary to prevent life-threatening exacerbations, but actual adherence averages only about 20%. A proof-of-concept study could clarify whether or not it is plausible that a treatment of interest could achieve ≥80% adherence. In a study of only ten participants who are given a new treatment, one result could be that none of the ten achieved clinically significant adherence. In this case, the treatment should be reconsidered. Another result could be that five of the ten achieved clinically significant adherence. In this case, it is plausible that the treatment could be beneficial. Another result could be that only two of the ten achieved clinically significant adherence. In this case, the treatment may need refinement to potentiate its effects, and possibly another proof-of-concept study before progressing to a planned trial. If potentially remediable reasons for non-response can be identified and built into the plan for the definitive behavioral trial, plausibility is increased, and progression to a planned trial without the second proof-of-concept study may be warranted. The value of this type of study is that it provides an easy, low-cost preliminary look. (*See Chapter 3: Behavioral Treatment Development.*)

A randomized pilot study can provide plausibility data for both a treated and comparator arm as long as a clinically significant target for improvement has been identified, a priori. For example, if a depression treatment has a clinically meaningful post-treatment target of <7 on the Hamilton Rating Scale for Depression, then any participants in the intervention group who meet this target provide evidence that the target is achievable, at least in some cases. If a high proportion of the intervention participants reach the target, this increases plausibility and makes it less likely that the successes are flukes. If the comparator arm also has a high proportion of successes, it may be too active for the planned behavioral trial. If it has a small proportion of successes, then it would be reassuring that it is an optimum comparator. The definition of "high proportion" is subjective but most frequently based upon the proportion of successes in other, established treatments for the disease or condition under study. (*See Chapter 5: Clinical Significance.*)

Unlike miniature efficacy trials, randomized plausibility studies do not provide false promises of efficacy, are not used in sample size calculations, judge success by clinical significance, and are strongly linked to planned trials. They simply show that it is plausible that a treatment could produce an improvement in health and should be investigated further to determine whether this plausible outcome can be translated into one that is efficacious.

Feasibility

There are a variety of questions that are important to be answered to assess the feasibility of a trial. But one of the most important of these is the feasibility of a recruitment plan. Recruitment failures are among the top reasons that clinical trials fail [3]. Preparation for a definitive *Phase II* or *Phase III* behavioral efficacy trial should include convincing support for the viability and success of the chosen recruitment approach.

An example of a recruitment feasibility study is presented in Table 7.2. Here the investigator needs to recruit 30 patients from clinical practice for a planned behavioral treatment provided in conjunction with the medical visit. They have two clinics available for recruitment. The question of interest is how long the recruitment period should continue to achieve the desired number of 30 patients. The study integrates

Table 7.2 Example of the results of a feasibility study examining time needed for recruitment

Source	Accessible/ Week	Eligible (55%)	Willing (70%)	Passed screen (90%)
Recruitment site #1	9	5.0	3.5	3.2
Recruitment site #2	7	3.9	2.7	2.4
Totals	**16**	**8.9**	**6.2**	**5.6**

Results:
Expected recruitment rate: 5.6/week
Number subjects needed: 30
Number weeks needed: 30/5.6 = 5.4 weeks   (double the estimate)

Time needed for recruitment: 5.4 Weeks x 2 = **12 Weeks**

electronic medical record data with newly collected data from a telephone survey. An algorithm is developed to identify patients at each of the two clinics with the appropriate diagnosis and without exclusion criteria. A period of 1 week is selected, and the electronic medical records provide a list of potentially eligible patients with appointments at the two clinics. These patients are called on the phone, the proposed study is described, their willingness to participate is assessed, and additional screening criteria are evaluated.

This study accomplishes several things. First, it identifies the number of accessible patients that attend each clinic, each week. In recruitment site #1, there are 9. Second, it identifies the percentage of accessible patients that are potentially eligible, based upon exclusion criteria. Across both recruitment sites, this percentage is 55% of those accessible. The telephone survey finds that of those who are potentially eligible, 70% would be "very interested" in participating across the two sites. Finally, a second screen to assess additional logistical barriers to participating reveals that 90% who are willing are indeed able to participate.

These numbers show that approximately 5.6 participants can be recruited per week for this study from these two clinics. Dividing the needed 30 participants by the weekly recruitment rate yields an estimate of 5.4 weeks needed for recruitment. Seasoned investigators realize that recruitment is always more difficult than expected, even given the best feasibility data. Therefore, the estimate of 5.4 weeks needed for recruitment is doubled to account for this expected difficulty. This produces a conservative estimate of a needed recruitment period of 12 weeks.

Are Miniature Efficacy Trials Still Justifiable?

Preliminary tests of behavioral interventions include investigations into plausibility and feasibility. Rigorous tests of efficacy are conducted with full-fledged, adequately powered *Phase II* behavioral trials with primary behavioral or surrogate outcomes and *Phase III* behavioral trials with primary chronic disease endpoints. This raises questions about the role of miniature efficacy trials in the process of preparing for a definitive behavioral trial.

Miniature efficacy trials are still being called viable pilot studies. For example, the National Institute of Mental Health issued a funding opportunity announcement (PAR-17-271) for "Pilot Effectiveness Trials for Post-Acute Interventions and Services to Optimize Longer-Term Outcomes." This is likely explained, in part, by the status quo, sustained by the belief that behavioral research should mirror medical research. But in this context, there is no mirror.

Phase II medical trials have different characteristics and purposes than concomitant miniature efficacy trials of behavioral interventions. *Phase II* medical trials pave the way for *Phase III* trials [e.g., 16, 17]. They have *surrogate outcomes* that can be studied with far fewer participants than are needed for *Phase III* trials with clinical endpoints. They are generally far smaller than the *Phase III* trials that follow them, but it is not unusual for them to study 200–300 participants. A positive outcome in many *Phase II* medical trials has been shown repeatedly to provide no guarantee that a subsequent *Phase III* trial will also have a positive outcome [18]. In contrast, miniature efficacy trials do not always precede a planned behavioral trial. They often evaluate efficacy on the *same* outcome that will be used as the primary outcome in a planned trial, thus undercutting the justification for a small sample size. They are far smaller than *Phase II* medical trials, often studying as few as 15–20 participants. They leap to claims of "preliminary evidence of efficacy" which are uncommon in *Phase II* medical trials.

In short, miniature efficacy trials do not mirror *Phase II* medical trials in either structure or function. They do not permit an inference about plausibility of benefit on health because they do not evaluate success based upon clinical significance. They do not permit an inference about efficacy because there is a poor connection between their results and the results of a fully powered efficacy trial. The only reason that remains to justify the value of miniature efficacy trials is preservation of the status quo.

Thus, it is time to change the status quo. It is time to retire the miniature efficacy trial because it has lost its purpose and credibility. It should be replaced with preliminary studies of plausibility and feasibility. Tests of efficacy should only be conducted with fully powered *Phase II* and *Phase III* behavioral trials. Support for making this shift comes from both biostatistics [7] and research guidelines [1]. Guidance for how to make this shift is provided by the revised ORBIT model. *(See Chapter 3: Behavioral Treatment Development.)*

SELECTED EXPERIENCE FROM BEHAVIORAL TRIALS

A Miniature Efficacy Trial's Short Hop

The large number of miniature efficacy trials that have been published in the behavioral intervention literature draws conclusions about potential efficacy with questionable support. Since very few have been followed by the publication of a definitive trial, the findings may be the *only* evidence ever published. They may be called "pilot" studies, but few of them fly very far.

An excellent example of the miniature efficacy trial tradition has been presented in a 2008 report by Markowitz and his colleagues [19]. It is a particularly good example because the first author is a renowned and productive psychiatric researcher. It demonstrates how this tradition has permeated the entire behavioral intervention research culture over the past few decades. It has not been limited to trainees or early career investigators who lacked experience with behavioral clinical trials.

Markowitz and colleagues reported the results of their study in a paper whose title begins with "Pilot Study." They enrolled 26 participants with primary dysthymic disorder and secondary alcohol abuse and randomly assigned them to 16 weeks of interpersonal therapy (IPT) or brief supportive psychotherapy (BSP). The abstract presents these results and conclusions:

> *"Participants in both treatments reported improved depressive symptoms and alcohol abstinence. IPT had a large and BSP a moderate effect size in depression, whereas BSP had a moderate and IPT a small effect size in percentage of days abstinent. This pilot study offers initial data on IPT and BSP for comorbid chronic depression and alcohol abuse/dependence. Results suggest IPT may have specific antidepressant benefits for dysthymic alcoholic participants but not in treating alcoholism."*

This abstract presents "initial" conclusions about the efficacy of IPT that were based on a miniature, underpowered efficacy trial. Their report says nothing about concrete plans for a more definitive efficacy trial. Nine years have elapsed since it was published, but there have been no reports on outcomes from a definitive efficacy trial. Searches of the NIH RePORTER and clinicaltrials.gov databases suggest that they have not conducted a definitive behavioral trial, and a Medline search suggests that their pilot study is still the only trial that anyone has ever conducted of IPT for treatment of primary dysthymia with secondary alcohol abuse.

Tentative conclusions can become conventional wisdom with the passage of time if they are neither challenged nor reinforced by newer and more rigorous research. This example is not intended to single out Dr. Markowitz and his colleagues or to imply that they did something that was out of step with research practices that are a widely accepted part of the status quo. It simply illustrates the fact that miniature, underpowered efficacy trials often become ends in themselves instead of helping to pave the way for definitive behavioral clinical trials. This can happen even when the investigator fully intends to follow through with a larger and more definitive trial, in the event that adequate funding cannot be obtained.

This example shows three problems with underpowered miniature efficacy trials. First, they ignore the imprecision of estimates of effect sizes drawn from underpowered studies that was so clearly illustrated by Kramer and colleagues [7]. Second, they draw conclusions and generalizations, whether tentative or not, about treatment efficacy and clinical applications. Third, the justification for a pilot study which should be based upon its importance for a subsequent planned definitive behavioral trial often does not exist.

This example shows that what has evolved in the behavioral clinical trial literature is a status quo that is simply bad science.

Contemporary Trends in Pilot and Feasibility Studies

A new open-access journal called *Pilot and Feasibility Studies* is, as its name implies, a good place to find contemporary examples of published feasibility and pilot studies. Many of them are true feasibility or pilot studies in the current sense of these terms, rather than miniature underpowered efficacy trials [e.g., 20]. However, relatively few of the studies that have been published thus far paved the way for a specific, planned, or proposed RCT. Some of these reports conclude that positive feasibility findings support the feasibility of a hypothetical future trial, without mentioning a specific proposal or any concrete plans for a definitive trial. Thus, it appears that some progress is being made in the design and conduct of feasibility and pilot studies but that there is not yet a consensus about the roles that these studies should or should not play in behavioral intervention research.

RECOMMENDATIONS

This chapter has made the argument that there is a need for a change in the status quo of how to prepare for definitive behavioral randomized clinical trials. To promote change in the status quo, recommendations include practices that should be stopped and practices that should begin.

Practices That Should Be Stopped

- Investigators should stop conducting miniature, underpowered efficacy trials. They are poor science. This is consistent with the reproducible science movement [21].

- Grant reviewers should stop asking for, and investigators should stop pretending that they can offer, so-called preliminary evidence of efficacy or a tacit guarantee that a proposed behavioral trial will turn out to support the investigator's primary hypothesis.

- Editors should not grant authors of "preliminary efficacy trial" reports special dispensation by publishing papers on behavioral trials that have grossly inadequate power, inadequate attention to fidelity of the treatment protocols, lack of detail about trial protocols, or other serious methodological weaknesses.

Practices That Should Begin

- Use the definitions for feasibility and pilot studies that are offered in the new CONSORT guidelines. Limit the term "feasibility study" to those that are connected to a specific, planned behavioral efficacy trial. Limit the term "pilot study" to studies with the special design feature of being a smaller version of a linked definitive trial, and have the goal of assessing the feasibility of some aspect of the proposed trial.

- Trainees and early-career investigators have to make the best use they can of small pilot study grants, career development awards, start-up funds, etc. Treatment development studies, proof-of-concept studies assessing plausibility, and feasibility studies assessing feasibility and acceptability are better investments than miniature efficacy trials.

- Justification for a definitive *Phase II* or *Phase III* behavioral clinical trial should rest on the importance of the research question, the credibility of the intervention, the plausibility of the research hypothesis, and the feasibility of implementation of the trial.

- When investigators conduct a pilot or feasibility study, they commit to a progression of studies. This progression is justified when the research question concerns a behavioral target or a surrogate outcome that is upstream from a clinically important outcome that the investigators hope to study in a subsequent, definitive behavioral clinical trial.

- Investigators should do whatever they can to ensure the feasibility of a planned or proposed behavioral clinical trial. But even when the way is paved with feasibility studies, they should recognize their fallibility and be prepared to troubleshoot unexpected problems and make midcourse corrections during the course of conducting definitive *Phase II* or *Phase III* behavioral trials.

- When the time is right to ask an efficacy or effectiveness question, the time is also right to conduct a full-fledged, well-designed, adequately powered *Phase II* or *Phase III* behavioral randomized clinical trial.

- Investigators, reviewers, and editors should be willing to tolerate the uncertainty of behavioral clinical trial outcomes. Many that are well worth conducting produce disappointing results. Failure is a distinct possibility, provides an opportunity for refinement, and should not undercut support for the research on promising behavioral interventions.

REFERENCES

1. Eldridge SM, Chan CL, Campbell MJ, Bond CM, Hopewell S, Thabane L, Lancaster GA, on behalf of the PAFS consensus group (2016) CONSORT 2010 statement: extension to randomised pilot and feasibility trials. Pilot Feasibility Stud 2:64. https://doi.org/10.1186/s40814-016-0105-8
2. Thabane L, Ma J, Chu R, Cheng J, Ismaila A, Rios LP, Robson R, Thabane M, Giangregorio L, Goldsmith CH (2010) A tutorial on pilot studies: the what, why and how. BMC Med Res Methodol 10:1. https://doi.org/10.1186/1471-2288-10-1
3. Williams RJ, Tse T, DiPiazza K, Zarin DA (2015) Terminated trials in the ClinicalTrials.gov results database: evaluation of availability of primary outcome data and reasons for termination. PLoS One 10:e0127242. https://doi.org/10.1371/journal.pone.0127242
4. Crutzen R, Viechtbauer W, Kotz D, Spigt M (2013) No differential attrition was found in randomized controlled trials published in general medical journals: a meta-analysis. J Clin Epidemiol 66:948–954
5. Crutzen R, Viechtbauer W, Spigt M, Kotz D (2015) Differential attrition in health behaviour change trials: a systematic review and meta-analysis. Psychol Health 30:122–134
6. Bellg AJ, Borrelli B, Resnick B, Hecht J, Minicucci DS, Ory M, Ogedegbe G, Orwig D, Ernst D, Czajkowski S, Treatment Fidelity Workgroup of the NIH Behavior Change Consortium (2004) Enhancing treatment fidelity in health behavior change studies: best practices and recommendations from the NIH Behavior Change Consortium. Health Psychol 23:443–451
7. Kraemer HC, Mintz J, Noda A, Tinklenberg J, Yesavage JA (2006) Caution regarding the use of pilot studies to guide power calculations for study proposals. Arch Gen Psychiatry 63:484–489
8. Kraemer HC (1992) Reporting the size of effects in research studies to facilitate assessment of practical or clinical significance. Psychoneuroendocrinology 17:527–536
9. Freedman B (1987) Equipoise and the ethics of clinical research. N Engl J Med 317:141–145
10. Colagiuri B, Schenk LA, Kessler MD, Dorsey SG, Colloca L (2015) The placebo effect: from concepts to genes. Neuroscience 307:171–190
11. Macklis RM (1993) Magnetic healing, quackery, and the debate about the health effects of electromagnetic fields. Ann Intern Med 118:376–383
12. Ma J, Rosas LG, Lv N (2016) Precision lifestyle medicine: a new frontier in the science of behavior change and population health. Am J Prev Med 50:395–397
13. Collins LM, Murphy SA, Nair VN, Strecher VJ (2005) A strategy for optimizing and evaluating behavioral interventions. Ann Behav Med 30:65–73
14. Czajkowski SM, Powell LH, Adler N, Naar-King S, Reynolds KD, Hunter CM, Laraia B, Olster DH, Perna FM, Peterson JC, Epel E, Boyington JE, Charlson ME (2015) From ideas to efficacy: the ORBIT model for developing behavioral treatments for chronic diseases. Health Psychol 34:971–982
15. Onken LS, Carroll KM, Shoham V, Cuthbert BN, Riddle M (2014) Reenvisioning clinical science: unifying the discipline to improve the public health. Clin Psychol Sci 2:22–34
16. Thomas NJ, Guardia CG, Moya FR, Cheifetz IM, Markovitz B, Cruces P, Barton P, Segal R, Simmons P, Randolph AG (2012) A pilot, randomized, controlled clinical trial of lucinactant, a peptide-containing synthetic surfactant, in infants with acute hypoxemic respiratory failure. Pediatr Crit Care Med 13:646–653
17. Miller KD, O'Neill A, Perez EA, Seidman AD, Sledge GW (2012) A phase II pilot trial incorporating bevacizumab into dose-dense doxorubicin and cyclophosphamide followed by paclitaxel in patients with lymph node positive breast cancer: a trial coordinated by the Eastern Cooperative Oncology Group. Ann Oncol 23:331–337
18. Bikdeli B, Punnanithinont N, Akram Y, Lee I, Desai NR, Ross JS, Krumholz HM (2017) Two decades of cardiovascular trials with primary surrogate endpoints: 1990–2011. J Am Heart Assoc 6:e005285. https://doi.org/10.1161/JAHA.116.005285

19. Markowitz JC, Kocsis JH, Christos P, Bleiberg K, Carlin A (2008) Pilot study of interpersonal psychotherapy versus supportive psychotherapy for dysthymic patients with secondary alcohol abuse or dependence. J Nerv Ment Dis 196:468–474
20. Hubbard G, O'Carroll R, Munro J, Mutrie N, Haw S, Mason H, Treweek S (2016) The feasibility and acceptability of trial procedures for a pragmatic randomised controlled trial of a structured physical activity intervention for people diagnosed with colorectal cancer: findings from a pilot trial of cardiac rehabilitation versus usual care (no rehabilitation) with an embedded qualitative study. Pilot Feasibility Stud 2:51. https://doi.org/10.1186/s40814-016-0090-y
21. Munafò MR, Nosek BA, Bishop DVM, Button KS, Chambers CD, Percie du Sert N, Simonsohn U, Wagenmakers E-J, Ware JJ, Ioannidis JPA (2017) A manifesto for reproducible science. Nat Hum Behav 1:0021. https://doi.org/10.1038/s41562-016-0021

Chapter 8
Protection of Random Assignment

"Daniel and his three companions were young Israelites who were taken to serve in the palace of the king of Babylon because they were of noble royal family, without physical defect, handsome, versed in wisdom, and competent. Daniel determined he would not defile himself with the King's food or wine. He asked the overseer:

> *'Please test us for 10 days and let us be given some vegetables*
> *to eat and water to drink. Then let our appearance be compared*
> *to the appearance of youths who are eating the King's choice food.'*

At the end of 10 days, their appearance seemed better and they were fatter than any of the youths who had been eating the King's food. So the overseer let them continue to eat vegetables and drink water instead of what the king provided."

Bible, Old Testament, Book of Daniel 1:16

Fundamental Point

Random assignment creates randomly equivalent treatment arms. This makes it possible to infer that any differences on the outcome are due to treatment and not to any known or unknown confounders. The single most important job of the behavioral trialist is to protect this random assignment in the design, operations, and analyses of the trial. This includes recruiting and retaining a target population that is likely to benefit, motivated to adhere to the treatment and trial protocols, and understands completely what is required for participation.

In the above passage from the Bible, the vitality of Daniel and his three friends after 10 days may have been due to the vegetables and water that they were given, or it may have been their pre-existing higher socioeconomic status, robust genetic endowment, tight social network, and/or a strong placebo effect. Alternative explanations for the benefit of a treatment are confounders which are nuisance "passen-

© Springer Nature Switzerland AG 2021
L. H. Powell et al., *Behavioral Clinical Trials for Chronic Diseases*,
https://doi.org/10.1007/978-3-030-39330-4_8

ger" variables that ride along with treatment and undermine the ability to make causal inferences. This chapter focuses on why random assignment is so powerful and should be protected. It presents a history of attempts to answer the question of whether or not a treatment works and the arrival at random assignment as the best way to make causal inferences. It defines confounding as an error of interpretation and the essential role of protecting the random assignment to avoid it. It then goes on to illustrate ways to protect random assignment in the design, conduct, and analyses of a trial, with particular attention to the central role of identifying a patient-centered target population, recruiting it, retaining it, and insuring that all randomized participants are included in the evaluation of trial results.

SCIENTIFIC PRINCIPLES

History of Random Assignment

Throughout the history of medicine, practitioners and patients alike have asked the question:

"Does this treatment work?"

Table 8.1, adapted from the excellent review by Bull [1], presents a variety of strategies that have been used to provide a conclusive answer to this question. The earliest approaches determined treatment effectiveness by some combination of experience, theory, and trial and error. But knowledge transfer using these methods was slow and inefficient, and it was difficult to disentangle treatment effects from extraneous influences. Rephrasing the question to include a comparator simplified the problem. The question of interest became:

"Does this treatment work better than X?"

The problem then became trying to figure out what the "X" should be. Historical controls compare patients before and after introduction of a treatment. But the treated patients differed not only on the treatment but also on the passage of time, opening the door to the possibility that it was some historical event(s), rather than the treatment, that accounted for results. Concurrent and matched controls compare patients who have the treatment to those without the treatment at the same moment in time and, in the case of matching, by selecting patients for comparison who are matched on known predictors of outcome. But even with matched comparisons, there are likely to be a variety of unknown pre-existing differences associated with the choice to undergo or forego treatment. Because they are unknown, they cannot be matched. ABA designs use subjects as their own controls and examine outcome when the treatment is given, withdrawn, and then given again. These designs can be

Table 8.1 Selected history of methods to identify effective treatments [1]

No Control

- The Egyptians applied their expertise in structural engineering to the treatment of accidental injuries. Success was unequivocal and easily tested by trial and error.
- The Greeks relied upon theory stemming from a general philosophy of nature. Hippocrates insisted that theory be combined with experience and reason, thus promoting a tension between trust in theory or trust in observation.
- In the Middle Ages, the intellectual atmosphere emphasized faith, authority, and idealism. This extended to medicine where in 1278 Bacon argued against experimentation because the "noble material in which one works demands no error."

Historical Control

- In 1537, Pare was treating men wounded in battle with the standard approach of burning wounds with boiling oil. When he ran out of the oil, he concocted a digestive which turned out to be more effective than the oil. He never again burned with oil.
- In 1870, Lister compared amputation in 35 cases before the use of antiseptics with 40 cases treated with antiseptics. Although mortality was only 15% with antiseptics vs. 43% without, Lister was hesitant to draw conclusions because of the small sample size.

Concurrent Control

- In 1600, the East India Company aimed to reduce the excessively high rate of scurvy in sailors on prolonged voyages by supplying only 1 of 4 ships with lemon juice. When sailors on the ship with lemon juice were almost free of scurvy, compared to the excessively high rate on the other 3 ships, the company provided lemon juice on all subsequent voyages.
- In 1747, Lind compared 10 sailors with scurvy on the same ship who were non-randomly allocated to 1 of 5 treatments. Only the 2 sailors receiving the treatment of oranges and lemons made an immediate recovery.

Subject as Own Control

- In 1676, Wiseman, the outstanding English surgeon of the century, treated patients who had leg edema with laced stockings. Using an ABA design, he showed that when the stocking was on, the edema remitted but when the stocking was removed, the edema returned.

Matched Case Control

- In 1865, Bennett examined a restorative treatment for pneumonia by analyzing carefully his patients with respect to sex, age, severity, and duration of illness and comparing them to similar participants in other series treated by more "heroic" methods.
- In 1896, Fibiger studied a serum for diphtheria in a treated and untreated series made comparable on age, symptoms, and severity. He then compared the results within age and severity subgroups and found that mortality was lower for those treated within each of the age and severity subgroups.
- In 1921, Chick and Dalyell treated one of a series of two twins admitted to the hospital for scurvy and rickets with vitamin therapy and then showed photographs of the twins displaying enormous improvement only in in those treated.

Random Assignment

- In 1931, Green studied 550 women with sepsis admitted to the hospital. Every other admission was given a treatment of Vitamins A and D. There was consistent improvement in those receiving the vitamins.
- In 1945, Porritt enlisted surgeons to explore the value of penicillin, relative to the standard of care, for soldiers wounded in North Africa. It was soon found that allocation of participants to trial arm was not impartial since surgeons were reluctant to withhold penicillin from the more seriously injured. Despite the direction of bias against penicillin, it showed a strong benefit, lending to the conclusiveness of the trial.

powerful demonstrations of efficacy but are limited to treatments that can be withdrawn completely and have outcomes that can change quickly. This is not the case for many behavioral treatments and chronic diseases.

There was a growing need for an ability to make more conclusive causal inferences that a treatment was the most plausible reason the treated improved and the untreated did not. This led to the strategy known as random assignment [2]. It appeared as early as 1662 (see box) in an argument between two practitioners, one dedicated to treatments supported by empirical observation and the other dedicated to treatments supported by accepted theory [3].

> **Randomized Experiment in 1662**
>
> *"Let us take out of the hospitals. ... 500 poor people that have fevers, pleurisies, etc. and divide them into half, let us cast lots that one half may be my share, the others to you. We shall see how many funerals both of us shall have."*
>
> Von Helmont, 1662

This interest grew throughout medical history [4–6]. But it wasn't until Sir RA Fisher, working in the area of agriculture in the 1920s, presented the statistical foundations of the randomized experiment that it became a prominent part of the scientific method. In the 1940s, the randomized design gained visibility in medicine primarily through the work of the English physician and scientist, Sir Austin Bradford Hill, who argued for well-designed experiments to eliminate nearly all extraneous causes and thus render the interpretation of a comparison more certain [7, 8]. By 1951 the randomized design had become the gold standard in medicine, evident by Sinclair's Cutter Lecture in Preventive Medicine at Harvard.

> *"The experimental method has brilliant discoveries to its credit, whereas the method of observation has achieved little." [9]*

Causal Inferences

The nineteenth-century philosopher of science, John Stuart Mill, outlined three criteria for inferring cause: (1) the cause precedes the effect; (2) the cause is related to the effect; and (3) no plausible alternative explanation exists for the effect other than the cause [10]. Sir Bradford Hill expanded these to nine criteria that determine whether or not a factor causes a disease [11]. "Hill's Criteria," fundamental to training in epidemiology, identify the randomized experiment as the criterion providing the strongest support for causation based upon its ability to rule out alternative explanations for results. With observational studies, it is difficult, if not impossible, to rule out alternative explanations even with sophisticated design and analytic strategies and particularly when potential causal factors are highly intercorrelated. No other design in science controls for the problem of alternative explanations, known more commonly as the problem of confounding, as well as the randomized trial. Observational studies with covariate adjustment remain "second-choice" options when a randomized trial is not possible.

The Problem of Confounding

Confounding is an error in interpretation. The error is assuming a treatment produced a result rather than some other factor that was correlated with the treatment and outcome. Bias, in contrast, is a technical problem that occurs during the trial and results in a spurious under- or over-estimation of the benefit of treatment. Bias can create confounding; confounding cannot create bias. Random assignment is the strongest way to prevent an error in interpretation due to confounding. Thus, it is the strongest way to make a causal inference that a treatment produced an effect.

The well-known maxim *correlation does not imply causation* reflects the fundamental underpinnings of confounding. A correlation between two variables does not indicate which variable came first and caused the other, nor does it rule out the alternative explanation that these two variables are only related due to their joint relationship to a third variable, the confounder. In the presence of highly complex tangles of causation that are characteristic of humans at risk for chronic diseases, it is possible that any association between treatment and outcome exists through the agency of a third variable. Sometimes this third variable is a mediator that is a part of the causal pathway by which the treatment influences the disease. But other times, this third variable is a nuisance "passenger" variable that simply rides along with the treatment. Observational studies attempt to deal with this problem in a number of ways, the most common of which is covariate adjustment in analyses. Clinical trials deal with this problem much more effectively in the design using random assignment.

For a variable to confound results from a clinical trial, it must satisfy three conditions. It must:

1. Be a risk factor for (i.e., correlated with) the outcome of interest;
2. Covary with the treatment under study; and
3. Not be a consequence of the treatment.

Figure 8.1 presents this visually. In Figure 8.1a, it is hypothesized that the treatment affects the disease. But in fact, the treatment is related to an extraneous risk factor

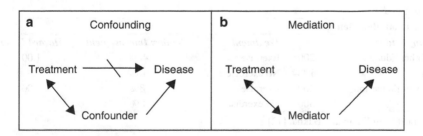

Fig. 8.1 Confounding (a) and mediation (b)

for the disease (i.e., a confounder), and it is this extraneous risk factor that influences the disease. In Figure 8.1b, a third factor meets the first two criteria for confounding; namely, it is related to both the disease and the treatment. But it is not independent of the treatment but rather a part of the causal pathway by which the treatment affects the disease. Thus, it is not a confounder but rather a mediator. It does not constitute an error in interpretation nor does it require design or statistical control. Statistical control for a mediator results in overcontrol and an underestimation of the true impact of the treatment on disease. It is extremely important to disentangle confounders from mediators in the design of a trial.

By way of a hypothetical example, consider a trial of the impact of exercise training on memory in 800 sedentary elderly presented in Table 8.2 (adapted from Wang and Bakhai (2006)) [12]. The 400 in the treated group receive an exercise intervention, and the 400 controls are a non-random concurrent group. Table 8.2a shows that there was an improvement in memory over time in both the exercise and no exercise groups, but the improvement was 33% greater in the exercise group (hazard ratio = 1.66, $p < 0.01$). Table 8.2b reveals the confounder. When the results were examined separately by educational level, there were more people with higher education in the exercise group ($N = 200$) than in the no exercise controls ($N = 100$). All participants in the higher educational stratum had a 40% improvement over time in memory, regardless of whether or not they exercised. All participants in the lower education stratum had only an 8% improvement over time in memory regardless of whether or not they exercised. Within each educational level, the risk of exercising vs. not exercising was exactly the same (hazard ratio = 1.0) suggesting that there was no relationship at all between exercise and memory when education was accounted for. The association between exercise and memory in Table 8.2a was spurious because of unrecognized confounding. Education met each of the 3 criteria for confounding: (1) there is a known association between higher education and exercise; (2) there is a known association between higher education and memory; and (3) since educational level was determined long before this exercise treatment

Table 8.2 Education confounds the relation between exercise and memory				
a. Confounder Not Identified				
	N	*Treatment*	*Memory Improvement*	*Hazard Ratio*
	400	Exercise	24%	1.66**
	400	No exercise	16%	
**p < 0.01*				
b. Confounder Identified				
Confounder	*N*	*Treatment*	*Memory Improvement*	*Hazard Ratio*
Higher Education	200	Exercise	40%	1.00
	100	No exercise	40%	
Lower Education	200	Exercise	8%	1.00
	300	No exercise	8%	
Adapted from Wang and Bakhai [12]				

was initiated, it could not be a result of exercise treatment and thereby could not mediate the causal pathway by which exercise enhances memory.

If the design of this study was a within-subject comparison of elderly before and after they underwent exercise training, confounders of concern would be the aging of the participants which could have suppressed a treatment effect or some historical event that could have either suppressed or potentiated the treatment effect. If the design of the study was to use a non-random control group that was matched to the treated group on key prognostic variables, such as education, confounding would remain a concern. Confounders are silent "riders" with treatment. They are not always known ahead of time. There is always the possibility that unknown prognostic variables accounted for results which, because they are unknown, could not be measured and incorporated into design and analyses using such strategies as matching, stratification, and covariate adjustment.

> **Tangles of Causation in Chronic Diseases**
>
> *"Human biology is far too incompletely understood and complex to reliably predict the clinical effectiveness of new treatments. . . Although advances in understanding genetics and disease mechanisms will improve ability to focus on populations more likely to need treatment and benefit from it, the randomized clinical trial will remain the ultimate gold standard for evaluating and quantifying the impact of new treatments."*
>
> Domanski, 2009 [13]

In summary, random assignment relieves the investigator of worrying about identifying all possible confounders and measuring them reliably. Random assignment relieves the investigator of worrying about whether or not a confounder potentiated, suppressed, or distorted the true effect of a treatment. If potential confounders are known, the investigator can hope to minimize their effects by stratifying random assignment or using regression models to adjust for them statistically. But it is the control not only for known, but more importantly for unknown confounders, that creates the power of the randomized design [12–18] and makes it the "Mercedes" of epidemiological designs. In Fisher's words:

> *"Randomization relieves the experimenter from the anxiety of considering and estimating the magnitude of the innumerable causes by which his data may be distributed." [19]*

Basic Elements of Random Assignment

Clinical trials come in all shapes and sizes, but their sine qua non is the element of random assignment [2]. This obviates the need for physical isolation in the laboratory to isolate treatment from the tangles of causation that are characteristic of chronic diseases [20].

Rationale

There are three key benefits achieved by random assignment [21]. First, it minimizes the impact of an incomplete understanding of confounders on the integrity of the trial. The treatment arms will have similar distributions of prognostic factors, including not only those that are known but also those that are unknown. Second, it avoids selection bias where participants of a particular kind are chosen to receive a particular form of treatment, either advertently or inadvertently. By definition, the use of chance in assigning subjects to treatment can have no such systematic bias. Third, it converts confounding variables into residual variation that is equally distributed between arms. This guarantees the validity of statistical tests of significance. Since the distribution of residual variation is equivalent between arms at baseline, any difference in this distribution at follow-up can be ascribed to treatment and expressed quantitatively, assuming sufficient sample size.

Process

In the simplest case, random assignment is a process by which there is a known likelihood of being assigned to trial arms. This assignment is not under the subject's or anyone else's control. If it were, the preference for a particular treatment would likely be correlated with a range of other characteristics associated with that preference, which are rarely understood in entirety.

The ideal process of random assignment insures that prospective participants are assigned to a trial arm on the basis of chance and that this assignment is unpredictable. This process has been described in detail in the CONSORT guidelines for reporting requirements [22]. Three different parts of the process need protection.

1. Allocation must be truly random. The most common method to ensure randomness is a computer random number generator. Allocation sequences based upon such non-random variables as date of hospital admission or date of birth are generally not considered to be random.

2. The allocation sequence must be concealed. The decision to accept or reject a potential participant must be made in ignorance of the next assignment sequence. This avoids advertent or inadvertent selection bias where certain types of patients have a greater probability of being allocated to a particular arm (e.g., healthier, greater need for treatment, etc.).

3. The people involved in generating the assignment to a trial arm should be different from the people involved in determining eligibility and implementing the treatment. This can be maximized by using external, third-party randomization systems.

If the random assignment process is compromised, the whole point of randomization is lost and selection bias offers an alternative explanation for

> "When randomization leaks, the entire trial runs down the drain."
> Mosteller [23]

results. In a study of 250 controlled trials, inadequate concealment of the allocation sequence resulted in a 30–40% inflation of the treatment effect [24]. The allocation process can become evident inadvertently through subconscious actions or advertently through some type of deciphering. It is human nature to want to demonstrate ingenuity by decoding a randomization scheme. It is human nature to want particular participants to get the treatment one "knows" to be more effective. It is human nature to want the results of the trial to reveal what one believes to be valid. But the price of these human tendencies is high. Articulation of the procedures for concealing the randomization process is now required by CONSORT guidelines [25–27]. Such safeguards aim to preserve quality by annoying human nature [28].

Limitations

Random assignment does not provide perfect control for confounding [20]. Consider the analogy of playing cards. The "luck of the draw" refers to fact that even with a well-shuffled deck, some players will be dealt a better hand than others. But over many hands, the quality of the cards will be equal across players. With random assignment in a clinical trial, distributions of factors that could affect the outcome will be balanced over repeated trials with repeated random assignment. But this is little comfort when repeated replications of a trial are considerably more difficult to accomplish than repeated playing of games of cards. The "luck of the draw" in any particular trial produces randomly equivalent arms which may still differ on important baseline prognostic factors (called sampling error by statisticians). The risk for such imbalance is increased when the sample size is small.

Traditionally, most trialists would argue that the primary analysis of a clinical trial is the simple comparison between arms on the primary endpoint, without any covariate adjustment [14]. This test answers the question of whether any participant who is randomly assigned to a treated group has an outcome that is likely to be better than that of any participant who is randomly assigned to a control group [29]. If the random assignment happens to result in an "unlucky hand" where there is baseline imbalance between treatment arms on one or more factors, not much can be done about it after the fact. At best, the primary analysis can be augmented by secondary sensitivity analyses controlling for any imbalance to create a more complete picture. It is obvious that clinical trials play an extremely conservative game.

But this traditional view is beginning to soften. If the question of interest is the effects of a treatment in combination with other prognostic factors, adjustment for these other prognostic factors can be justified [30]. Such factors must be predictors of outcome, proposed a priori, have a strong rationale, be limited in number, and be as uncorrelated to each other as possible [29, 30]. If the sample size is small and the risk of imbalance due simply to the "luck of the draw" is high, prognostic factors that could confound results could be specified a priori and proposed as covariates in the primary analysis plan. There is little downside to this approach, particularly for

small sample sizes. If a potential prognostic factor turns out
to be a unrelated to the outcome, covariate adjustment
will be useless [29, 30]. But in
the event of an "unlucky hand,"
the opportunity to adjust for
pre-specified potential confounders provides a safeguard
that is superior to other alternatives such as stratified randomization, which is severely
limited in small sample sizes,
or the need to repeat the trial in
hopes of a "better hand."

> ## Covariate Adjustment in a Primary Analysis of a Clinical Trial
>
> An "unlucky hand" in a clinical trial is when random assignment creates treatment arms that differ at baseline on important predictors of outcome. The risk for this is increased when the sample size is small. A priori identification of key predictors, and pre-specification of a primary analysis plan that adjusts for them, has no downside and could cushion the otherwise severe blow of an unlucky hand [30].

There is widespread agreement that the temptation to adjust post hoc for unlucky baseline differences between randomized arms should be resisted. Such a post hoc test is equivalent to making a bet on a horse when he approaches the finish line rather than before the race begins [29]. So it all comes back to an a priori identification of a small number of important prognostic factors that could turn out to be imbalanced between arms and thus confound results. This is a safeguard that offers considerable benefit with minimal risk. In the case of an "unlucky draw," a priori specification of potential confounders could save a trial.

Post-Randomization Exclusions

Protection of random assignment goes beyond insuring quality of the process of randomization at baseline. It is also about preserving that balance throughout the duration of the trial. On the operational side, this means not excluding any random-ized participant for any of the following reasons.

1. *Discovery of ineligibility.* This can occur when a participant is deemed to be eligible and randomized, only to find out later that they are not truly eligible. If, for example, the trial is aimed at determining the best treatment for participants with a recent heart attack and it is subsequently discovered that a participant, now randomized, never had a heart attack, the temptation is to exclude him/her post-randomization.

2. *Development of a competing risk.* A randomized participant may be free of disqualifying competing events at the time of randomization but one emerges after randomization. For example, a participant randomized to weight loss treatment in a behavioral trial may be subsequently diagnosed with an advanced and aggressive malignancy. This competing condition could promote weight loss that was unrelated to the trial treatment. Rather than risk a spurious benefit of weight loss from treatment, the temptation is to exclude the participant.

3. *Non-adherence*. A randomized participant may fail to adhere to the treatment as outlined in the trial protocol. Indeed, a participant may never even show up for the first treatment contact. The temptation is to exclude this participant on the basis of never having received any treatment.

4. *Missing or poor quality data*. If outcome data are compromised or missing for a potential participant, it is tempting to eliminate this participant to obtain an accurate understanding of the value of treatment on the outcome of interest.

It is obvious that there are competing tensions between detection of a treatment benefit and protection of random assignment. In the past, detection of a treatment benefit appears to have been the priority. In a report of 110 trials conducted between 1990 and 1991 in obstetrics/gynecology, 55% reported post-randomization exclusion of randomized subjects, and 29% reported exclusions of more than 10% of the original randomized cohort [31]. This is likely to be an underestimate because the trials with no exclusions in this report were of lower quality, suggesting that they may have underreported them.

There is now wide consensus in the clinical trial community that avoidance of confounding through protection of random assignment should be given the highest priority in primary analyses. If there are a number of these special problems, random assignment will distribute them approximately equally across treatment arms. In secondary analyses, it is possible to explore the robustness of primary findings by, for example, excluding participants with special circumstances. With luck, the secondary analysis will not differ from the primary analysis. If it does, avoidance of confounding takes primacy over all other concerns.

Intent-to-Treat Analyses

On the analysis side, the equilibrium achieved at baseline between randomized groups is preserved with intent-to-treat analyses. Under intent-to-treat, trial participants are analyzed as members of the group to which they were randomized regardless of their adherence to, or receipt of, the intended treatment [32]. Eliminating participants who were randomized but not treated, or moving participants between treatment groups according to the treatment they actually received, violates the intent-to-treat principle [32]. The question answered by intent-to-treat is the benefit of a *program* of offering a particular treatment. This includes not only its biopsychosocial effects but also the ability to administer it and the participant's ability to adhere to it.

Clinicians often have difficulty with intent-to-treat analyses because they are in pursuit of understanding whether or not a treatment works in those who undergo it. Per-protocol analyses which evaluate only the subgroup of participants who actually received the treatment are often paired with intent-to-treat analyses to provide a complete evaluation. However, the limitation of per-protocol analyses is that they break the equilibrium between groups and require adjustment for potential confounders. This is the reason that the intent-to-treat analysis, which preserves the random assignment, is the primary analytic approach for a clinical trial and per-protocol analyses serve as informative secondary analyses.

Ethics

Questions about the ethics of random assignment emerged during the HIV epidemic. When people were dying every day, was it ethical to randomize them to a placebo pill when the alternative was a potentially lifesaving therapy? The answer is, of course, no. When faced with imminent mortality, throw caution to the wind and try anything.

But in less extreme situations where the value of a new treatment is uncertain, or the relative merits of existing treatments are in dispute, empirical support takes precedence over trial and error. A clinical trial is undertaken when there is genuine uncertainty about the value of a treatment [33]. This uncertainty, or lack of equipoise, occurs at both the community and investigator level. Equipoise is pivotal to the question of the ethics of random assignment in a clinical trial. One does not randomize to something vs. nothing. One randomizes to two options which could be two "somethings" or two "nothings." *(See Chapter 10: Preferences, Equipoise, and Blinding.)*

Acceptance of uncertainty about the therapeutic merits of a treatment, combined with the value of objective, empirical evidence to reduce that uncertainty, is the ethical underpinning of a randomized trial. Alternatives to the randomized trial exist but should not be seen as easier routes to valid answers. They are, and will continue to be at least in the near future, second-choice methodologies used only when random assignment is impossible. A randomized clinical trial is not perfect. But there is no other study design that is so elegant in the simplicity with which it can make causal inferences [34]. To paraphrase Churchill, replacing "democracy" with "randomized controlled trials:"

> *"Randomized controlled trials are fallible and far from perfect; the only good thing that we can say about them is that there are no better alternatives." [35]*

CHALLENGES FOR BEHAVIORAL TRIALS

The Dangers of Confounding

An appreciation of the dangers of confounding provides the strongest and most basic rationale for protecting random assignment. But in the behavioral clinical trial literature, these dangers tend to be underappreciated. Most behavioral randomized trials are designed as experiments. Confounding is defined as a type of construct validity where true treatment benefits are confused with non-specific factors such as experimenter expectancy [20, 36]. The value of random assignment is to avoid selection bias.

The epidemiologic literature has a broader conceptualization of the definition, causes, and control of confounding. It is defined as an error of interpretation; not a bias. It is best controlled by balancing trial arms using random assignment. But even when random assignment is carried out perfectly, confounding can create a problem if the randomized treatment arms are imbalanced at baseline due to sampling error. Moreover, even if the trial arms are balanced perfectly at baseline, confounding can set in after the trial is underway if there is differential attrition resulting in post-randomization imbalance between trial arms.

A broad appreciation of the dangers of confounding that emerge when trial arms become imbalanced helps with the design of a behavioral trial in a number of important ways. It: (1) encourages interest in identifying potential confounders; (2) minimizes the false security that random assignment alone solves imbalance problems; (3) provides justification for stratified random assignment and pre-specified subgroup analyses; (4) provides a rationale for pre-specified covariate adjustment; and (5) fosters respect for the value of intent-to-treat analyses.

Tension Between Internal and External Validity

In behavioral clinical trials, it is common to test interventions in real-world settings with diverse populations, minimal exclusions, and suboptimal follow-ups to achieve wide generalizability of benefit [37]. These trials pursue external validity, sometimes at the expense of internal validity.

If an intervention has unknown efficacy because it has not been tested under internally valid testing conditions, interpretation of the results of effectiveness testing can be clouded. When an intervention of unknown efficacy fails in effectiveness testing, it is not known whether it would not work under any circumstances or whether its signal was overwhelmed by the noisy conditions under which it was tested. If a treatment does not work under any circumstances, a reasonable course of action would be to abandon it. If it works in trials with strong internal validity but does not work in trials with strong external validity, a reasonable course of action would be to refine it to adapt to the noisy conditions rather than to abandon it.

The tension between internal and external validity has created confusion between ecologically valid treatments (e.g., treatments conducted in real-world settings) and internally valid trial design (e.g., eligibility criteria that maximize successful follow-up). Interventions designed to be implemented in real-world settings can be tested in efficacy trials with strong internal validity to establish a causal relationship. This includes interventions implemented in highly controlled settings by highly trained personnel and ecologically valid interventions conducted in real-world settings by diverse change agents. But inclusion of participants who are unlikely to complete a follow-up based upon medical, logistical, or motivational reasons compromises the random assignment and thereby compromises the internal validity and ability to make causal inferences. This extends to any type of intervention and any type of trial design. This problem is not solved by increasing the sample size.

In progressive, translational research, the tension between internal and external validity does not exist. Efficacy is a prerequisite for effectiveness [17]. A progression of questions is answered in a progression of studies which progress from strong internal to strong external validity. An efficacy trial with strong internal validity establishes a causal relationship. A series of effectiveness trials study the extent to which the causal relationship holds over diverse persons, settings, and treatments [20].

Representative Target Populations

A well-specified hypothesis focuses on a well-specified target population [38]. It is generally accepted that all people with a particular disease or condition comprise the target population for a clinical trial, with exclusions based only upon medical and logistical concerns. This approach is encouraged by the National Institutes of Health where funding is contingent upon making eligibility available to all who have the disease of interest, unless there is a strong argument for exclusion of specific subgroups.

While this assumption works well for drug trials where the target biologic mechanism tends to be consistent across diverse groups, it runs into several problems in behavioral trials. First, if eligibility extends to all at medical risk, those who do not have an elevation in the behavioral target of the intervention might be included. Second, not all those at medical risk may have interest in undergoing a behavioral intervention which requires some level of individual agency. Making eligibility for a behavioral trial based only upon medical risk is akin to a "one size fits all" approach which is not only naïve [39] but also makes considerable demand on a behavioral treatment. Many with low motivation for a behavioral treatment will simply self-select out of the invitation to participate. Others will participate, sometimes with reluctance, but are often the source of retention problems and extraordinary investigator efforts to prevent them.

People who have low motivation to make behavioral changes are not good candidates for behavioral interventions that require active individual agency. This is demonstrated persuasively by the results of smoking cessation studies. Stages of change theory defines *pre-contemplators* as people who do not intend to make changes now or in the near future [40]. This theory encourages inclusion of pre-contemplators in clinical trials and advocates for tailoring treatment materials to the stage of change.

Table 8.3 Pre-contemplators in behavioral trials for smoking cessation

Prevalence	22–60% of those at risk for a disease
Behavior	Most resistant, least active
Dropout Rate	Higher than those at other stages
Outcome Assessment	Lower completion than those at other stages
Efficacy	– Half as likely to benefit as those at other stages – Benefit no different from controls
Progression of Stage of Change	– "Pre-contemplation" is a stable pattern – Slight progression but no different from controls

Table 8.3 summarizes what they actually do in smoking studies [41–44]. Pre-contemplators comprise 22–60% of trial participants, are the most resistant to treatment, have higher dropout rates, derive benefit that is no different from controls, and show little evidence of moving from their pre-contemplation stage during treatment to a more motivated stage.

The pre-contemplators appear to be voting with their feet. Tailoring to move them to a more motivated stage of change is relatively ineffective. Their inclusion in a *Phase II* or *Phase III* behavioral confirmatory trial has limited justification. Rather than including them in these trials in pursuit of enhancing generalizability to all who have a disease or condition, it may be better to seek a closer alignment between patient motivation and the nature of the treatment. Those with low motivation to change behavior could be given the opportunity to self-select out of confirmatory trials and be redirected toward interventions that are targeted specifically at motivational factors.

The consequence of non-adherence in a clinical trial is that it makes randomized arms look more alike, thereby reducing the effect size [17]. This is illustrated dramatically in Fig. 8.2 which presents data from the Physicians' Health Study, a trial examining the benefit of aspirin on CHD mortality [45]. The figure compares the power to detect a 15% difference in mortality between aspirin or placebo arms, by sample size and level of adherence. The first and third bars compare power when adherence is 100% in both arms but the sample size is reduced by 67% in the third bar. The impact of a reduced sample size on power is minimal, dropping from 90% with the sample size of 33,000 to 85% with a sample size of 22,000.

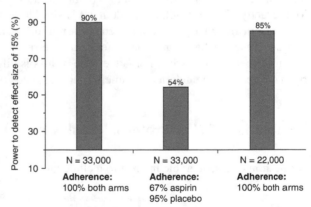

Fig. 8.2 The power to detect a 15% difference in mortality by sample size and adherence in the Physicians' Health Study[45]

The impact of non-adherence to treatment is much greater. The first and second bars have the same sample size of 33,000, but the first has 100% adherence in both arms, and the second has 67% adherence to aspirin and 95% adherence to placebo. Power drops to 54% when non-adherence is a problem. This runs the risk that despite the huge sample size, there will be inadequate power to detect a 15% difference in mortality between arms. This trial would likely be inconclusive, and the question posed unanswered because of bias stemming from non-adherence.

An inconclusive trial resulting from a bias in procedures is a clear and present danger and a dreaded outcome of any clinical trial. Sample size calculations generally include estimates for dropout rates but fail to include estimates for rates of non-adherence to the treatment arms. At best, non-adherence is reflected in the estimate of the magnitude of the effect. This puts considerable demand on a behavioral treatment to show efficacy in a substantial proportion of participants, despite non-adherence. Attention is urgently needed to define the appropriate target population for a behavioral trial which is sensitive to diverse patient preferences.

Differential Treatment Demands

In behavioral trials, the randomized arms tend to offer different treatments which often make differential demands upon participants and invite differential adherence and dropout. Greater adherence in one arm than the other may result when a behavioral treatment is too demanding or a comparator arm is too underwhelming to command much attention. This is a stark contrast to a drug trial where the treatments look exactly alike, the adherence demand is similar, and, barring any unique side effects from the active pill, dropouts tend to be non-differential. If post-randomization non-adherence or losses are non-differential, the result is lower power to detect a treatment benefit. But when non-adherence or loss is differential, baseline equilibrium created by the random assignment is altered, and confounding can set in.

Temptation of "Per-Protocol" Analyses

A question of considerable interest to a clinician is:

"Does this treatment work in those who adhered to it?"

To answer this question, one must conduct a *per-protocol* analysis (also called *responder-only* or *on-treatment* analysis.). This type of analysis compares the subgroup of those randomized to active treatment who actually adhered to the treatment protocol to various approaches to comparator groups (e.g., those in the treatment arm who did not adhere to the protocol; controls who did adhere to the control protocol, etc.). The problem with such analyses is that they break the comparability created by randomization and open the door to confounding. The beauty of the randomized trial is therefore lost, and the design becomes one that is similar to a prospective observational study where statistical control for confounders is essential but suboptimal because unknown confounders cannot be controlled.

Students of epidemiologic methods are taught the dangers of per-protocol analyses using the famous example presented in Fig. 8.3. Data are from the Coronary Drug Project which compared the value of clofibrate, a lipid-lowering drug, to placebo on 5-year mortality in 3892 men with a recent heart attack [46]. This was a null trial reporting no difference between the randomized arms on mortality. Since the protocol for adherence to the trial pills was demanding (participants had to take between one and three capsules, three times per day), non-adherence, defined as taking less than 80% of prescribed pills, occurred in 33% of participants in both trial arms. It was thus reasonable to ask whether or not the drug improved mortality in the 66% who actually took the drug as prescribed.

The answer to this question was provided by a per-protocol analysis in which adherers were compared to non-adherers within the clofibrate group. The results, presented on the left in Fig. 8.3, show a big difference on mortality suggesting that the drug worked in those who actually took it as prescribed. But what makes this example so famous is that the investigators did the same thing in the placebo group and found the

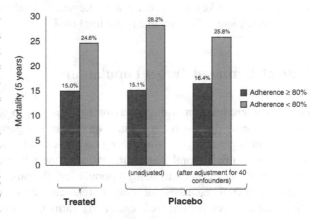

Fig. 8.3 Comparison between adherence ($\geq 80\%$) and non-adherence ($<80\%$) within the treated and placebo arms of the Coronary Drug Project [46]. No difference on overall trial result: 18% mortality in those treated with clofibrate; 19.5% mortality in placebo (ns)

same result (Fig. 8.3, middle). Those who actually took the placebo capsules as prescribed had lower mortality than those who did not. Since the randomization, and thus the comparability between groups, was broken, there was an obvious need to adjust statistically for baseline factors that differed between adherers and non-adherers in the placebo group. Adjustment for 40 factors that could confound the relationship produced similar results (Fig. 8.3, right). Those who adhered to placebo still had lower mortality than those who did not, after adjustment for a wide variety of known confounders.

It is clear from this example that unmeasured and/or unknown confounders which may reflect general health consciousness were responsible for the results. Random assignment provided balance on these unknown confounders. The investigators concluded that it was difficult if not impossible to find a valid comparator for the subgroup of adherers in the treated arm because reasons for non-adherence are not well understood, may differ across arms, and thus create imbalance which cannot be handled statistically [46].

OVERCOMING THESE CHALLENGES IN A BEHAVIORAL TRIAL

A valid result in a clinical trial is based, in part, upon obtaining complete and accurate follow-up information for a representative, randomized cohort [17]. The following are some key areas that can be targeted to inform representativeness and achieve complete follow-up in a behavioral trial.

Patient-Centered Target Populations

Patient-centeredness provides behavioral treatments to those who need and want them. It is easier to assess need than want. Need is generally defined as medical need. Want is generally subordinate to need. But despite investigator enthusiasm for the merits of a behavioral treatment, not everyone who needs it wants it. When the priority is on a representative target population, the push is to get potential participants into a trial regardless of their preferences. When the priority is on a close alignment between patient preference and treatment, patient-centered eligibility criteria, recruitment, and informed consent should be used.

Patient-Centered Eligibility

Eligibility criteria for a behavioral efficacy trial are a combination of eligibility to achieve the target population to whom one wants to generalize and eligibility based upon the requirements of the trial protocol (see box). The target population is fixed, and these criteria do not vary throughout behavioral treatment development. They aim to identify a population who is able to benefit medically without compromising safety, representative of those with the disease on such characteristics as gender, ethnicity, age, and socioeconomic status, and able and motivated to undergo a behavioral treatment. The trial protocol requirements vary depending upon the goal of the study. In an efficacy trial where the premium is on internal validity, requirements include an ability to complete the protocol based upon an absence of competing medical risks or logistical barriers, a willingness to be randomized, and a willingness to adhere to trial and treatment protocols. Because trial protocol eligibility produces the subset of the target population who is willing and able to participate in a clinical trial, generalizability is compromised. In effectiveness trials where the premium is on external validity, these criteria are often relaxed. Because trial pro-

Two types of eligibility criteria in an efficacy trial		
ELIGIBILITY CRITERION	**TARGET POPULATION**	**TRIAL PROTOCOL**
MEDICAL	Able to benefit medically	Able to complete follow-up
DEMOGRAPHIC	Representative of the population at risk	Absence of barriers to protocol implementation
BEHAVIORAL	Motivated to undergo behavioral treatment	Motivated to adhere to treatment and trial protocols
LOGISTICAL		Able to receive intervention

tocol eligibility is relaxed in these studies, which tend to take "all comers" regardless of their ability to complete the trial protocol, internal validity is compromised. The importance of these respective goals, but the difficulty in achieving all of them in the same trial, is the basis for progressive translational research.

Patient-centered eligibility focuses on the criteria used to identify the target population. Most eligibility criteria for a behavioral clinical trial exclude patients for medical or logistical contraindications. But they vary in their approach to behavioral eligibility. Patient-centered eligibility is sensitive to patient preferences. These preferences can be assessed indirectly using run-in periods or directly using specific questions.

Run-in periods make behavioral eligibility contingent on performance of actual behaviors essential to trial evaluation. They tend to focus on such trial protocol requirements as self-monitoring, completion of selected assessments, and/or attendance at scheduled visits. But they can also be an indirect measure of motivation. The more extensive the run-in, the more motivated a prospective participant must be to complete it successfully. Eligibility based upon successful completion of a run-in has been shown to enhance adherence to treatment and reduce attrition from a trial [47–49].

It is more difficult to make eligibility contingent upon answers to questions that assess motivation or intention. Indeed, motivation may be an intrapersonal characteristic that may or may not be known even to the prospective participant. Motivation may be best judged by an informed prospective participant. A specific list of all of the actions and behaviors that are required by a treatment may help the prospective participant better understand the time commitment involved and whether it can be accomodated given the demands already faced in his/her life. Single questions predict treatment success and can be used to initiate discussions about fit. For example, a pre-contemplator will state that they have no interest in making any changes now or in the near future. A person who is destined for success at weight loss may be identified by a single question about his/her degree of confidence in sustaining physical activity [50, 51].

Patient-centered eligibility aims to produce a target population that not only needs, but also wants, a behavioral intervention. This accurately reflects those to whom the results of a behavioral trial can be generalized. A *Phase II* or *Phase III* behavioral efficacy trial is confirmatory. It is a place to evaluate how well a treatment works in those who are well aligned with it. It is not a place to enhance motivation to try it. This latter goal is important but better placed in early treatment development activities, such as those proposed by the ORBIT model [52]. A target population that needs and wants a behavioral treatment will maximize the internal validity of the trial by minimizing differential dropout, minimizing confounding, and reducing the need for per-protocol analyses. It is also likely that it will maximize the overall success rate for behavioral trials.

Patient-Centered Recruitment

Prospective participants for a clinical trial make decisions based upon whether they need and want a particular treatment and whether they want to participate in a trial. This calculus involves a variety of considerations including, for example, strength of preference for a treatment, likelihood of getting it in the trial, burden imposed by trial participation, and the life context within which participation is set. Patient-centered recruitment encourages prospective participants to consider all of these criteria carefully when making a decision about whether or not to participate in a behavioral trial.

Successful recruitment in a clinical trial is characterized by meeting recruitment goals on time, maximizing the diversity of participants who are at risk for the disease, and recruiting those who are well aligned with the treatment. There is a large literature on overcoming barriers to recruitment. Table 8.4 provides a selective summary, identifying four key barriers: access, burden, distrust, and ambivalence. The challenge of reaching the target population tends to be overcome by using multiple methods, including internet and social media approaches and the innovative use of approaches that have been successful in the marketing literature. The challenge of the burden of participation can be overcome by making use of the internet and electronic medical records to simplify recruitment and treatment and by reducing extensive assessment batteries. The challenge of distrust is most effectively overcome by drawing on community-based participatory approaches which create partnerships with trusted community leaders, organizations, and individuals.

But the "elephant in the room" that receives far less attention is how to recruit the prospective participant who is ambivalent (i.e., has mixed feelings about participating) or reluctant (i.e., hesitant to participate). The most common approach is the

Table 8.4 Recruitment challenges and ways to overcome them		
Barrier	**Challenge**	**Approach**

Access [53–59]	Patient-centered information does not reach the target population	• Recruitment materials:
		  – Professionally designed
		  – Use marketing principles
		• Multiple recruitment methods
		• Personalized telephone follow-up

Burden [53, 59–64]	Enrollment and intervention are time and resource intensive	• Recruit using internet, phone, social media, mobile devices, electronic medical records, registries • Intervene with minimal inconvenience using technology, flexible schedules, convenient locations, compensation for time and travel, and limited assessment batteries

Distrust [59, 65–69]	Special populations distrust research and researchers	• Community-based participatory approaches
		  – Community advisory board
		  – Community health workers
		  – Community recruitment and treatment sites (e.g., barber shops, churches)

Ambivalence [17, 70, 71]	Recruitment demands reduce time needed to convert reluctance into participation	• Realistic recruitment plans based upon prior recruitment feasibility study • Run-in periods before randomization to assess adherence • Sequential recruitment process providing opportunity to consider pros and cons of participation

"hard sell," fostered by the reality, in most trials, of recruitment that lags behind milestones and the pressure put on recruiters to recruit more and faster. Under this pressure, reluctance and ambivalence tends to be converted by taking a "pro-enrollment" position which reinforces the pros for participating and problem-solves around the cons. Unfortunately, the "hard sell" approach may result in a Pyrrhic victory characterized by a short-term gain followed by a long-term loss. A participant may agree to enroll, only to vote with his/her feet later by not adhering to the treatment and weakening its effect size, and/or by dropping out and compromising the randomization. This is particularly problematic for a behavioral trial where something about the arm to which one is randomized encourages differential dropout.

An alternative to this "hard sell" approach to converting ambivalence is the innovative method provided by Goldberg and Kiernan [71]. Through the vehicle of a group-based orientation session held several weeks prior to randomization, a prospective participant is provided with the opportunity to explore his/her ambivalence by helping him/her understand what is involved in participation, what is

required by the science of the trial, and how realistic it is for the prospective participant to meet the requirements of the trial. During the orientation, staff use motivational interviewing techniques to provide the prospective participant with the
opportunity to articulate explicitly the pros and cons of being randomized to the
treatment arm and, equally important, the comparator arm. The group makes it possible for potential participants to listen to each other's pros and cons, thus fleshing
out a full range of reasons. Prospective participants are then explicitly asked to
reflect on the pros and cons over the upcoming week before deciding whether they
want to continue by moving to baseline assessment. In a descriptive study of this
approach in a behavioral weight management trial [71], 71% of the 228 who attended
the orientation session went on to be randomized into the trial. Of the 162 who were
randomized, 159 (98%) completed the 6-month follow-up, and 156 (96%) completed the final 18-month follow-up. There was no differential dropout by trial arm.

By giving prospective participants the time to evaluate the pros and cons of participation, there will be a certain percentage who will opt out. In the Goldberg and
Kiernan study above, this was 29% of those who expressed initial interest. When
given the time to make this decision without pressure from the investigators, they
decided that they were not well aligned with the trial. Generalizability of results
from this trial will be to those who need and want the treatments under consideration. Acceptance of a decision not to participate in some who express initial interest is a way to show respect for potential participants. Moreover, those who decide
that they are well aligned with the trial will be less likely to drop out or fail to adhere
to the protocols, maximizing a conclusive result. More empirical studies are needed
in this important area.

Patient-Centered Consent

Informed consent procedures were instituted to protect participants from getting
involved in studies in which they are unaware of the risks [72]. But often informed
consent procedures are cryptic, excessively long, and confusing. They may cover all
of the legal bases, but the price is in prospective participant comprehension. Patient-
centeredness maximizes the ability of prospective participants to understand fully
what they are getting themselves into before, rather than after, they are randomized.

An excellent example of how to do this comes from the literature on placebo effects
[73]. A clinical trial evaluated the value of arthroscopic surgery for knee osteoarthritis. Participants were randomized to one of three arms. Two arms were for real surgeries, but the third arm was for a sham surgery that simulated the actual activities
involved in the real surgeries. Under the guidance of Baruch Brody, the clinical trial
ethicist, prospective participants underwent standard informed consent procedures.
But in addition, they were asked to write, in their own hand, the following.

> *"On entering this study, I realize I may receive only placebo surgery. I further realize that
> this means that I will not have surgery on my knee joint. This placebo surgery will not
> benefit my knee arthritis." [73]*

The results of this trial both at the 1-year and the 2-year follow-ups were that all three arms showed benefit on a subjective measure of pain and an objective measure of physical function. There was no difference in benefit across the three arms. The sham surgery was as effective as the real surgeries.

This informed consent procedure resulted in 44% of the eligible prospective participants declining to participate. This high rate of nonparticipation suggests that participants completely understood that they had a one-third chance of getting sham surgery without any known benefit. In the calculus of their decision-making, these patients may have decided that a 33% chance of getting a sham treatment was not worth the demand of the trial protocol to undergo a surgery that simulated in every detail what would have been required by a real surgery.

Of the 56% who did participate, there was greater than 90% completion of the 2-year follow-up assessments in all three arms. The patient-centered informed consent protected the random assignment and thus the internal validity of the trial. But there was no benefit of surgery over sham. In the calculus of their decision-making, the participants may have been more willing to take the 66% chance of getting the real surgery relative to the nonparticipants. But if these "risk takers" also happened to be more susceptible to the placebo effect (i.e., an unknown confounder), a selection bias resulting from the rigor of the control group could have attenuated detection of a true benefit from the arthroscopic surgery. If the goal of the trial was to disentangle non-specific from active treatment components, the rigorous sham control was the optimum choice. But if the goal was to evaluate the benefit of the surgery on outcomes, selection bias could have underestimated the true benefit if those most likely to respond to surgery, but not placebo, did not participate. A comparator that was linked closely to this goal of the trial, such as current drug treatment for knee pain, may have been a better choice. *(See Chapter 6: The Choice of a Comparator.)*

Other techniques that have been used to maximize prospective participant understanding of what is involved in a trial include the use of participant-centered videotapes explaining the trial [74], short, simple descriptions (e.g., *A placebo pill is an inert or inactive pill, like a sugar pill, without any medication in it.*) [75], and a request to have the prospective participant reiterate out loud, or in their own handwriting, what is involved in the trial from his/her perspective [73]. The point of all of these techniques is to insure that prospective participants fully understand the nature of the trial and what they are expected to do, thereby maximizing the chance that once they are randomized they will stick with it and random assignment will be protected.

Patient-Centered Retention

There is some imprecision in the way retention issues are described. Retention can refer to adherence/compliance to a treatment protocol or to a trial protocol. It can be phrased in the positive (i.e., adherence, compliance) or in the negative (i.e., dropout, withdrawal, non-adherence). For purposes of this discussion, retention, attrition, and dropouts refer to the trial protocol, while adherence and compliance refer to the treatment protocols. Low retention jeopardizes the random assignment and opens the door to confounding. Non-adherence to the treatments weakens the efficacy of the intervention and thus reduces the effect size of the trial.

Recruitment and retention are linked. The broader the eligibility criteria for a trial, the greater the risk of poor retention. The push to recruit can result in successfully meeting recruitment goals, but if it results in poorer than expected retention, the success is short-lived. The goal is to find ways to achieve recruitment success while also retaining those recruited. Once a participant is enrolled, retention is essential for protecting randomization.

A number of strategies have been identified to enhance retention (Table 8.5). Although all are important, perhaps the most important is the participant experience. In most behavioral or prevention-oriented trials where the discomfort from a disease is minimal, adherence to a trial protocol may become relatively unimportant when faced with more immediate problems that compete for attention such as schedule conflicts, family demands, transportation problems, lack of time, and too

Table 8.5 Common retention strategies

Focus of Strategy	Description
Design of trial [76–78]	– Minimize time commitment for intervention and assessments – Avoid uncomfortable, invasive tests
Recruitment [38, 76, 79]	– Obtain permission to contact family – Involve family in consent – Screen out those unable to adhere to protocol – Include a run-in to assess motivation, commitment, availability
Follow-up [38, 62, 76, 77, 79]	– Increasing financial rewards for each follow-up visit – Provide transportation or reimburse for its cost – Maintain regular contact with participant: mobile phone, newsletters, trial results – Maintain continuous community contact: trial procedures, trial results, risks vs benefits
Participant Experience [38, 80]	– Show gratitude – Provide support – Provide opportunities for meaningful social activity – Facilitate positive experiences

much stress [81]. Participant perception of the trial being associated with warm, supportive people, enjoyable activities, and pleasurable emotions may be the most powerful way to enhance retention. Budgeting time and resources for these activities proves to be well worth the effort.

Secondary "Per-Protocol" Analyses

Protection of random assignment translates into an analytic strategy called *intent-to-treat* in which all randomized participants are included regardless of their level of participation. This can present a "perfect storm" for the behavioral trialist caused by three interrelated "squalls." (1) The demand for participant volition combined with long follow-ups raises the risk of non-adherence and dropouts. (2) Analyses of results using all who were initially randomized, regardless of the dose of treatment received, weaken the efficacy of a treatment and undercut power to detect a benefit. (3) Some questions of interest require a different analytic strategy, such as *How much benefit is there for those able to adhere to the treatment?* This "perfect storm" can be resolved by establishing primary and secondary analyses. Priority in any clinical trial, regardless of the context, is to get a conclusive result on the primary outcome. This is accomplished by minimizing the possibility of confounding through the protection of random assignment and analyzing results as "intent-to-treat." But this may be a Faustian bargain. It may be equivalent to selling one's soul by sacrificing a question of interest in pursuit of methodological purity. Clinicians and policy-makers may need to make decisions based upon evidence about whether or not a treatment works in those who choose to adhere to it.

Secondary analyses can explore "per-protocol" effects of treatment in those who adhered to it. Because such analyses break the balance achieved by randomization, they are subject to confounding which requires appropriate covariate adjustment and clear interpretations that acknowledge the problems of unmeasured and unknown confounding. Alternatively, incorporation of a measure of adherence in the assessment protocol, and testing adherence by treatment interactions in multivariate models, can help to estimate the magnitude of the effect of adherence, as well as the differential effect of adherence by trial arm, on the outcome [81]. These secondary analyses, however, are hypothesis generating. A new test of this treatment, after it has been refined to improve adherence, would be needed using intent-to-treat analyses as the primary analytic strategy.

The combination of a primary "intent-to-treat" analysis with a secondary "per-protocol" analysis provides a thorough understanding of trial results [82]. But even this approach is not without its limitations [83]. However, the designation of primary and secondary analyses resolves the temptation to forego the methodologic beauty of the randomized design in pursuit of a question that is important but more difficult to answer.

SELECTED EXPERIENCE FROM BEHAVIORAL TRIALS

Behavioral Eligibility in a Successful Behavioral Clinical Trial

The Diabetes Prevention Program (DPP) was among the greatest successes ever achieved by a behavioral clinical trial [84]. In this trial of insulin-resistant patients, a lifestyle intervention reduced the incidence of diabetes by 58% compared to placebo pill and by 31% compared to metformin, the drug of choice.

What is often not recognized, however, is that the population under study was highly selected [85, 86]. Of the 158,000 people screened at 27 clinical centers, 30,986 were deemed to qualify based upon objective evidence of being insulin resistant. Of these, 3234 were randomized into one of three arms. Eligible participants were nondiabetic but with a high risk of progressing to Type II diabetes during the trial follow-up period. Ineligible participants had conditions which increased risk of adverse events from the interventions, shortened life expectancy, interfered with the conduct of the trial, or affected the assessment of Type II diabetes. The trial population turned out to be 2.1% of those screened and 10.4% of those who were screened and found to be insulin resistant.

Eligibility also included behavioral eligibility. To get into the trial, prospective participants had to successfully complete four screening steps that took place over 4–13 weeks, and were ordered by progressive levels of difficulty and expense. At Step 1, a simple fasting or casual glucose measurement was undertaken. At Step 2, an oral glucose tolerance test was administered after a 12–14-hour fast in which no smoking, exercise, or any unusual activity was permitted. At Step 3, a 3-week run-in was undertaken to assess adherence to placebo pills and willingness to undergo detailed record-keeping of diet and physical activity. At Step 4, a pregnancy test for women and a final checklist for eligibility were used to determine eligibility for randomization.

It is likely that the 10.4% of insulin-resistant participants in this trial were a highly selected and highly motivated subgroup of all participants at risk. They underwent progressive tests over 4–13 weeks giving them ample time to consider both the pros and cons of participating in both the trial and in the treatment, if they were randomized to receive it. At the stage where a causal inference about the efficacy of a treatment is needed, the DPP investigators protected the random assignment and thus the internal validity of the trial by selecting motivated participants whose alignment with the treatment was demonstrated by their success with a prolonged run-in.

Despite this selectivity, the DPP has had far-reaching implications and is a testament to progressive translational research. It opened the door to a large number of effectiveness studies that evaluated the DPP program in such community settings as the YMCA, churches, and medical clinics for the underserved. It formed the basis for success at achieving third-party reimbursement for the costs of undergoing this program.

Some have argued that the "trickle down" model of translating efficacy trial findings into practice is flawed, and use this as a justification for broad eligibility criteria which result in great diversity in participants [37]. But the DPP has shown the flaw in this argument. This efficacy trial did indeed "trickle down" to effectiveness studies and clinical practice. This is an excellent example of the spirit of progressive translational research where the best candidates for evaluation in effectiveness studies are those interventions that have been shown to be efficacious.

Failure to Protect Random Assignment

In the early 1980s, there was mounting evidence that periods of emotional stress precede acute ischemic heart disease episodes. Therefore, Frasure-Smith and Prince [87] reasoned that monitoring stress in post-heart attack patients and, when stress was high, sending a nurse to the home to intervene as needed could be a simple and cost-effective approach to the prevention of recurrent events. They randomized 769 post-heart attack men to treatment or standard care, conducted a 1-year nurse intervention, and followed participants for an average of 5 years to examine mortality and cardiovascular recurrences [87, 88].

Figure 8.4 presents the design of the trial. The IRB required informed consent to be obtained *after* participants were randomized to a trial arm to make it possible for prospective participants to have an accurate understanding of what was required for participation. Thus, participants provided consent to participate in the arm to which they were randomized. This approach resulted in a large dropout rate and, perhaps more importantly, a differential dropout rate.

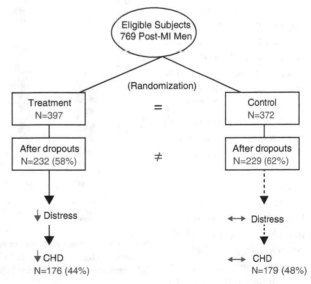

Fig. 8.4 Dropouts in the Ischemic Heart Disease Life Stress Monitoring Program [88]

Approximately 40% of the randomized participants dropped out before the treatment began, thus compromising the balance achieved by the initial randomization. But different types of people dropped out of each of the treatment arms. In the treated arm, more participants of lower socioeconomic status dropped out, possibly because of the requirement that nurses come to the home. In the control arm, more participants of higher socioeconomic status dropped out, possibly because they saw participation as a waste of time.

Differential dropout opened the door to confounding between treatment arm and socioeconomic status. Participants in the treated arm were of higher socioeconomic status, and participants in the control arm were of lower socioeconomic status (Fig. 8.5).

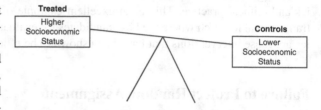

Fig. 8.5 Confound between treatment arm and socioeconomic status in the Ischemic Heart Disease Life Stress Monitoring Program [88]

During the course of the 5-year follow-up, more participants were lost from each arm, ending up with only 44% and 48% of the original randomized participants in the treated and control arms, respectively.

The results of the trial on mortality at the end of the program year are portrayed in the two bars at the left in Fig. 8.6. There were almost twice as many cardiac deaths in the controls as there were in the treated ($p = 0.07$) [87]. But the large and differential dropout rates provided an alternative explanation: men of higher socioeconomic status had lower mortality than men of lower socioeconomic status [89]. Because of the confounding between treatment arm and socioeconomic status, and the inability to control for this

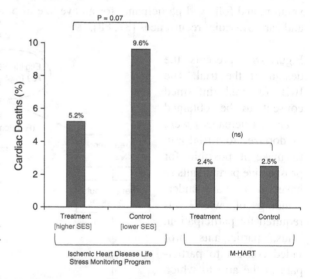

Fig. 8.6 Comparison of cardiac deaths in men in the Ischemic Heart Disease Life Stress Monitoring Program [88] and the M-HART trial [90]

confounder because of missing data, the trial was inconclusive.

It was important, however, to answer the question of the efficacy of this innovative treatment which was tailored, low cost, and simple to implement. This was the rationale for conducting a replication of the trial to obtain a more conclusive answer to the question of the efficacy of this treatment. The M-HART trial randomized 1376 post-heart attack men and women [90]. This time around the investigators were successful in preserving the randomization by following up all of the 1376 participants. The results on mortality in the men only are presented in the two bars on the right in Fig. 8.6. There was no impact on mortality ($p = 0.94$) [90]. This suggests that the benefit seen in the men in the earlier trial was likely due to confounding by socio-economic status rather than to the efficacy of the treatment.

More importantly for purposes here, it illustrates why the most important job of a behavioral trialist is to protect the random assignment. Clinical trials examining important disease endpoints draw upon considerable resources in terms of investigator, staff, and participant time and money. This large expenditure of resources puts the onus on the investigator to get a conclusive answer, regardless of whether the answer is positive or negative. When confounding provides a viable alternative explanation for results, the trial is inconclusive. This type of problem generally can only be fixed by more expenditure of time and resources in a replication.

The Power of "Per-Protocol" Secondary Analyses

In the mid-2000s, the American College of Cardiology, the American Heart Association, the European Society of Cardiology, and the Canadian Cardiovascular Society adopted recommendations that exercise be considered for medically stable patients with systolic heart failure. But the safety and effectiveness of exercise in patients whose life-threatening illness was characterized by fatigue and shortness of breath upon exertion were based upon a limited number of small studies. The HF-ACTION trial was designed to provide a more definitive evaluation of efficacy and safety of exercise in patients with systolic heart failure [91]. Between 2003 and 2007, 2331 medically stable patients with systolic heart failure were randomized at 82 centers in the United States, Canada, and France and followed for a median of 2.5 years to ascertain the impact of aerobic exercise on the combined primary endpoint of all-cause mortality or all-cause hospitalization. Patients were randomized into usual care or usual care plus exercise. To enhance implementation of exercise at home, patients in the exercise arm were given a heart rate monitor and either a stationary bike or a treadmill. The target training regimen was exercise five times/week for 40 minutes at a heart rate of 60–70% of heart rate reserve. The assumptions in the sample size calculations were to provide 90% power to detect an 11% reduction in the primary endpoint.

The exercise prescription was a challenge in this patient population. At all time points, 60% of the patients in the treatment arm were not exercising at goal [91].

This high non-adherence rate was a major contributor to HF-ACTION being a null trial (Fig. 8.7a). In the investigators' words:

"Despite extensive efforts, adherence to the exercise training regimen may have diminished the study's ability to detect a significant effect of exercise on the primary outcome." [91]

In subsequent papers, the investigators evaluated the safety and efficacy of exercise in the 40% who met exercise goals. This was the "per-protocol" question. It was of considerable clinical importance but was unanswered by the primary results of the trial which were based upon intent-to-treat analyses.

The answer was provided by a retrospective analysis of the prospective data [92]. In this analysis, 959 participants (83% of the total) who were randomized to the exercise arm and were free of a primary event during the first 3 months were included. The randomized clinical trial design was abandoned, and the design of this study was to categorize the sample into five levels of exercise achieved using MET-hours/week. Because the comparison was within only one of the randomized arms, the design became similar to a

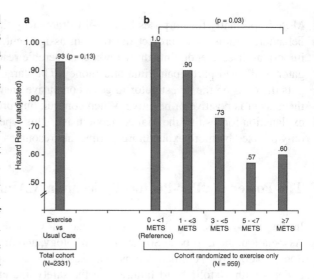

Fig. 8.7 Reduction in risk of all-cause mortality or hospitalization: (a) between exercise and usual care in the total cohort and (b) by METS of exercise/week in the exercise arm only

prospective study, and confounding could create an alternative explanation for any results found. The investigators identified 60 candidate baseline variables, constructed 5 complete datasets that featured different assumptions for missing variables, and arrived at 19 covariates that were associated with the primary outcome and therefore adjusted in the analyses. In Fig. 8.7b, the results of the per-protocol analysis are presented. An inverse J-shaped distribution between level of exercise and the primary endpoint was observed. Benefit appeared to occur at moderate levels of exercise, achieved by about 4 MET-hours/week of exercise, the equivalent of walking at 1.7 mph for 26 minutes four times/week. This moderate exercise goal is important because it could enhance motivation to adhere to exercise in a vulnerable heart failure population.

But the "per-protocol" analysis had limitations. The most important limitations were the risk of selection bias and confounding by unmeasured variables. In the investigators' words:

"Participants who expressed interest in exercise may have been healthier, adhered better to any medical treatment, more physically able, and more likely to undertake an exercise regimen . . .

Although we controlled for many possible confounders, models may not have included all variables related to adherence or clinical endpoints . . .

A sufficiently powered prospective trial that randomly assigned subjects to different exercise levels is warranted to establish a causal relationship."

The combination of the "intent-to-treat" and "per-protocol" analyses provided a complete picture of the value of exercise in systolic heart failure patients. It was safe, and, in those who are able and willing, it *may* provide benefit on definitive clinical outcomes. This conclusion was convincing. The HF-ACTION investigators joined with leaders of the largest professional societies in cardiology to incorporate, into ACC/AHA guidelines, light to moderate exercise as a Class I recommendation for patients with systolic heart failure [93]. The inclusion of exercise into guidelines resulted in success in achieving expanded coverage by Medicare and Medicaid for exercise training to beneficiaries with stable, chronic systolic heart failure [94].

RECOMMENDATIONS

The most important job of the behavioral trialist in a confirmatory *Phase II* or *Phase III* efficacy trial is to protect the random assignment for the purpose of controlling confounding and maximizing causal inferences. Several recommendations can encourage success.

The Primacy of a Conclusive Result

The primary consideration in a clinical trial should always be to get a conclusive result [17]. The essential rationale for protecting random assignment is to obtain a conclusive result. An inconclusive result occurs when there is an alternative explanation for the outcome of a trial [95]. The risk of confounding is great in the presence of the background noise that surrounds most trials in humans. Contrast this to the experimental control that is possible with laboratory studies. Even if key confounders are identified, the possibility that unmeasured confounders loom in the background remains. This is why measuring, stratifying, and adjusting for potential confounders in analyses is a poor solution that provides false security. These approaches are useful adjuncts to random assignment but do not supplant it. Random assignment, avoidance of post-randomization exclusions and biases, minimizing losses and withdrawals, and analyzing using the intent-to-treat principle may not be a perfect approach to control confounding, but it is the best available. Therefore, the maxim in clinical trial methodology holds:

"Once randomized, always analyzed."

The Target Population for a Behavioral Clinical Trial

The future of behavioral treatments, and the trials designed to assess their efficacy, is rapidly moving toward precision lifestyle medicine [96–99] which goes beyond *one size fits all* in favor of tailoring a behavioral treatment to those patients most likely to benefit from it. Those most likely to benefit are those who are willing to participate actively.

A patient-centered target population for a behavioral trial is a population that both needs and wants the behavioral intervention. This shows respect for those patients who prefer drug management, or no management at all, relative to the prospect of having to change their behavior. Such respect can come from shifting the status quo away from representativeness based upon only on medical considerations and moving toward a new status quo that aims to generalize to those who can benefit medically and are motivated behaviorally.

Respect also comes from sensitivity to the complex calculus a prospective patient undergoes when considering the pros and cons of participation in a behavioral trial. This is not an easy decision. It requires consideration of one's preference for treatment(s), the randomness of actually getting it, the constraints imposed by the trial evaluation, and the life context within which participation will be placed.

We have to live with the fact that not all of the participants who could benefit medically and behaviorally will be participants in behavioral efficacy trials. The spirit of translational research accepts this fact and pushes for effectiveness studies with more representative participants at later stages in the translational spectrum. This progression relaxes trial protocol criteria and includes more participants who generally do not like to participate in clinical trials. But this progression does not influence the target population to whom results should be generalized.

The target population for a behavioral treatment should be identified early in treatment development and be consistent across the translational spectrum. It should represent those who both need and want a behavioral treatment. If a closer link between a behavioral treatment and participants likely to benefit from it were made, it is likely that behavioral treatments would be more relevant and behavioral trials would have a greater record of success.

Attention to Retention

A *Phase III* behavioral trial with a chronic disease endpoint is likely to have a long follow-up period. As the length of follow-up increases, the risk of non-adherence and dropout increases. This is a particular problem for prevention trials where participants often do not experience any symptoms. It is not uncommon that once a life event occurs, it takes precedence and the participant is at risk for non-adherence to the treatment and/or dropping out of the trial.

Behavioral trials should pay close attention to retention. As Delia West has observed in her lectures on retention, once a participant is randomized, they are *"yours to raise."* Perhaps we know more about "raising" than we think. Immediate positive reinforcers are more powerful incentives for behavior than distal negative reinforcers. This translates into the participant experience with the trial. Every contact, whether it is for treatment or some part of an outcome assessment, should be as enjoyable as possible. Intervention protocols should be simple. Assessment protocols should be minimal and easy to complete. Everything about the trial should be associated with immediate positive benefits from the participant's perspective. This may be as important as money and more important than concern about some future medical event.

Large budgets for retention activities should be a part of all behavioral trials. These budgets should go beyond holiday and birthday cards and provide immediate benefits in terms of logistical assistance, social interactions, appreciation incentives, food, and the time needed to develop relationships of mutual respect. All staff that have contact with participants should be hired based upon their superior interpersonal skills. Respecting the participant is protecting the random assignment. This is the most important goal of the behavioral trialist.

Investigate Non-Adherence

It is a false dichotomy to argue for either "intent-to-treat" or "per-protocol" analyses. It is poor trial design to lead with "per-protocol" or responder-only analyses. Behavioral trials would be most persuasive if they integrated both of these types of analyses. The preservation of "intent-to-treat" as the primary analysis is a commitment to understanding if a relationship between a treatment and an outcome is causal. But this does not mean that adherence should be ignored.

The best approach to non-adherence is, of course, to minimize it. Exploration of ways to minimize non-adherence is an ideal goal for early intervention development studies. But despite these efforts, non-adherence is always going to occur. Estimates of non-adherence should be incorporated into sample size calculations, similar to what is done with estimates for dropout rates. Non-adherence should be studied carefully during a trial by collecting both qualitative and quantitative data, using adherence as a covariate in secondary analyses, and/or pairing the primary analysis with "per-protocol" analyses [32, 81]. Greater sophistication in solving this problem may come from methods to estimate a "complier average causal effect" which are in development.

REFERENCES

1. Bull JP (1959) The historical development of clinical therapeutic trials. J Chron Dis 10:218–248
2. Armitage P (1982) The role of randomization in clinical trials. Stat Med 1:345–352
3. Van Helmont JB (1662) Oriatrike or Physik Refined. In Debus AG (1968) The chemical dream of the renaissance. Heffer, London
4. Peirce CS, Jastrow J (1884) Fifth memoir: on small differences of sensation. Ntl Acad Sci 3:73–83
5. Yule G (1924) The function of statistical method in scientific investigation. Industrial Health Research Board Report 28. His Majesty's Stationery Office, London
6. Eliot MM (1925) The control of rickets: preliminary discussion of the demonstration in New Haven. JAMA 85:656–663
7. Hill AB (1952) The clinical trial. New Engl J Med 247:113–119
8. Hill AB (1953) Observation and experiment. New Engl J Med 248:995–1001
9. Sinclair HM (1951) Nutritional surveys of population groups. New Engl J Med 245:39–47
10. Mill JS (1843) A system of logic ratiocinative and inductive. Being a connected view of the principles of evidence and the methods of scientific investigation. Book I. In Robson JM (ed). The collected works of John Stuart Mill (1974). University of Toronto Press, Toronto
11. Hill AB (1965) The environment and disease: association or causation. Proc Roy Soc Med 58:295–300
12. Wang D, Bakhai A (2006) Clinical trials: a practical guide to design, analysis, and reporting. Remedica, London
13. Domanski M, McKinlay S (2009) Successful randomized trials. A handbook for the 21st century. Lippincott Williams & Wilkins, Philadelphia
14. Friedman LM, Furberg CD, DeMets D, Reboussin DH, Granger CB (2015) Fundamentals of clinical trials, 5th edn. Springer, Cham
15. Rothman KJ, Greenland S, Lash TL (2008) Modern epidemiology, 3rd edn. Lippincott Williams & Wilkins, Philadelphia
16. Szklo M, Nieto FJ (2019) Epidemiology: beyond the basics, 4th edn. Jones & Bartlett Learning, Burlington
17. Hennekens CH, Buring JE, Mayrent SL (1987) Epidemiology in medicine. Little Brown, Boston
18. Susser M (1973) Causal thinking in the health sciences: Concepts and strategies of epidemiology. Oxford University Press, New York
19. Fisher RA (1951) The design of experiments, 6th edn. Hafner, New York
20. Shadish WR, Cook TD, Campbell DT (2002) Experimental and quasi-experimental designs for generalized causal inference. Houghton Mifflin, Boston
21. Byar DP, Simon RM, Friedewald WT, Schlesselman JJ, DeMets D, Ellenberg JH, Gail MH, Ware JH (1976) Randomized clinical trials--perspectives on some recent ideas. N Engl J Med 295:74–80
22. Moher D, Hopewell S, Schulz KF, Montori V, Gotzche PC, Devereaux PJ, Elbourne D, Egger M, Altman DG (2010) CONSORT 2010 explanation and elaboration: updated guidelines for reporting parallel group randomised trials. BMJ 340:c869. https://doi.org/10.1136/bmj.c869
23. Mosteller F, Gilbert JP, McPeek B (1980) Reporting standards and research strategies for controlled trials. Control Clin Trials 1:37–58

24. Schulz KF, Chalmers I, Hayes RJ, Altman DG (1995) Empirical evidence of bias. Dimensions of methodological quality associated with estimates of treatment effects in controlled trials. JAMA 273:408–412
25. CONSORT Group (2010) CONSORT checklist. www.consort-statement.org
26. Schulz KF, Altman DG, Moher D, CONSORT Group (2010) CONSORT 2010 statement: updated guidelines for reporting parallel group randomized trials. Ann Intern Med 152:726–732
27. Zwarenstein M, Treweek S, Gagnier JJ, Altman DG, Tunis S, Haynes B, Oxman AD, Moher D, and for the CONSORT and Pragmatic Trials in Healthcare (Practihc) groups (2008) Improving the reporting of pragmatic trials: an extension of the CONSORT statement. BMJ 337:a2390. https://doi.org/10.1136/bmj.a2390
28. Schulz KF (1995) Subverting randomization in controlled trials. JAMA 274:1456–1458
29. Kraemer HC (2015) A source of false findings in published research studies: adjusting for covariates. JAMA Psychiatry 72:961–962
30. Pocock SJ, Assmann SE, Enos LE, Kasten LE (2002) Subgroup analysis, covariate adjustment and baseline comparisons in clinical trial reporting: current practice and problems. Stat Med 21:2917–2930
31. Schulz KF, Grimes DA, Altman DG, Hayes RJ (1996) Blinding and exclusions after allocation in randomised controlled trials: survey of published parallel group trials in obstetrics and gynaecology. BMJ 312:742–744
32. Detry MA, Lewis RJ (2014) The intention-to-treat principle: how to assess the true effect of choosing a medical treatment. JAMA 312:85–86
33. Freedman B (1987) Equipoise and the ethics of clinical research. N Eng J Med 317:141–145
34. Green SB, Byar DP (1984) Using observational data from registries to compare treatments: the fallacy of omnimetrics. Stat Med 3:361–373
35. Hollon SD, Wampold BE (2009) Are randomized controlled trials relevant to clinical practice? Can J Psychiatry 54:637–643
36. Cook TD, Campbell DT (1979) Quasi-experimentation: Design and analysis issues for field settings. Houghton Mifflin, Boston
37. Glasgow RE, Lichtenstein E, Marcus AC (2003) Why don't we see more translation of health promotion research to practice? Rethinking the efficacy-to-effectiveness transition. Am J Public Health 93:1261–1267
38. Areán PA, Kraemer HC (2013) High-quality psychotherapy research: From conception to piloting to national trials. Oxford University Press, New York
39. Brownell KD, Wadden TA (1992) Etiology and treatment of obesity: understanding a serious, prevalent, and refractory disorder. J Consult Clin Psychol 60:505–517
40. Prochaska JO, DiClemente CC, Norcross JC (1992) In search of how people change: Applications to addictive behaviors. Am Psychol 47:1102–1114
41. Hall SM, Tsoh JY, Prochaska JJ, Eisendrath S, Rossi JS, Redding CA, Rosen AB, Meisner M, Humfleet GL, Gorecki JA (2006) Treatment for cigarette smoking among depressed mental health outpatients: a randomized clinical trial. Am J Public Health 96:1808–1814
42. Prochaska JJ, Hall SE, Delucchi K, Hall SM (2014) Efficacy of initiating tobacco dependence treatment in inpatient psychiatry: a randomized controlled trial. Am J Public Health 104:1557–1565
43. Prochaska JJ, Hall SE, Hall SM (2009) Stage-tailored tobacco cessation treatment in inpatient psychiatry. Psychiatr Serv 60:848. https://doi:10.1176/appi.ps.60.6.848
44. Prochaska JJ, Velicer WF, Prochaska JO, Delucchi K, Hall SM (2006) Comparing intervention outcomes in smokers treated for single versus multiple behavioral risks. Health Psychol 25:380–388

45. The Steering Committee of the Physicians Health Study Research Group (1988) Preliminary report: findings from the aspirin component of the ongoing Physicians' Health Study. N Engl J Med 318:262–264
46. Coronary Drug Project Research Group (1980) Influence of adherence to treatment and response of cholesterol on mortality in the Coronary Drug Project. N Engl J Med 303:1038–1041
47. Adamson J, Cockayne S, Puffer S, Torgerson DJ (2006) Review of randomised trials using the post-randomised consent (Zelen's) design. Contemp Clin Trials 27:305–319
48. Fabricatore AN, Wadden TA, Moore RH, Butryn ML, Gravallese EA, Erondu NE, Heymsfield SB, Nguyen AM (2009) Attrition from randomized controlled trials of pharmacological weight loss agents: a systematic review and analysis. Obes Rev 10:333–341
49. Lang JM (1990) The use of a run-in to enhance compliance. Stat Med 9:87–93
50. Kong W, Langlois MF, Kamga-Ngandé C, Gagnon C, Brown C, Baillargeon JP (2010) Predictors of success to weight-loss intervention program in individuals at high risk for type 2 diabetes. Diabetes Res Clin Pract 90:147–153
51. Teixeira PJ, Going SB, Houtkooper LB, Cussler EC, Metcalfe LL, Blew RM, Sardinha LB, Lohman TG (2004) Pretreatment predictors of attrition and successful weight management in women. Int J Obes Relat Metab Disord 28:1124–1133
52. Czajkowski SM, Powell LH, Adler N, Naar-King S, Reynolds KD, Hunter CM, Laraia B, Olster DH, Perna FM, Peterson JC, Epel E, Boyington JE, Charlson ME (2015) From ideas to efficacy: the ORBIT model for developing behavioral treatments for chronic diseases. Health Psychol 34:971–982
53. Bailey JV, Pavlou M, Copas A, McCarthy OL, Carswell K, Rait G, Hart G, Nazareth I, Free CJ, French R, Murray E (2013) The Sexunzipped trial: optimizing the design of online randomized controlled trials. J Med Internet Res 15:e278. https://doi.org/10.2196/jmir.2668
54. Boyd A, Tilling K, Cornish R, Davies A, Humphries K, Macleod J (2015) Professionally designed information materials and telephone reminders improved consent response rates: evidence from an RCT nested within a cohort study. J Clin Epidemiol 68:877–887
55. Dickson S, Logan J, Hagen S, Stark D, Glazener C, McDonald AM, McPherson G (2013) Reflecting on the methodological challenges of recruiting to a United Kingdom-wide, multi-centre, randomised controlled trial in gynaecology outpatient settings. Trials 14:389. https://doi.org/10.1186/1745-6215-14-389
56. Gupta A, Calfas KJ, Marshall SJ, Robinson TN, Rock CL, Huang JS, Epstein-Corbin M, Servetas C, Donohue MC, Norman GJ, Raab F, Merchant G, Fowler JH, Griswold WG, Fogg BJ, Patrick K (2015) Clinical trial management of participant recruitment, enrollment, engagement, and retention in the SMART study using a Marketing and Information Technology (MARKIT) model. Contemp Clin Trials 42:185–195
57. Hadidi N, Buckwalter K, Lindquist R, Rangen C (2012) Lessons learned in recruitment and retention of stroke survivors. J Neurosci Nurs 44:105–110
58. Hartlieb KB, Jacques-Tiura AJ, Naar-King S, Ellis DA, Jen KL, Marshall S (2015) Recruitment strategies and the retention of obese urban racial/ethnic minority adolescents in clinical trials: the FIT families project, Michigan, 2010–2014. Prev Chronic Dis 12:E22. https://doi.org/10.5888/pcd12.140409
59. Johnson DA, Joosten YA, Wilkins CH, Shibao CA (2015) Case study. Community engagement and clinical trial success: outreach to African American women. Clin Transl Sci 8:388–390
60. Blake K, Holbrook JT, Antal H, Shade D, Bunnell HT, McCahan SM, Wise RA, Pennington C, Garfinkel P, Wysocki T (2015) Use of mobile devices and the internet for multimedia informed consent delivery and data entry in a pediatric asthma trial: study design and rationale. Contemp Clin Trials 42:105–118
61. Cermak SA, Stein Duker LI, Williams ME, Lane CJ, Dawson ME, Borreson AE, Polido JC (2015) Feasibility of a sensory-adapted dental environment for children with autism. Am J Occup Ther 69:6903220020. https://doi.org/10.5014/ajot.2015.013714

62. Giuffrida A, Torgerson DJ (1997) Should we pay the patient? Review of financial incentives to enhance patient compliance. BMJ 315:703–707

63. Brown SD, Lee K, Schoffman DE, King AC, Crawley LM, Kiernan M (2012) Minority recruitment into clinical trials: experimental findings and practical implications. Contemp Clin Trials 33:620–623

64. Kiernan M, Phillips K, Fair JM, King AC (2000) Using direct mail to recruit Hispanic adults into a dietary intervention: an experimental study. Ann Behav Med 22:89–93

65. Batliner T, Fehringer KA, Tiwari T, Henderson WG, Wilson A, Brega AG, Albino J (2014) Motivational interviewing with American Indian mothers to prevent early childhood caries: study design and methodology of a randomized control trial. Trials 15:125. https://doi.org/10.1186/1745-6215-15-125

66. Clark F, Pyatak EA, Carlson M, Blanche E, Vigen C, Hay J, Mallinson T, Blanchard J, Unger JB, Garber SL, Diaz J, Florindez L, Atkins M, Rubayi S, Azen SP, PUPS Study Group (2014) Implementing trials of complex interventions in community settings: the USC-Rancho Los Amigos Pressure Ulcer Prevention Study (PUPS). Clin Trials 11:218–229

67. Cruz TH, Davis SM, FitzGerald CA, Canaca GF, Keane PC (2014) Engagement, recruitment, and retention in a trans-community, randomized controlled trial for the prevention of obesity in rural American Indian and Hispanic children. J Prim Prev 35:135–149

68. Jimenez DE, Reynolds CF 3rd, Alegría M, Harvey P, Bartels SJ (2015) The Happy Older Latinos are Active (HOLA) health promotion and prevention study: study protocol for a pilot randomized controlled trial. Trials 6:579. https://doi.org/10.1186/s13063-015-1113-3

69. Koziol-McLain J, Vandal AC, Nada-Raja S, Wilson D, Glass NE, Eden KB, McLean C, Dobbs T, Case J (2015) A web-based intervention for abused women: the New Zealand *isafe* randomised controlled trial protocol. BMC Public Health 15:56. https://doi.org/10.1186/s12889-015-1395-0

70. Bakari M, Munseri P, Francis J, Aris E, Moshiro C, Siyame D, Janabi M, Ngatoluwa M, Aboud S, Lyamuya E, Sandström E, Mhalu F (2013) Experiences on recruitment and retention of volunteers in the first HIV vaccine trial in Dar es Salam, Tanzania - the phase I/II HIVIS 03 trial. BMC Public Health 13:1149. https://doi.org/10.1186/1471-2458-13-1149

71. Goldberg JH, Kiernan M (2005) Innovative techniques to address retention in a behavioral weight-loss trial. Health Educ Res 20:439–447

72. National Commission for the Protection of Human Subjects of Biomedical Behavioral Research (1978) The Belmont report: ethical principles and guidelines for the protection of human subjects of research. ERIC Clearinghouse, Bethesda

73. Moseley JB, O'Malley K, Petersen NJ, Menke TJ, Brody BA, Kuykendall DH, Hollingsworth JC, Ashton CM, Wray NP (2002) A controlled trial of arthroscopic surgery for osteoarthritis of the knee. N Engl J Med 347:81–88

74. Hays JL, Hunt JR, Hubbell FA, Anderson GL, Limacher MC, Allen C, Rossouw JE (2003) The Women's Health Initiative recruitment methods and results. Ann Epidemiol 13:S18–S77

75. Kaptchuk TJ, Friedlander E, Kelley JM, Sanchez MN, Kokkotou E, Singer JP, Kowalczykowski M, Miller FG, Kirsch I, Lembo AJ (2010) Placebos without deception: a randomized controlled trial in irritable bowel syndrome. PLoS One 5:e15591. https://doi.org/10.1371/journal.pone.0015591

76. Crichton GE, Howe PR, Buckley JD, Coates AM, Murphy KJ, Bryan J (2012) Long-term dietary intervention trials: critical issues and challenges. Trials 13:111. https://doi.org/10.1186/1745-6215-13-111

77. Hulley SB, Cummings SR, Browner WS, Grady DG, Newman TB (2013) Designing clinical research, 4th edn. Lippincott Williams & Wilkins, Philadelphia

78. Siddiqi AE, Sikorskii A, Given CW, Given B (2008) Early participant attrition from clinical trials: role of trial design and logistics. Clin Trials 5:328–335

79. Idoko OT, Owolabi OA, Odutola AA, Ogundare O, Worwui A, Saidu Y, Smith-Sanneh A, Tunkara A, Sey G, Sanyang A, Mendy P, Ota MO (2014) Lessons in participant retention in the course of a randomized controlled clinical trial. BMC Res Notes 7:706. https://doi.org/10.1186/1756-0500-7-706

80. Rucker-Whitaker C, Flynn KJ, Kravitz G, Eaton C, Calvin JE, Powell LH (2006) Understanding African-American participation in a behavioral intervention: results from focus groups. Contemp Clin Trials 27:274–286

81. Gross D, Fogg L (2004) A critical analysis of the intent-to-treat principle in prevention research. J Primary Prevention 25:475–489

82. Feinstein AR (1991) Intent-to-treat policy for analyzing randomized trials: statistical distortions and neglected clinical challenges. In: Cramer JA, Spilker B (eds) Patient compliance in medical practice and clinical trials. Raven, New York

83. Sheiner LB, Rubin DB (1995) Intention-to-treat analysis and the goals of clinical trials. Clin Pharmacol Ther 57:6–15

84. Knowler WC, Barrett-Connor E, Fowler SE, Hamman RF, Lachin JM, Walker EA, Nathan DM, Diabetes Prevention Program Research Group (2002) Reduction in the incidence of type 2 diabetes with lifestyle intervention or metformin. N Engl J Med 346:393–403

85. Diabetes Prevention Program Research Group (1999) The Diabetes Prevention Program. Design and methods for a clinical trial in the prevention of type 2 diabetes. Diabetes Care 22:623–634

86. Diabetes Prevention Program Research Group (2000) The Diabetes Prevention Program: baseline characteristics of the randomized cohort. Diabetes Care 23:1619–1629

87. Frasure-Smith N, Prince R (1985) The Ischemic Heart Disease Life Stress Monitoring Program. Impact on mortality. Psychosom Med 47:431–445

88. Frasure-Smith N, Prince R (1989) Long-term follow-up of the Ischemic Heart Disease Life Stress Monitoring Program. Psychosom Med 51:485–513

89. Powell LH (1989) Unanswered questions in the Ischemic Heart Disease Life Stress Monitoring Program. Psychosom Med 51:479–484

90. Frasure-Smith N, Lespérance F, Prince RH, Verrier P, Garber RA, Juneau M, Wolfson C, Bourassa MG (1997) Randomised trial of home-based psychosocial nursing intervention for patients recovering from myocardial infarction. Lancet 350:473–479

91. O'Connor CM, Whellan DJ, Lee KL, Keteyian SJ, Cooper LS, Ellis SJ, Leifer ES, Kraus WE, Kitzman DW, Blumenthal JA, Rendall DS, Miller NH, Fleg JL, Schulman KA, McKelvie RS, Zannad F, Piña IL, HF-ACTION Investigators (2009) Efficacy and safety of exercise training in patients with chronic heart failure: HF-ACTION randomized controlled trial. JAMA 301:1439–1450

92. Keteyian SJ, Leifer ES, Houston-Miller N, Kraus WE, Brawner CA, O'Connor CM, Whellan DJ, Cooper LS, Fleg JL, Kitzman DW, Cohen-Solal A, Blumenthal JA, Rendall DS, Piña IL, HF-ACTION Investigators (2012) Relation between volume of exercise and clinical outcomes in patients with heart failure. J Am Coll Cardiol 60:1899–1905

93. Yancy CW, Jessup M, Bozkurt B, Butler J, Casey DE Jr, Drazner MH, Fonarow GC, Geraci SA, Horwich T, Januzzi JL, Johnson MR, Kasper EK, Levy WC, Masoudi FA, McBride PE, McMurray JJ, Mitchell JE, Peterson PN, Riegel B, Sam F, Stevenson LW, Tang WH, Tsai EJ, Wilkoff BL, American College of Cardiology Foundation, American Heart Association Task Force on Practice Guidelines (2013) 2013 ACCF/AHA guideline for the management of heart failure: a report of the American College of Cardiology Foundation/American Heart Association Task Force on Practice Guidelines. J Am Coll Cardiol 62:e147–e239

94. Centers for Medicare and Medicaid Services (2014) Decision memo for cardiac rehabilitation programs - chronic heart failure (CAG-00437N). US Department of Health & Human Services. http://www.cms.gov/medicare-coverage-database/details/nca-decision-memo.aspx?

95. McCambridge J, Kypri K, Elbourne D (2014) In randomization we trust? There are overlooked problems in experimenting with people in behavioral intervention trials. J Clin Epidemiol 67:247–253

96. Ashley EA (2015) The precision medicine initiative: a new national effort. JAMA 313:2019–2020
97. Khoury MJ, Evans JP (2015) A public health perspective on a national precision medicine cohort: balancing long-term knowledge generation with early health benefit. JAMA 313:2117–2118
98. Ma J, Rosas LG, Lv N (2016) Precision lifestyle medicine: a new frontier in the science of behavior change and population health. Am J Prev Med 50:395–397
99. Brewin CR, Bradley C (1989) Patient preferences and randomised clinical trials. Br Med J 299:313–315

Chapter 9
Outcomes

"Truth is ever to be found in simplicity,
and not in the multiplicity and confusion of things."
Isaac Newton

Fundamental Point

Selecting a single clinically meaningful, objectively assessed primary outcome is essential for evaluating whether a behavioral intervention improves health. Inclusion of multiple secondary outcomes, including moderators, mediators, and mechanisms, is more useful in earlier stages of treatment development where the risk of unintended adverse consequences and responder burden is lower than it is for definitive clinical trials.

The objective of all confirmatory *Phase II* and *Phase III* behavioral trials is to estimate the likelihood that the intervention(s) under study will improve a future health outcome. This future health outcome is the primary outcome for the trial. It is a decision that is made early in the design phase and drives many subsequent design decisions. This chapter focuses on considerations that guide the selection of a primary outcome, ways to avoid biased assessment, and the balance between multiple secondary outcomes and the risk of unintended consequences from them. Simplicity, objectivity, pre-specification, and clinical relevance are characteristics of outcome assessment in confirmatory behavioral trials. Exploration of moderators, mediators, and mechanisms are more appropriate for earlier stages of behavioral treatment development.

© Springer Nature Switzerland AG 2021   209
L. H. Powell et al., *Behavioral Clinical Trials for Chronic Diseases*,
https://doi.org/10.1007/978-3-030-39330-4_9

SCIENTIFIC PRINCIPLES

A study that is specifically designed to confirm the efficacy or effectiveness of one or more treatments is called a clinical trial. Results are expected to provide an unbiased estimate of a typical individual's response to a treatment or management strategy. For results to be persuasive and influence clinical practice, policy, or public health, the trial must pose a significant clinical question and answer it without bias in the selection of participants, allocation of them to treatments, delivery of the interventions, and assessment of outcomes. The choice of a clinically meaningful primary outcome and an unbiased method for its ascertainment is among the most important considerations for credibility in the eyes of the research community, patients, providers, and policy-makers.

There is an intimate connection between the aims of a behavioral clinical trial and the choice of outcomes for it. What would be a good choice for an outcome in one type of trial could be a poor choice in another type of trial. Therefore, it is useful to define types of outcomes and types of trials for the purpose of informing the subsequent discussion. A summary of these definitions is presented in Table 9.1.

Types of Outcomes

A *primary outcome* is the dependent variable that the investigator deems to be the most important for determining the efficacy or effectiveness of an intervention. Providers, payers, and patients are most often interested in actual disease outcomes such as survival, disability, hospitalization, or progression of disease [1].

Surrogate outcomes are assumed to be highly associated with the primary health outcome of interest [2]. They are often utilized for practical reasons such as reduced sample size, shorter follow-up duration, or cost [3]. Increasingly, the scientific community has become skeptical of the ability of surrogate outcomes to reflect accurately disease outcomes such as survival or disease progression [4]. There are numerous examples of critical failures [5], the most important being an inflation of effect sizes [6].

Secondary outcomes are all other measures. *Intermediate outcomes* are a type of secondary outcome that focuses on the pathway by which a behavioral treatment is hypothesized to improve a health outcome. *(See Chapter 4: Hypothesized Pathway and Bias.)* An intermediate outcome in a *Phase III* trial can be a primary outcome in a *Phase II* trial. For example, because treating depressive symptoms is important in its own right, a *Phase II* trial of depression management would have depressive symptoms as its primary outcome. But depressive symptoms also increase

Table 9.1 Key definitions	
Types of Outcomes	
Primary Outcome	The measure that determines the efficacy or effectiveness of a behavioral intervention. It is the outcome that is used to estimate sample size and the resulting statistical power in a trial
Surrogate Outcome	A measure that is associated with the primary outcome but is more easily accessible and therefore often used as a substitute for the primary outcome, particularly in smaller, early phase studies
Intermediate Outcomes	Mediators in the pathway by which a behavioral treatment is hypothesized to improve a primary outcome
Secondary Outcomes	All outcomes that are not primary or intermediate
Exploratory Outcomes	Outcomes that do not have a hypothesis associated with them but are included simply to discover potential associations. If associations are found, they would then need to be tested with pre-specified hypotheses
Types of Behavioral Trials	
Efficacy Trial	A confirmatory trial designed to test whether or not a behavioral treatment improves a disease or health condition when implemented in a selected population under controlled circumstances to maximize internal validity
Effectiveness Trial	A confirmatory trial designed to test whether or not a behavioral treatment improves a disease or health condition when implemented in a diverse population in real-world community or clinical settings to maximize external validity
Definitive or Confirmatory Trial	A trial designed to test a hypothesis about the efficacy or effectiveness of a fixed treatment on a definitive health outcome, rather than to explore benefit of various dimensions of that treatment
Phase II Trial	A confirmatory trial designed to test whether or not a behavioral treatment improves a primary outcome that is a behavioral risk factor, biological mediator, or surrogate outcome. It can be an end unto itself or provide the justification for a *Phase III* efficacy trial
Phase III Trial	A confirmatory trial designed to test whether or not a behavioral treatment improves a primary outcome that is a clinically important disease or health condition

cardiovascular risk. A *Phase III* trial of depression management to reduce cardiac risk would have depressive symptoms as an intermediate outcome and major cardiac events as a primary outcome.

Exploratory outcomes provide the opportunity to explore hunches. They are not hypothesis driven, they should not be analyzed with statistical hypothesis testing, and any positive associations should be confirmed in subsequent trials with pre-specified hypotheses.

Types of Trials

An *efficacy trial* is a confirmatory trial of the efficacy of a behavioral treatment on a selected population under controlled conditions. The priority is on high internal validity. An *effectiveness trial* is a confirmatory trial of the effectiveness of a behavioral treatment delivered to a diverse population under the "real-world" conditions usually seen in clinical practice or community settings. Its priority is on external validity. Recent research has suggested that trials often have elements of both efficacy and effectiveness. Thus, it may be more accurate to view efficacy and effectiveness as a continuum rather than a dichotomy. A rating system has been proposed where a trial can be evaluated on the efficacy/effectiveness continuum using four criteria: participants, setting, flexibility of interventions, and clinical relevance [7]. *(See Chapter 2: The Quality of a Behavioral Trial.)*

A *definitive or confirmatory behavioral trial* is a trial that tests a specific hypothesis about the impact of a behavioral treatment on an important health outcome for the purpose of influencing clinical practice or policy. It is distinguished from an exploratory trial where the purpose is to explore various dimensions of the treatment. In the context of the drug approval process, the equivalent term is a *pivotal trial,* defined as one that fulfills the criteria for approval from a regulatory agency. To avoid regulatory implications in this discussion, the term "pivotal" has been replaced with "definitive" and "confirmatory."

Definitive or confirmatory behavioral trials are most often *Phase III efficacy trials* which are designed to establish the efficacy of a behavioral treatment on a clinically meaningful improvement in a disease outcome. A *Phase II efficacy trial* is one that targets a behavioral, biomedical, or surrogate outcome. If it is conducted in the service of determining readiness to conduct a *Phase III* efficacy trial, it is not a definitive trial but one that is a predecessor to a definitive trial. If it is conducted as an end unto itself without pushing toward a subsequent *Phase III* efficacy trial, it would be a definitive trial. An example of a definitive *Phase II* trial would be in the area of smoking cessation. The link between smoking and lung cancer is so strong that research has turned away from the need to document benefits of smoking cessation on lung cancer and toward finding behavioral treatments that are successful in producing sustained cessation. In this case, an example of a definitive *Phase II* trial would be a smoking treatment with the primary outcome of smoking recidivism.

Pre-Specification

A fundamental principle of outcome assessment in a clinical trial is pre-specification. Design, execution, and interpretation of clinical trial results require pre-specification of the primary outcome at the earliest planning stage, including the method of assessment and the times at which it will be ascertained. Pre-specification minimizes the temptation to claim efficacy based upon an unexpected significant result which could be due to chance alone. Pre-specification of a clinically significant target on the primary outcome is a crucial element of the estimation of the sample size. *(See Chapter 5: Clinical Significance.)* Secondary outcomes, particularly intermediate outcomes, should also be pre-specified to enhance the weight given to positive results. However, the clinical importance of a positive secondary outcome when the primary is null is questionable [8].

CHALLENGES FOR BEHAVIORAL TRIALS

Multiple Outcomes

Some health problems that behavioral treatments are well-suited to alleviate have multiple, clinically valid dimensions, expressed differentially as the disorder progresses and assessed by a variety of methods. For example, dementia and Alzheimer's disease involve a progressive deterioration of cognitive function and at least ten different scales for assessing function, symptoms, and quality of life [9]. Similarly, some behavioral treatments are complex and have multiple components with multiple dimensions by which they can be evaluated. In these instances it can be difficult to avoid evaluating behavioral treatments with multiple instruments to assess the full spectrum of possible treatment effects.

When the choice is to assess all of the dimensions of the outcome and/or treatment, the assessment battery is characterized by multiplicity of measures (M&M's). There are several problems with this. First, it requires a large sample size to correct the Type I error rate for taking multiple looks at the data and insure adequate power to detect differences on each of the multiple outcomes [8, 10]. Second, it increases the risk of "cherry picking" by choosing to focus only on the subset of outcomes that proved to be most favorable. This scientifically misleading practice is one of the reasons that results from trials cannot be replicated [11]. Third, it increases the risk of undue participant burden which can easily translate into dropouts from the trial and/or non-adherence to the trial or intervention protocols. An excellent discussion of the many issues surrounding multiple outcomes is provided by the Food and Drug Administration [12].

Subjective Outcomes in Single-Blind Designs

Subjective primary outcomes are common in behavioral trials because behavioral treatments can play a major role in subjective dimensions of health such as quality of life. Subjective patient-reported outcomes are patients' reports of the status of their own health, without interpretation by a clinician or anyone else [13]. They include (1) simple measures such as symptom frequency, intensity, or duration; (2) more complex measures such as functional capacity; (3) health-related quality of life which generally involves physical, psychological, and social domains; (4) pain intensity; and (5) judgments of perceived improvement. Because these tend to be subjective self-reports, they are influenced by such factors as deception [14], response style [15], and social desirability [16]. In a clinical trial, "faking good" in responses to a subjective self-report is a danger since participants often want to please those who provided them with treatment.

Double-blind designs provide design control for any bias in subjective assessments resulting from pre-existing expectations of benefit. Since participants, investigators, and research staff are all blinded to treatment assignment, and the treatments being compared appear to be identical, it is difficult for expectancy bias to creep in. Behavioral trials generally do not have the option of using double-blind designs because treatments being compared are not identical and participants know to which treatment they have been assigned. Behavioral trials are, at best, single-blind where the outcomes assessors are blinded to the treatment status of the participants they are assessing.

When a subjective primary outcome is used in a single-blind design, there is a risk of biased assessment where the evaluation reflects not only the benefit of the treatment but also expectations about that benefit, which are often differential by trial arm. The implication of this confounding is that the treatment effect sizes tend to be inflated [17]. Although various strategies have been used to promote equipoise in patients and staff and to blind outcomes assessors to treatment status, they can be imperfect. Investigators, staff, and participants may have reason to prefer one treatment over another. Participants may wish to please or punish investigators after receiving a particular treatment for which they have pre-existing preferences. This is likely the reason that the Medicare Advisory Council has less confidence in depression trials that are single-blinded than those that are double-blinded [18]. This means that this Advisory Council and, by extension, third-party payers, place more confidence in drug treatments for depression, which are evaluated in double-blinded trials, than they do in behavioral treatments for depression such as cognitive behavior therapy, which are evaluated in single-blinded trials.

The onus is on behavioral trials to compensate for design limitations whenever possible by maximizing the use of objective primary outcomes such as death or disease recurrence in *Phase III* efficacy trials. When subjective, patient-reported outcomes are used with a single-blinded design, the onus is on the investigator to avoid bias with rigorous trial operations. These are, however, at best, "second string" compensations for what is viewed widely as an inherent design limitation. *(See Chapter 10: Preferences, Equipoise, and Blinding.)*

Ceiling Effects

Behavioral clinical trials use a behavioral treatment to improve a chronic disease outcome. The target of the behavioral treatment is a behavioral risk factor. The chronic disease outcome is some measure of health in need of improvement. Ceiling effects can occur when either participants enrolled in the trial are not at behavioral risk or they are relatively healthy already and cannot improve much on a primary health outcome. Treating people for a risk factor, or a health problem, they do not have runs the risk of underestimating the value of a behavioral treatment. Rather than the treatment being inefficacious, it is only inefficacious when given to those who do not need it.

An excellent example of this is a multi-site trial of 2328 post-myocardial infarction patients who were offered psychological rehabilitation featuring stress, depression, and anxiety management to prevent a recurrent cardiac event [19]. Superficially the trial was impressive. It had a multi-site design, large sample size, and objective screening for the presence of a prior myocardial infarction. However, none of the patients were evaluated for the presence of psychological distress, depression, or anxiety. Instead, they were believed to have these problems because they had a heart attack, and the need for treatment was implied. At baseline, only 33% of the patients had clinically significant anxiety and only 19% had clinically significant depression. At the 6-month follow-up, the prevalence of these psychological problems was unchanged. The result was a null trial on the primary outcome of cardiovascular recurrence. A likely reason for the null finding is that a large majority of patients did not need this type of treatment. Moreover, those who did need it did not improve. Thus, a ceiling effect combined with a weak treatment undercut the ability to evaluate the hypothesis that this psychological rehabilitation reduced the cardiac recurrence rate. The treated were not "sick" and therefore could not be "cured."

Assessment Reactivity

Assessment reactivity is an emerging concept that describes the act of measuring as an unintended treatment effect (see

> "What we observe is not nature itself,
> but nature exposed to our method of questioning."
> Werner Heisenberg

box). The idea that observations can have unintended consequences is not new. The Hawthorne effect was named after a series of studies on the work environment at the Hawthorne Works in Cicero, Illinois in the 1920s. Various changes in the work environment had been shown to produce increases in worker productivity. But on reanalyses, some of the data suggested that this increased productivity may have been less a function of various changes in the work environment and more a function of the workers' awareness that they were being observed [20].

Assessment reactivity can be triggered by assessments conducted during screening, diagnosis, baseline evaluation, and follow-up evaluation. It can affect such diverse factors as mood, craving, motivation, self-efficacy, and behavior. Assessment reactivity confounds any benefit of a treatment with reactivity to the assessments. It can promote unwanted attrition if participants respond negatively to the nature or number of outcome assessments or perceive them to be irrelevant [21].

An excellent example of assessment reactivity has been provided by the Screening, Motivational Assessment, Referral, and Treatment in Emergency Departments (SMART-ED) randomized trial [22]. Screening for substance use in emergency rooms provides a moment of opportunity for a brief intervention. But it is possible that the process of screening, in itself, is an intervention that could obscure the value of a brief intervention. To answer this question, the behavioral trial had three arms: usual care, brief intervention only, and screening only. The results showed a reduction in the number of hair samples positive for drug abuse in both the brief intervention only, and screening only, conditions and no difference between them. This suggested that assessment by itself was an intervention that was powerful enough to reduce substance use [23].

A systematic review of studies evaluating the influence of the measurement process on outcomes was inconclusive, but the number of studies was small and they were generally of inadequate quality [24]. However, there is enough evidence to warrant a conservative approach to the number and intrusiveness of outcome assessments in confirmatory behavioral trials. This can minimize confounding between treatment effects, which can be replicated in clinical practice, and assessment effects, which cannot.

OVERCOMING THESE CHALLENGES IN A BEHAVIORAL TRIAL

Single Primary Outcome

The general dictum in a confirmatory *Phase II* or *Phase III* behavioral trial is to favor simplicity over complexity. This simplicity takes the form of one primary question. It is framed in the form of a test of the hypothesis that an intervention will have a beneficial impact on a clinical event such as improvement in survival or disease, or on a patient-reported outcome such as improvement in symptoms or quality of life [25]. The primary outcome must be persuasive to clinicians based upon its visibility, utility, and immediate implication for clinical practice.

In the early phases of treatment development, explorations of potent treatment components and their impact on various dimensions of behavior, biomarkers, surrogates, and mechanisms is appropriate and necessary. But when a definitive efficacy trial is the goal, these early explorations are in the service of optimizing the intervention, simplifying the assessment protocol, providing persuasive preliminary studies, and producing a confirmatory behavioral trial characterized by simplicity. *(See Chapter 3: Behavioral Treatment Development.)*

Even in areas where a diagnosis is made using a complex set of symptoms, there is movement toward simplification of outcome assessment when conducting a clinical trial. For example, clinical guidelines for the assessment of neuropathic pain recommend assessments across six domains: intensity; physical functioning; emotional functioning; patient improvement and satisfaction; symptoms and adverse events; and patient disposition [26]. Despite this, a systematic review of randomized trials for neuropathic pain revealed that 87% used only intensity of pain as the primary outcome [27].

Pre-specified Primary Outcome

The primary outcome must be pre-specified before the trial begins, included in the trial protocol, and registered in ClinicalTrials.gov [28]. Details should include its clinical significance, the exact method and instrument used to assess it, the timing and frequency at which it is to be collected, and how the data will be used in the primary analysis. Pre-specification prevents "cherry picking" from among a variety of outcomes for the purpose of claiming benefit of a treatment.

In the ORBIT model for behavioral treatment development, the primary outcome is specified much earlier than when a definitive confirmatory trial is being planned. Specification of the primary outcome for an ultimate *Phase III* trial in the early design phase of treatment development makes it possible to identify less costly, more accessible surrogate outcomes that can be used to judge the success of various treatment approaches as they are being developed. *(See Chapter 3: Behavioral Treatment Development.)*

Objective Outcomes

An objective primary outcome is one that is not under the influence of a participant or a research team. When the outcome is an event that depends upon the interpretation of medical records, tests, or images, the common practice is to establish an adjudication committee who first develop a protocol for adjudication and then assign each case to two committee members for independent, blinded review. Any disagreements are resolved by a third committee member. Although this process can be tedious and generally requires compensation for committee members, it increases confidence in the interpretation of primary results and can lead to the identification of more events than are detected by clinic staff alone [29].

When the primary outcome is a biomarker, the most rigorous way to promote objectivity is to send samples to independent laboratories without disclosing the rationale or the fact that the subjects are in a clinical trial. For other types of outcomes, the widely-accepted practice is to blind outcomes assessors to the trial arm to which the participant is assigned. But this can be difficult to achieve in practice when outcomes assessors have verbal interactions with participants who, despite being told not to, often describe experiences specific to one trial arm. It is particularly important that all staff, especially those involved in assessing or adjudicating outcomes, be trained in procedures to protect data quality, including reducing unnecessary communication with participants, separation of operations functions on a need-to-know basis, and utilizing diagnostic services from sources not involved in the trial. The SPIRIT 2013 Statement provides a good discussion of these issues [30]. In addition, to enhance the rigor of the trial, it is useful to increase the sophistication of the investigators and staff in the principles of preferences, equipoise, and blinding. *(See Chapter 10: Preferences, Equipoise, and Blinding.)*

Patient-Reported Outcomes

Patient-reported outcomes (PROs) are particularly important for evaluating the effects of behavioral treatments. They are vital for assessing aspects of health that cannot be determined through physical or biological tests, and include the presence, frequency, and intensity of physical symptoms such as pain, insomnia, and vertigo and psychological symptoms such as anxiety, depression, and phobia. Since individuals differ in the way they describe their condition, standardized instruments have been developed which provide norms for healthy individuals against which severity can be assessed.

Because of the importance of PROs, the Food and Drug Administration has published guidelines for their use in medical product development [31]. This excellent reference describes theoretical and practical considerations for choosing an existing instrument or, when one is not available, creating a specialized instrument. It emphasizes five requirements for a useful PRO (see box).

> **Five Requirements for a Useful Patient-Reported Outcome [31]**
>
> 1. A model by which a treatment is hypothesized to affect a patient-reported outcome
> 2. A clear conceptual framework that specifies the relationships among concepts, assessment domains, and items in the instrument
> 3. Documented psychometric properties including reliability, content validity, construct validity, and responsiveness to change
> 4. A definition of a responder
> 5. Documentation of any modifications of an instrument for a specific purpose

An equally important development is the National Institutes of Health Patient-Reported Outcomes Measurement Information System (PROMIS) [32]. Through the use of item response theory and computer adaptive testing, PROMIS draws on an item bank to create scales that evaluate a wide range of physical, behavioral, and mental conditions, translated into several languages. Some of its most promising attributes are the small number of items needed to assess a construct which translates into a lower response burden for participants in a clinical trial, improved precision resulting from the accumulation of data across a large number of studies, and the availability of normative values for diverse populations and important subgroups. A potential limitation of PROMIS is that most of the measures have not been validated for their ability to register change in response to an intervention. When this validation does not exist, it should be studied in early phase developmental studies before the measure is used in a confirmatory *Phase II* or *Phase III* behavioral trial.

Composite Outcomes

When used appropriately, composite outcome measures can be an excellent approach for minimizing needed sample size and/or trial duration while evaluating a comprehensive health outcome. For example, in the Look AHEAD trial, the primary outcome was the first occurrence of nonfatal myocardial infarction, nonfatal stroke, hospitalization for angina, or cardiovascular death [33]. The justification for combining these events into a composite was based upon the fact that they were all manifestations of underlying vascular disease. This made it unlikely that different components would be affected in opposite directions, leading to a null trial.

But there is no free lunch with composite outcomes [34]. First, each component of a composite may not have the same importance. In the ACCORD trial, for example, the primary composite outcome, which included death, was null but the intensive intervention group had significantly more deaths [35]. Because death was a more serious outcome than other parts of the composite, it justified the decision to terminate the trial early. Second, the various components of a composite may not occur at the same frequency or be ascertained with equal ease. Whereas death is absolute, diagnosis of a myocardial infarction requires validation by patterns of symptoms and evolving enzyme biomarkers. Biased subjective assessment of some components of the composite could neutralize the effects of an intervention on the more objective components. Third, some components of the composite may not be subject to change following a behavioral intervention. An excellent example is the Framingham score. Although the composite score accounts for 56% of cardiovascular disease mortality, some of the components (i.e., family history, age) are not modifiable [36]. Fourth, various components of a composite could tap into separate biological pathways which may be influenced differentially by a behavioral treatment. For example, the Framingham score includes smoking as part of its composite. If a diet intervention does not influence smoking, its inclusion in the composite would weaken the resulting effect size in a clinical trial.

Minimal Clinically Important Difference

After selecting a primary outcome, it is important to determine how strong an impact a behavioral treatment must have on it to judge that the treatment is efficacious. The most common approach is to use statistical significance to evaluate the probability that the observed difference between a treatment and comparator is consistent with a null hypothesis of no benefit. However, small differences that are not informative clinically can reach statistical significance if the sample size is sufficiently large. Therefore, evaluations of efficacy should not rely exclusively upon statistical significance but should also consider whether or not the improvement is of clinical significance. *(See Chapter 5: Clinical Significance.)*

Clinical significance can be arrived at in a number of ways. When the primary endpoint is a disease rate, it is a widespread practice to select an arbitrary target, such as a 10% or 20% difference between treated and comparator conditions. This target generally is justified as clinically meaningful based upon the success rate of current treatments, its consistency with past successful trials, its ability to resonate with the clinical trial community or providers in practice, and its relevance for third-party payers.

When the primary endpoint is a continuous outcome, it is common to use the standards set by Cohen [37] to determine whether the difference between treated and comparator conditions, translated into standard deviation (sd) units, is small (0.2 sd), medium (0.5 sd), or large (0.8 sd). This approach is popular, despite the fact that Cohen himself cautioned against it [37].

Sometimes the clinically significant target is arrived at by delta inflation which is essentially performing sample size calculations in reverse. In light of financial, time, and logistical constraints, investigators first determine the number of participants that is feasible to enroll in a trial, then they calculate the effect size they can detect using that sample size. This approach tends to overestimate the true effect size, underestimate the power of the trial to detect a treatment benefit, result in a high prevalence of null trials, lead to premature abandonment of promising treatments, waste resources, and raise questions about clinical trial ethics [38].

The Minimal Clinically Important Difference (MCID) is the smallest difference in the domain of interest that patients or providers perceive as beneficial and that would mandate, in the absence of troublesome side effects and excessive cost, a meaningful change in the patient's management [39]. This takes a clinical, rather than a statistical, perspective on efficacy, considering patients' as well as clinicians' perspectives on a goal for a treatment. When an MCID is a primary endpoint in a behavioral trial, it serves as the basis for sample size calculations. When an MCID has been defined for secondary or intermediate outcomes, it generally is not used as the basis for sample size calculations but can, nonetheless, inform the power to detect statistically a fuller range of clinical improvement. The rationale and approach used to determine the MCID should be documented in the trial protocol.

Minimal Clinically Important Difference for Dichotomous Outcomes

Phase III efficacy trials generally have primary endpoints that are dichotomous disease endpoints that did or did not occur, such as death, stroke, recurrence, hospitalization, or surgery. The simplest way to determine an MCID for these events is to reference the status quo. Can the new treatment do as well or better than other treatments for the same disorder, other trials of the same intervention, or recommendations from clinical guidelines? For example, Powell et al. [40] developed a lifestyle intervention for patients with the metabolic syndrome where the primary target was to achieve remission of the metabolic syndrome in ≥50% of treated patients after 2 years. The choice of a positive response in ≥50% of participants was based upon three criteria. (1) The average rate of adherence to drug therapy, the standard treatment for the metabolic syndrome, is less than 50% regardless of drug class [41]. The most successful lifestyle trial for the metabolic syndrome to date achieved 47% remission at 2 years [42]. The threshold for judging success in weight loss interventions, defined by the Food and Drug Administration, was the ability to achieve a clinically significant weight loss of ≥5% of baseline body weight in ≥35% of participants [43].

A clinically meaningful metric for judging the efficacy of a treatment from a population perspective is the Number Needed to Treat (NNT) [44–46]. Since only some patients respond to any treatment, some are unaffected, and some may be harmed, the NNT defines the number of patients that need to be treated in order to achieve benefit in one patient. It is computed as the inverse of the absolute risk reduction (ARR): ARR = Comparator event rate – Treated event rate

---

Number Needed to Treat (NNT)

A lifestyle treatment for the metabolic syndrome achieved remission in 20% in the comparator condition and 50% in the treated condition.

$$\text{The ARR} = 0.2 - 0.5 = 0.3$$
$$\text{The NNT} = 1/0.3 = 3.3.$$

The interpretation is that approximately 3.3 patients must be given the lifestyle treatment to achieve remission in one of them.

(ignoring the signs). NNT = 1/ARR (see box). If the NNT is integrated with the cost of treatment, it can provide a justification based upon cost-effectiveness [47]. If the cost of embedding a treatment within a particular healthcare context is fixed at a targeted dollar amount, above which it cannot be supported regardless of its efficacy, that cost can be translated into the maximum acceptable number needed to treat and thus serve as the minimal clinically important difference.

Minimal Clinically Important Difference for Continuous Outcomes

Often in behavioral trials, a primary endpoint is a continuous outcome such as blood pressure, glucose, depression, or severity of pain. If the behavioral trial is a *Phase II* behavioral efficacy trial, conducted in the service of pushing toward a *Phase III* behavioral efficacy trial, a determination of the MCID is based upon the difference needed to affect the ultimate clinical endpoint. *(See Chapter 5: Clinical Significance.)*

If the behavioral trial is a terminal *Phase II* or a *Phase III* efficacy trial with a continuous primary endpoint, there are three common ways to estimate the MCID: consensus, anchoring, and distribution-based methods. Because each has strengths and limitations, use of more than one method can produce a more robust range of values for the MCID [48–50].

The consensus method seeks agreement among stakeholders such as researchers, clinicians, and patients concerning a clinically significant target for improvement in a specific disorder. This target is often articulated in clinical practice guidelines or identified in psychometric studies of the assessment measure of interest. If guidelines or cutpoints do not exist, consensus can be achieved through Delphi methods [51] which query researchers, clinicians, and/or patients iteratively until agreement is achieved. This method is potentially useful when patient perspectives differ from those of clinicians [52]. MCIDs have been published for a wide variety of instruments and populations including the patient perspective on clinically significant improvement in depression on the Beck Depression Inventory-II [53] and the clinician perspective on clinically significant improvement in depression on the Montgomery-Asberg Depression Rating Scale [54]. These standards can be useful as a general guide, but MCIDs may vary in important subgroups of patients based upon such things as socioeconomic differences, severity of the disorder, and/or cultural beliefs.

The ENRICHD clinical trial used consensus methods to determine the MCID for alleviation of depression. The trial aimed to determine the impact of treatment for depression in survivors of a heart attack on a reduced cardiovascular recurrence rate [55]. Thus, the question of how to determine whether or not depression was alleviated was crucial to testing the central hypothesis under investigation. Consensus was evaluated in two ways. First, psychometric studies and clinical guidelines indicated that a score on the Beck Depression Inventory of ≤ 7 was the gold standard for alleviation of depression. *(See Chapter 5: Clinical Significance.)* Second, senior therapists both within and outside of the trial were consulted and consensus reached that an average improvement of 2 points on the Hamilton Depression Rating Scale would indicate an alleviation of depression. The results of the trial showed that, on average, participants randomized to the depression treatment arm did not achieve a clinically significant improvement on depression using either of the MCID criteria. Thus, the null result of this trial on the primary outcome of a recurrent heart attack was likely due, in large part, to the fact that the depression treatment did not achieve the MCID based upon either of the two consensus methods used.

Anchor-based methods link values on a new scale, often a patient-reported outcome, to an "anchor" that is an established gold standard based upon such criteria as expert ratings. This makes it possible to determine clinically significant improvement on the new scale by referencing it to clinically significant improvement on the gold standard. Distribution-based methods use the statistical characteristics of the normal distribution of a stable sample of healthy subjects to judge a clinically significant deviation from that range, often equivalent to a z-score of 1.96 which is equivalent to the 97.5 percentile. Since both approaches are limited by the need for judgment in determining clinically relevant cutpoints, they are most robust when used together and arrive at similar MCIDs [48, 56, 57].

The Clinical Antipsychotic Trials of Intervention Effectiveness Schizophrenia Trial used both the anchor- and distribution-based methods to determine the MCID for the Positive and Negative Syndrome Scale (PANSS) in 1442 patients with schizophrenia [56]. The anchor method linked clinician-rated scores on a 1–7 scale to PANSS score ranges, judged clinically significant improvement to be a 1-point change on the clinician rating, and produced a PANSS MCID equal to a 15.3 point (34.0%) change from baseline. The distribution method showed that a z-score of 1.96 on the normal distribution of the PANSS in 707 stable patients corresponded to an MCID equal to a 16.5 point (36.2%) change from baseline. The convergence of results from these two methods enhances confidence that an MCID of approximately 15 points or 34% improvement over the baseline values is a clinically significant improvement following treatment [56].

Moderators, Mediators, and Mechanisms

M&M's

There is a well-established tradition, indeed imperative, to evaluate moderators, mediators, and mechanisms in behavioral clinical trials [58]. This often results in assessment batteries characterized by a multiplicity of measures (M&M's). It has been argued that moderator and mediator

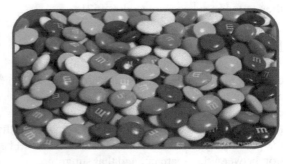

investigations can help to bridge the large gap between theory and practice [59]. This tradition emanates from experimental clinical and social psychology where the aim is to explore and discover relationships. While this is justified and needed in the early phases of treatment development, when it is extended to confirmatory behavioral trials, it contributes to M&M outcome assessment.

Definitive *Phase II* and *Phase III* behavioral trials characterized by M&M's can impose significant burden on both participants and staff. During recruitment,

M&M's can undercut interest in participating in the trial. After entry into a trial, the burden is doubled. Not only do participants have to implement a behavioral treatment, but they also have to undergo to an extensive assessment protocol. This can easily translate into a reduction in participant commitment, non-adherence to the treatment, dropout from the trial, and, as such, place the primary aim of evaluating the efficacy of the treatment on a primary outcome in jeopardy [60]. When participant time is limited, priority should be placed on the treatment rather than on completing extensive M&M outcome assessments.

An excellent example is provided by the ENRICHD clinical trial [55]. The approximately 40 investigators from 8 clinical sites developed an ambitious assessment protocol which made it possible to answer a number of secondary questions in which specific investigators had an interest, as well as explore a variety of mediators, moderators, and mechanisms [61]. Although all of the investigators were pleased that their "pet" research questions would be answered in the trial, once recruitment started, problems emerged. After the first 600, of the 2481 total, were enrolled, recruitment was falling behind schedule, and the investigators realized that one reason for this was the extensive test battery, which was a burden on prospective participants and staff. The investigators decided to reduce the assessment battery by more than 60%.

M&M's in definitive clinical trials are reflective of a "one fell swoop" approach to research where all relevant questions about a behavioral treatment are attempted to be answered in a single trial. A progressive, translational science approach features early explorations of moderators, mediators, and mechanisms, which then provide a springboard for the development of a more focused, optimized, and simplified treatment that is ready for testing in a confirmatory trial. Attention to M&M's in early phase studies, and less attention in later phase studies, is consistent with progressive science where early tests drive the formulation of new simplified hypotheses that are then tested in subsequent studies [62].

Moderators

A significant moderator of a behavioral treatment indicates that it works better for one subgroup than it does for another. The problem for confirmatory behavioral trials is that they are powered, and sample size is determined, on the assumption that, on average, all participants will respond. If there is reason to believe that a behavioral treatment will work better for one subgroup than another, then this should be the primary hypothesis and the trial which should be powered to detect the interaction between the treatment and that subgroup.

In clinical trial methodology, moderator effects are called subgroup hypotheses. They are: (a) specified in advance of data collection; (b) based upon reasonable expectations; and (c) limited in number [25]. In general, subgroup hypotheses are not encouraged in a clinical trial because their existence weakens the overall effect size and increases risk of a null trial. Differences in subgroups are difficult to detect statistically unless the trial was powered to find them. Failure to find them in trials that are not powered to detect them does not mean they do not exist. In a null trial, post hoc identification of subgroups who did respond to the intervention should be interpreted with considerable caution. At best, they provide the basis for a new trial that targets only the subgroup that responded to determine if the original subgroup finding can be replicated in a trial designed to directly test that hypothesis.

The tradition to study moderators in confirmatory behavioral trials comes from a failure to distinguish among the different purposes of randomized designs. Randomized designs can be used to explore, refine, and confirm. The ideal place to study moderators is in refinement studies. Identification of significant moderators early in treatment development makes it possible to optimize the treatment by studying ways to enhance response in all subgroups. This refinement then leads to a confirmatory behavioral trial which assumes that, on average, all participants will respond. *(See Chapter 2: Quality of a Clinical Trial; Chapter 3: Behavioral Treatment Development.)*

Mediators

Mediators are links in an explanatory chain that connects a behavioral treatment to a health outcome. In conceptual models that explain a behavioral risk factor or a chronic disease, there is often a network of multilevel, bidirectional mediators at a variety of ecological levels ranging from the biological to the contextual. But in a confirmatory behavioral trial, this complex set of mediators is translated into a simple, selected pathway by which a behavioral treatment is hypothesized to influence a behavioral risk factor or chronic disease event. The hypothesis is that the elements of the pathway must improve for the treatment to be successful at altering a primary endpoint. If they do not improve, the treatment has failed. Thus, the strongest justification for mediators is for those that are necessary for improving an outcome and, as such, part of the hypothesized pathway. Other mediators that are aimed at exploring the range of benefits that a behavioral treatment may have should be kept to a minimum.

The distinction between a general mediator and a mediator in the hypothesized pathway can be appreciated by considering the example of turning on a light switch to illuminate a room [63]. The hypothesis is that turning on the switch causes the room to light up. Although there are other ways (i.e., mediators of outcome) to light up a room, such as the morning sunrise or lighting a fire in a fireplace, they are ignored in this hypothesis. If the hypothesis is not supported and the "treatment" (i.e., the light switch) is unsuccessful at solving the problem (i.e., illuminating a room), one goes back to the hypothesized pathway to find the culprit, examining the light bulb, the plug, the circuit, and the passage of electricity through the circuit. Other ways to solve the problem (i.e., to light up the room) are mediators (i.e., a fire in the fireplace) but not of interest for this particular treatment (i.e., the light switch).

Because behavioral factors can improve health by many pathways, the best we can do in a clinical trial is hypothesize one mediational pathway and test whether the results of the clinical trial support it. Explorations of other possible pathways and their interconnected, bidirectional links are well suited for early phase exploratory studies and can be a critical basis for the choice of the pathway to be tested. But when it comes to a confirmatory clinical trial, investigators must "stick their necks out," test a hypothesized pathway, and limit measurement to those mediators in it. *(See Chapter 4: Hypothesized Pathway and Bias.)*

Mechanisms

Hopes of gaining significant insights into mechanisms of change from ancillary data collected in confirmatory clinical trials should be reconsidered. Alan Kazdin made a sobering observation.

> *"After decades of psychotherapy research, we cannot provide an evidence-based explanation of how or why even our most well studied interventions produce change; that is, the mechanism(s) through which treatments operate." [64]*

Mechanism is a vague term that can apply to mechanisms of behavior change or biobehavioral mechanisms by which a definitive health outcome is influenced. Mechanistic experiments are a crucial part of intervention development. Grounding a behavioral treatment in basic mechanisms of behavior change can strengthen it. Understanding biologic mechanisms by which a behavioral treatment influences a disease provides a strong rationale for readiness to conduct an efficacy trial. These explorations are vital background for a definitive clinical trial. But they should precede it and be independent of it.

SELECTED EXPERIENCE FROM BEHAVIORAL TRIALS

Obfuscation from M&M's

The Multimodal Treatment Study of children with attention-deficit hyperactivity disorder (ADHD) provides an excellent example of the adverse effects of M&M's in outcomes assessment batteries in a behavioral trial [65]. This was a four-arm trial that compared: (1) medical management with methylphenidate, a central nervous system stimulant sold under the trade name Ritalin; (2)

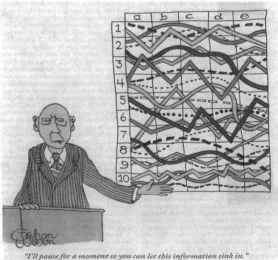

"I'll pause for a moment so you can let this information sink in."

behavioral treatment; (3) combined medical and behavioral treatment; and (4) usual care delivered in the community. It was intended to answer three questions [66].

1. *How does medical management compare to behavioral treatment?*

2. *Are there additional benefits when these two treatments are combined?*

3. *What is the effectiveness of carefully delivered treatments relative to treatments implemented in routine community care?*

The follow-up was 14 months. No primary outcome was specified. The assessment battery included 90 different assessments (see box). Children were evaluated by self-reports, observations by trained individuals placed in classrooms, and reports by parents and teachers. When there was a discrepancy among parent, teacher, and trained assessor ratings, all were interviewed by study staff to ascertain the rationale for their ratings. The drug dosage in the medical management condition was titrated to the individual patient using an algorithm developed in a previous study. The behavioral treatment was "one size fits all."

Highlights of the findings at 14 months showed that all groups underwent significant reductions in symptoms in most areas but there were significant differences

> ### 90 Assessment Measures in the Multimodal Treatment Study
>
> - Three domains of *symptoms* (ADHD, disruptive, internalizing) provided by parents, teachers, and children.
> - Three domains of *functional impairment* (parent-child interactions, peer relations, academic achievement) provided by parents, teachers, and classroom observers.
> - Assessments of:
>   - Internalizing (anxiety and sadness) ratings provided by parents, teachers, and children;
>   - Social skills ratings provided by parents, teachers, and children;
>   - Parent child relations rated by parents;
>   - Academic achievement assessed by 26 standardized tests;
>   - Factor scores that combined domains and scores within domains.

in degree of change. Results on the key questions of interest can be summarized as follows:

How does medical management compare to behavioral treatment?

- For ADHD core symptoms (inattention, hyperreactivity/impulsivity), medical management was better than behavioral treatment.

- For non-ADHD symptoms and positive functioning (oppositional behavior, peer relations, internalizing, and academic achievement), there was no difference between medical management and behavioral treatment.

Are there additional benefits when these two treatments are combined?

- For ADHD core symptoms, combined was no different than medical management but better than behavioral treatment.

- For non-ADHD symptoms and positive functioning, combined was better than medical management and behavioral treatment.

What is the effectiveness of carefully delivered treatments relative to treatments implemented in routine community care?

- For ADHD core symptoms, medical management and combined were better than usual community care.

- For non-ADHD symptoms and positive functioning, combined was better than usual community care, but medical management and behavioral treatment were not better.

The conclusion of the trial was to prescribe Ritalin for children with ADHD symptoms:

> *"We conclude that for ADHD symptoms, carefully crafted medication management, maintained through 14 months, was superior to behavior treatment alone and to routine usual care in the community." [65]*

This conclusion received substantial media attention and influenced US treatment guidelines to feature medication as a first-line treatment for children with ADHD. However, in a 3-year follow-up, no differences remained among the four arms of the trial [67]. In an 8-year follow-up, participants in all three arms fared worse than the usual community care group on 91% of the variables tested [68].

Simplified, the combined treatment which featured medical management combined with behavioral treatment appeared to be superior on most dimensions assessed. But the multiplicity of measures and the failure to specify a primary outcome promoted obfuscation of the relative effectiveness of the four treatment strategies, facilitated "cherry picking" the positive results from the medical management condition, and minimized the potential advantage of adding behavioral treatment to medication management. The lack of a clearly specified primary outcome allowed for extensive data dredging, capitalizing on the ambiguity resulting from the M&M's.

It is unknown whether reports and behaviors at many levels were biased by assessment reactivity stemming from the Hawthorne effect or social desirability. An understanding of assessment reactivity in behavioral clinical trials is fragmented and deserves much more systematic research attention. In the meantime, a cautious approach to M&M's maximizes the possibility that assessment strategies detect the influence of the interventions without bias.

In retrospect, it may have been wise in this behavioral trial to focus on a single aspect of ADHD, such as behavior at school, rather than including all aspects of ADHD as a primary endpoint. Alternatively, the science in the field may not have progressed far enough to select a single aspect. In this case, the scientific need may be for studies aimed at refining assessment, the results of which could facilitate the design of a simplified and focused *Phase III* efficacy trial aimed at influencing clinical practice.

It is clear, however, that the M&M's in this trial resulted in many children being prescribed drugs without the benefit of also receiving a behavioral treatment. Enthusiasm for M&M's makes it possible for investigators to mix together a variety of important, and not so important, scientific questions and focus on those answers in which they have a vested interest. It is hoped that this example makes it clear that this practice can come at the cost of finding optimum treatments.

Ceiling Effect in a *Phase III* Behavioral Clinical Trial

Phase II and *Phase III* confirmatory behavioral clinical trials must establish a primary outcome that is a clinically significant barometer of the effectiveness of a treatment. This outcome must be subject to improvement in response to a behavioral intervention. An estimate of the event rate on this outcome in the comparator condition drives the estimation of needed sample size. Eligibility criteria typically exclude patients who are unable to undergo the treatment or who have comorbidities or logistical barriers that would confound the interpretation of results.

These principles were applied in the Look AHEAD trial [33]. Look AHEAD was an important follow-up to the Diabetes Prevention Program, a lifestyle intervention that was successful in preventing diabetes in patients who were insulin resistant [69]. Look AHEAD sought to determine whether a similar intensive lifestyle intervention that focused on weight loss in people who were already diabetic would reduce subsequent cardiovascular events, compared to a comparator receiving diabetes support and education. The primary outcome was a composite of acute cardiac events and stroke assessed over 13.5 years and estimated to be approximately 2% per year for the comparator, based upon event rates observed among participants with similar profiles enrolled in the Atherosclerosis Risk in Communities Study and the Cardiovascular Health Study [70]. Results after 9.6 years showed that the event rate in the control group was only 0.7% per year, far below what was expected [71]. This led to a null trial that was terminated early based upon futility.

Whenever a large multi-center trial is terminated for futility, post hoc evaluations to determine why are needed [72]. Among the most persuasive explanations is that the eligibility criteria yielded unusually healthy patients with diabetes. Patients were excluded if they were unable to successfully complete a maximal graded exercise tolerance test showing that it was safe to exercise. Although the physical activity target was 175 minutes of moderate intensity activity per week, participants were asked to walk at a brisk pace for at least 50 minutes per week. Few primary care physicians require an exercise test before prescribing moderate exercise in patients with diabetes [72].

The futility in the Look AHEAD trial appears to be due, in part, to an exceedingly healthy population which made it impossible to detect benefit on the primary outcome due to a ceiling effect. Safety concerns went well beyond those in place in clinical practice and produced a trial that was underpowered to detect a health benefit in the healthy.

Questionable Value of Moderators and Mediators

A trial to assess the best setting for treating children diagnosed with oppositional defiant disorder randomized children to either a community or clinic setting [73]. In anticipation of moderator and mediator analyses, data collection featured an array of measures including the Columbia Impairment Scale, a teacher report form, the Trauma Events Screening Inventory, the Beck Depression Inventory, the Family Environment Scale, an assessment of attention-deficit hyperactivity disorder, oppositional defiant disorder history, and a variety of demographic characteristics.

A detailed analysis revealed only two moderators. For short-term outcomes, higher baseline impairment was associated with worse externalizing and disruptive behaviors when treatment was in the community rather than the clinic setting. For long-term outcomes, children from families with low levels of family conflict had worse externalizing behavior if treated in the community rather than the clinic setting. Both of these moderators were assessed during routine intake and diagnosis and required no additional data collection. No significant relationships were identified by the multiple instruments administered in anticipation of moderator and mediator analyses.

Efforts to evaluate moderators and mediators in confirmatory clinical trials have rarely resulted in the development of more effective interventions. In a search of the literature, not one instance could be found where moderators and mediators were evaluated in a clinical trial, used to refine an intervention, and produced improved outcomes in a follow-up trial [60]. Instead, investment of resources in anticipation of moderator and mediator analyses appears to support primarily academic pursuits.

RECOMMENDATIONS

Simplicity is a virtue. It is emulated in art, science, literature, design, technology, and folk wisdom (see box). It is therefore not surprising that simplicity is also a virtue in clinical trial design. It is characteristic of wisdom, clarity, depth of understanding, clear thinking, sophistication, and progression.

The primary recommendation from this chapter is a simple one. It is to embrace simplicity in the design of a definitive *Phase II* or *Phase III* behavioral trial. To achieve this simplicity, it is necessary to do exploratory, developmental, and refinement work up front, and have the patience, perseverance, and willingness to fail along the way.

Simplicity is most evident in the choice of outcomes for a behavioral trial. In pursuit of simplicity, the following are recommended.

> ## Simplicity
>
> *"Simplicity is the ultimate sophistication."*
>   Leonardo da Vinci
>
> *"The art of being wise is the art of knowing what to overlook."*
>   William James
>
> *"I would have written a shorter paper but I did not have enough time."*
>   Mark Twain
>
> *"Knowledge is a process of piling up facts; wisdom lies in their simplification."*
>   Martin H. Fischer
>
> *"Don't use a lot when a little will do."*
>   Proverb
>
> *"Less is more."*
>   Andrea del Sarto
>
> *The KISS principle: Keep it simple stupid.*
>
> *"Everything should be made as simple as possible, but not simpler."*
>   Albert Einstein
>
> *"Simple can be harder than complex. You have to get your thinking clean to make it simple."*
>   Steve Jobs
>
> *The first principle of Japanese flower arranging is minimalism. Know what to leave out.*

1. Stick your neck out. Prespecify one clinically meaningful, objectively determined, primary outcome. Preferably, it will be one that is in common use in clinical practice. Be accountable by registering this outcome in ClinicalTrials.gov before beginning a trial.

2. Seek clinical significance. Seek a level of change on the primary outcome that is clinically, not just statistically, significant. Embrace the concept of a minimal clinically important difference.

3. Place time, energy, and emphasis in a behavioral trial on the quality and fidelity of administration of the behavioral treatment, adherence, and retention rather than the pursuit of ancillary data. Be willing to cut down an assessment protocol mid-trial if such symptoms as stalled recruitment, non-adherence, and missing data begin to creep in.

4. Avoid the tendency toward M&M's. Limit the collection of moderator, mediator, and mechanism data to those that are essential to the interpretation of primary results. Limit the collection of data on secondary outcomes to those that are of the highest priority.

5. The act of observing changes the observed. Little is known about the strength of bias imposed by assessment reactivity. If it is suspected before a trial, add an assessment-only arm. If it is suspected during the trial, eliminate those assessments that appear to trigger the most reactivity.

6. There is an interdependence between exploration and confirmation. Exploration studies precede confirmatory studies. Explorations are the seeds that bear the fruit of a confirmatory causal association. Seeds must be planted *before* expecting to see the fruit.

REFERENCES

1. Kolodziej M, Klein I, Reisman L (2013) A new value proposition. Nat Med 19:1365. https://doi.org/10.1038/nm1113-1365
2. Temple RJ (1995) A regulatory authority's opinion about surrogate endpoints. In: Nimmo W, Tucker G (eds) Clinical measurement in drug evaluation. Wiley, New York
3. Department of Health and Human Services, Food and Drug Administration (1992) New drug, antibiotic, and biological drug product regulations: accelerated approval. Fed Regist 57:13234–13242
4. D'Agostino RB (2000) Debate: the slippery slope of surrogate outcomes. Curr Control Trials Cardiovas Med 1:76–78
5. Svensson S, Menkes DB, Lexchin J (2013) Surrogate outcomes in clinical trials: a cautionary tale. JAMA Intern Med 173:611–612
6. Ciani O, Buyse M, Garside R, Pavey T, Stein K, Sterne JAC, Taylor RS (2013) Comparison of treatment effect sizes associated with surrogate and final patient relevant outcomes in randomised controlled trials: meta-epidemiological study. BMJ 346. https://doi.org/10.1136/bmj.f457
7. Wieland LS, Berman BM, Altman DG, Barth J, Bouter LM, D'Adamo CR, Linde K, Moher D, Mullins CD, Treweek S, Tunis S, van der Windt DA, Zwarenstein M, Witt C (2017) Rating of included trials on the efficacy-effectiveness spectrum: development of a new tool for systematic reviews. J Clin Epidemiol 84:95–104
8. Freemantle N (2001) Interpreting the results of secondary end points and subgroup analyses in clinical trials: should we lock the crazy aunt in the attic? BMJ 322:989–991
9. Sheehan B (2012) Assessment scales in dementia. Ther Adv Neurol Disord 5:349–358
10. Gracely E (2008) So, why do I have to correct for multiple comparisons? Concepts and commentary on Turk et al. Pain 139:481–482
11. Ioannidis JPA (2005) Why most published research findings are false. PLoS Med 2:e124. https://doi.org/10.1371/journal.pmed.0020124
12. U.S. Department of Health and Human Services (2017) Multiple endpoints in clinical trials. Draft guidance for industry; 4353–4354 [2017-00695]. https://www.fda.gov/downloads/Drugs/GuidanceComplianceRegulatoryInformation/Guidances/ucm536750
13. U.S. Department of Health and Human Services (2009) Patient-reported outcome measures: use in medical product development to support labeling claims. Guidance for Industry, December. https://www.fda.gov/ucm/groups/fdagov-public/@fdagov-drugs-gen/documents/document/ucm193282
14. Stone AA, Shiffman S, Schwartz JE, Broderick JE, Hufford MR (2002) Patient non-compliance with paper diaries. BMJ 324:1193–1194
15. Bolt DM, Lu Y, Kim JS (2014) Measurement and control of response styles using anchoring vignettes: a model-based approach. Psychol Methods 19:528–541
16. Stirratt M, Dunbar-Jacob J, Crane HM, Simoni JM, Czajkowski S, Hilliard ME, Aikens JE, Hunter CM, Velligan DI, Huntley H, Ogedegbe G, Rand CS, Schron E, Nilsen WJ (2015) Self-report measures of medication adherence behavior: recommendations on optimal use. Transl Behav Med 5:470–482
17. Wood L, Egger M, Gluud LL, Schulz KF, Jüni P, Altman DG, Gluud C, Martin RM, Wood AJ, Sterne JA (2008) Empirical evidence of bias in treatment effect estimates in controlled trials with different interventions and outcomes: meta-epidemiological study. BMJ 336:601–605
18. U.S. Department of Health and Human Services, Medicare Evidence Development and Coverage Advisory Committee (2016) Treatment resistant depression. https://www.cms.gov/Regulations-and-Guidance/Guidance/FACA/downloads/id71c
19. Jones DA, West RR (1996) Psychological rehabilitation after myocardial infarction: multicentre randomised controlled trial. BMJ 313:1517–1521

20. Landsberger HA (1958) Hawthorne revisited. Management and the worker, its critics, and developments in human relations in industry. Cornell University, Ithaca
21. McCambridge J, Kalaitzaki E, White IR, Khadjesari Z, Murray E, Linke S, Thompson SG, Godfrey C, Wallace P (2011) Impact of length or relevance of questionnaires on attrition in online trials: randomized controlled trial. J Med Internet Res 13:e96. https://doi.org/10.2196/jmir.1733
22. Donovan DM, Bogenschutz MP, Perl H, Forcehimes A, Adinoff B, Mandler R, Oden N, Walker R (2012) Study design to examine the potential role of assessment reactivity in the Screening, Motivational Assessment, Referral, and Treatment in Emergency Departments (SMART-ED) protocol. Addict Sci Clin Pract 7:16. https://doi.org/10.1186/1940-0640-7-16
23. Bogenschutz MP, Donovan DM, Mandler RN, Perl HI, Forcehimes AA, Crandall C, Lindblad R, Oden NL, Sharma G, Metsch L, Lyons MS, McCormack R, Macias-Konstantopoulos W, Douaihy A (2014) Brief intervention for patients with problematic drug use presenting in emergency departments: a randomized clinical trial. JAMA Intern Med 174:1736–1745
24. McCambridge J, Butor-Bhavsar K, Witton J, Elbourne D (2011) Can research assessments themselves cause bias in behaviour change trials? A systematic review of evidence from solomon 4-group studies. PLoS One 6:e25223. https://doi.org/10.1371/journal.pone.0025223
25. Friedman LM, Furberg CD, DeMets D, Reboussin DM, Granger CB (2015) Fundamentals of clinical trials, 5th edn. Springer, Cham
26. Turk DC, Dworkin RH, Allen RR, Bellamy N, Brandenburg N, Carr DB, Cleeland C, Dionne R, Farrar JT, Galer BS, Hewitt DJ, Jadad AR, Katz NP, Kramer LD, Manning DC, McCormick CG, McDermott MP, McGrath P, Quessy S, Rappaport BA, Robinson JP, Royal MA, Simon L, Stauffer JW, Stein W, Tollett J, Witter J (2003) Core outcome domains for chronic pain clinical trials: IMMPACT recommendations. Pain 106:337–345
27. Mehta P, Claydon L, Hendrick P, Winser S, Baxter GD (2015) Outcome measures in randomized-controlled trials of neuropathic pain conditions: a systematic review of systematic reviews and recommendations for practice. Clin J Pain 2015:169–176
28. Zarin DA, Tse T, Williams RJ, Carr S (2016) Trial reporting in ClinicalTrials.gov: the final rule. N Engl J Med 375:1998–2004
29. Mahaffey KW, Harrington RA, Akkerhuis M, Kleiman NS, Berdan LG, Crenshaw BS, Tardiff BE, Granger CB, DeJong I, Bhapkar M, Widimsky P, Corbalon R, Lee KL, Deckers JW, Simoons ML, Topol EJ, Califf RM, for the PURSUIT Investigators (2001) Systematic adjudication of myocardial infarction end-points in an international clinical trial. Curr Control Trials Cardiovasc Med 2:180–186
30. Chan AW, Tetzlaff JM, Altman DG, Laupacis A, Gøtzsche PC, Krleža-Jerić K, Hróbjartsson A, Mann H, Dickersin K, Berlin J, Doré C, Parulekar W, Summerskill W, Groves T, Schulz K, Sox H, Rockhold FW, Rennie D, Moher D (2013) SPIRIT 2013 statement: defining standard protocol items for clinical trials. Ann Intern Med 158:200–207
31. Burke LE, Kennedy DL, Miskala PH, Papadopoulos EJ, Trentacosti AM (2008) The use of patient-reported outcome measures in the evaluation of medical products for regulatory approval. Clin Pharmacol Ther 84:281–283
32. Riley WT, Pilkonis P, Cella D (2011) Application of the National Institutes of Health Patient-Reported Outcome Measurement Information System (PROMIS) to mental health research. J Ment Health Policy Econ 14:201–208
33. Look AHEAD Research Group, Wing RR, Bolin P, Brancati FL, Bray GA, Clark JM, Coday M, Crow RS, Curtis JM, Egan CM, Espeland MA, Evans M, Foreyt JP, Ghazarian S, Gregg EW, Harrison B, Hazuda HP, Hill JO, Horton ES, Hubbard VS, Jakicic JM, Jeffery RW, Johnson KC, Kahn SE, Kitabchi AE, Knowler WC, Lewis CE, Maschak-Carey BJ, Montez MG, Murillo A, Nathan DM, Patricio J, Peters A, Pi-Sunyer X, Pownall H, Reboussin D, Regensteiner JG, Rickman AD, Ryan DH, Safford M, Wadden TA, Wagenknecht LE, West DS, Williamson DF, Yanovski SZ (2013) Cardiovascular effects of intensive lifestyle intervention in type 2 diabetes. N Engl J Med 369:145–154
34. Tomlinson G, Detsky AS (2010) Composite end points in randomized trials: there is no free lunch. JAMA 303:267–268

35. The ACCORD Study Group, Gerstein HC, Miller ME, Genuth S, Ismail-Beigi F, Buse JB, Goff DC Jr, Probstfield JL, Cushman WC, Ginsberg HN, Bigger JT, Grimm RH Jr, Byington RP, Rosenberg YD, Friedewald WT (2011) Long-term effects of intensive glucose lowering on cardiovascular outcomes. N Engl J Med 364:818–828

36. Brindle PM, McConnachie A, Upton MN, Hart CL, Davey Smith G, Watt GC (2005) The accuracy of the Framingham risk-score in different socioeconomic groups: a prospective study. Br J Gen Pract 55:838–845

37. Cohen J (1988) Statistical power analysis for the behavioral sciences, 2nd edn. Lawrence Erlbaum Assoc, Mahwah

38. Aberegg SK, Richards DR, O'Brien JM (2010) Delta inflation: a bias in the design of randomized controlled trials in critical care medicine. Crit Care 14:R77. https://doi.org/10.1186/cc8990

39. Jaeschke R, Singer J, Guyatt GH (1989) Measurement of health status: ascertaining the minimal clinically important difference. Control Clin Trials 10:407–415

40. Powell LH, Appelhans BM, Ventrelle J, Karavolos K, March ML, Ong JC, Fitzpatrick SL, Normand P, Dawar R, Kazlauskaite R (2018) Development of a lifestyle intervention for the metabolic syndrome: discovery through proof-of-concept. Health Psych 37:929–939

41. De Geest S, Sabate E (2003) Adherence to long-term therapies: evidence for action. Europ J Cardiovasc Nursing 2:323. https://doi.org/10.1016/S1474-5151(03)00091-4

42. Esposito K, Marfella R, Ciotola M, Di Palo C, Giugliano F, Giugliano G, D'Armiento M, D'Andrea F, Giugliano D (2004) Effect of a Mediterranean-style diet on endothelial dysfunction and markers of vascular inflammation in the metabolic syndrome: a randomized trial. JAMA 292:1440–1446

43. Colman E (2012) Food and Drug Administration's obesity drug guidance document: a short history. Circulation 125:2156–2164

44. Wen L, Badgett R, Cornell J (2005) Number needed to treat: a descriptor for weighing therapeutic options. Am J Health Syst Pharm 62:2031–2036

45. Stang A, Poole C, Bender R (2010) Common problems related to the use of number needed to treat. J Clin Epidemiol 63:820–825

46. McAlister FA (2008) The "number needed to treat" turns 20--and continues to be used and misused. CMAJ 179:549–553

47. Fairman KA, Davis LE, Kruse CR, Sclar DA (2017) Financial impact of direct-acting oral anticoagulants in medicaid: budgetary assessment based on number needed to treat. Appl Health Econ Health Policy 15:203–214

48. Revicki D, Hays RD, Cella D, Sloan J (2008) Recommended methods for determining responsiveness and minimally important differences for patient-reported outcomes. J Clin Epidemiol 61:102–109

49. Copay AG, Subach BR, Glassman SD, Polly DW Jr, Schuler TC (2007) Understanding the minimum clinically important difference: a review of concepts and methods. Spine J 7:541–546

50. Gatchel RJ, Mayer TG, Choi Y, Chou R (2013) Validation of a consensus-based minimal clinically important difference (MCID) threshold using an objective functional external anchor. Spine J 13:889–893

51. Black N, Murphy M, Lamping D, McKee M, Sanderson C, Askham J, Marteau T (1999) Consensus development methods: a review of best practice in creating clinical guidelines. J Health Serv Res Policy 4:236–248

52. Karow A, Naber D, Lambert M, Moritz S, the EGOFORS Initiative (2012) Remission as perceived by people with schizophrenia, family members, and psychiatrists. Eur Psychiatry 27:426–431

53. Button KS, Kounali D, Thomas L, Wiles NJ, Peters TJ, Welton NJ, Ades AE, Lewis G (2015) Minimal clinically important difference on the Beck Depression Inventory-II according to the patient's perspective. Psychol Med 45:3269–3279

54. Duru G, Fantino B (2008) The clinical relevance of changes in the Montgomery-Asberg Depression Rating Scale using the minimum clinically important difference approach. Curr Med Res Opin 24:1329–1335

55. Berkman LF, Blumenthal J, Burg M, Carney RM, Catellier D, Cowan MJ, Czajkowski SM, DeBusk R, Hosking J, Jaffe A, Kaufmann PG, Mitchell P, Norman J, Powell LH, Raczynski JM, Schneiderman N, the Enhancing Recovery in Coronary Heart Disease Patients Investigators (ENRICHD) (2003) Effects of treating depression and low perceived social support on clinical events after myocardial infarction: the Enhancing Recovery in Coronary Heart Disease Patients (ENRICHD) Randomized Trial. JAMA 289:3106–3116

56. Hermes EDA, Sokoloff DM, Stroup TS, Rosenheck RA (2012) Minimum clinically important difference in the Positive and Negative Syndrome Scale with data from the CATIE schizophrenia trial. J Clin Psychiatry 73:526–532

57. Wright A, Hannon J, Hegedus EJ, Kavchak AE (2012) Clinimetrics corner: a closer look at the minimal clinically important difference (MCID). J Man Manip Ther 20:160–166

58. Kraemer HC, Wilson T, Fairburn CG, Agras WS (2002) Mediators and moderators of treatment effects in randomized clinical trials. Arch Gen Psychiatry 59:877–883

59. Hinshaw SP (2007) Moderators and mediators of treatment outcome for youth with ADHD: understanding for whom and how interventions work. J Pediatr Psychol 32:664–675

60. Kaufmann PG (2009) Psychosocial interventions in breast cancer: to light a candle. Cancer 115:5617–5619

61. ENRICHD (2011) Enhancing Recovery in Coronary Heart Disease Patients (ENRICHD) protocol, Version 7.0. https://biolincc.nhlbi.nih.gov/studies/enrichd/

62. Popper KR (1959) The logic of scientific discovery. Basic Books, New York

63. Shadish WR, Cook TD, Campbell DT (2002) Experimental and quasi-experimental designs for generalized causal inference. Houghton Mifflin, Boston

64. Kazdin A (2007) Mediators and mechanisms of change in psychotherapy research. Ann Rev Clin Psychol 3:1–27

65. Hinshaw SP, Arnold LE for the MTA Cooperative Group (2015) ADHD, multimodal treatment, and longitudinal outcome: evidence, paradox, and challenge. Wiley Interdiscip Rev Cog Sci 6:39–52

66. MTA Cooperative Group (2004) National Institute of Mental Health Multimodal Treatment Study of ADHD follow-up: 24-month outcomes of treatment strategies for attention-deficit/hyperactivity disorder. Pediatrics 113:754–761

67. Jensen PS, Arnold LE, Swanson JM, Vitiello B, Abikoff HB, Greenhill LL, Hechtman L, Hinshaw SP, Pelham WE, Wells KC, Conners CK, Elliott GR, Epstein JN, Hoza B, March JS, Molina BSG, Newcorn JH, Severe JB, Wigal T, Gibbons RD, Hur K (2007) 3-year follow-up of the NIMH MTA study. J Am Acad Child Adolesc Psychiatry 46:989–1002

68. Molina BSG, Hinshaw SP, Swanson JM, Arnold LE, Vitiello B, Jensen PS, Epstein JN, Hoza B, Hechtman L, Abikoff HB, Elliott GR, Greenhill LL, Newcorn JH, Wells KC, Wigal T, Gibbons RD, Hur K, Houck PR, MTA Cooperative Group (2009) The MTA at 8 years: prospective follow-up of children treated for combined-type ADHD in a multisite study. J Am Acad Child Adolesc Psychiatry 48:484–500

69. Knowler WC, Barrett-Connor E, Fowler SE, Hamman RF, Lachin JM, Walker EA, Nathan DM, Diabetes Prevention Program Research Group (2002) Reduction in the incidence of type 2 diabetes with lifestyle intervention or metformin. N Engl J Med 346:393–403

70. Look AHEAD clinical trial protocol, 7th revision (2009). https://www.div12.org/wp-content/uploads/2015/04/Look-AHEAD-Protocol

71. Brancati FL, Evans M, Furberg CD, Geller N, Haffner S, Kahn SE, Kaufmann PG, Lewis CE, Nathan DM, Pitt B, Safford MM, Look AHEAD Study Group (2012) Midcourse correction to a clinical trial when the event rate is underestimated: the Look AHEAD (Action for Health in Diabetes) Study. Clin Trials 9:113–124

72. Barrett-Connor E (2013) Looking back on the look AHEAD trial. https://www.acc.org/latest-in-cardiology/articles/2014/07/18/18/22/looking-back-on-the-look-ahead-trial

73. Shelleby EC, Kolko DJ (2015) Predictors, moderators, and treatment parameters of community and clinic-based treatment for child disruptive behavior disorders. J Child Fam Stud 24:734–748

Chapter 10
Preferences, Equipoise, and Blinding

"So many professional scientists suffer from prejudices. Independence from prejudices is, in my opinion, the mark of distinction between a mere artisan and a real seeker after truth."

Albert Einstein 1944 [1]

Fundamental Point

Investigator preference for, and confidence in, a specific trial result is a post-randomization expectancy bias which can trigger unintended interventions, treatment crossovers, co-intervention bias, and ascertainment bias. Because double-blind design control for preferences and expectations is generally not possible in a behavioral trial, the onus is on the behavioral trialist to protect the trial from expectancy bias. Trial leaders should adopt an objective mindset characterized by freedom from preferences for a particular trial result, and by equipoise or true uncertainty about what the result will be. This mindset will trickle down to all trial operations. Further protection against expectancy bias is provided by a push to extend the blind in as many ways as possible and by efforts to identify risk of bias early and often enough to provide time for remediation.

Unique challenges for behavioral clinical trials are posed by expectancy bias resulting from the lethal combination of visible treatment status and visible beliefs about these treatments. In contrast to double-blind drug trials where pre-existing beliefs are neutralized by treatments that look identical, behavioral trials evaluate randomized arms that often look different, thus limiting options for design control of biases resulting from preferences. Blinding outcomes assessors is a necessary, but insufficient, approach to minimize expectancy bias in a behavioral trial. Three additional targets should be considered. The mindset of the principal investigator should be scientific and objective, characterized by equipoise and freedom from a preference for a particular trial result. Design control can be maximized by a push to extend the

© Springer Nature Switzerland AG 2021
L. H. Powell et al., *Behavioral Clinical Trials for Chronic Diseases*,
https://doi.org/10.1007/978-3-030-39330-4_10

blind to as many entities as possible, by the use of neutral names for trial arms, and by blinding to trial hypotheses but not to aims. Prevention and early detection of adverse implications of expectancy bias can be accomplished by ongoing assessment of risk of bias in such areas as differential retention, adherence, and co-interventions.

SCIENTIFIC PRINCIPLES

Scientific Mindset

The mindset of the scientist is a combination of objectivity and openness. The objective, critical judgment side is the Sancho to the open and idealistic side of the Don Quixote [3].

> *"Belief and commitment are states of the human mind. Scientific value is independent of the mind that creates it and depends only on the support that a conjecture has in facts."*
> Lakatos 1977 [2]

The objective side of the scientist is to be skeptical and eschew belief. Although it is part of being human to have beliefs, opinions, and preconceptions, when they are unsubstantiated by evidence, they are considered to be nonscience. In science, belief is the enemy of rationality and tested truths are the prize.

The softer side of the scientist is openness to experience. This side takes pleasure in the discovery of new truths, enjoys exploring new ways to express them, and is driven by the journey to find the grail in an unexplored land [4]. This softer side is open to any and all possibilities with minimal preconceptions.

A scientific mindset in a clinical trialist balances objectivity and openness. Objectivity is a healthy skepticism about the value of a new treatment. Openness is the promise that the new treatment offers. This delicate balance can be compromised in a clinical trial. It is natural for an investigator to have a *preference for* or a *belief about* the benefit of a particular treatment, particularly in light of promising preliminary data and/or a long-term investment in that treatment. These beliefs are intuitive and often a somewhat vague sense of the probability of

Scientific Mindset	Unscientific Mindset
Skepticism	Belief
Openness	Preconceptions
Curiosity	Expectations
Discovery	Preferences
Objectivity	Prejudice
Uncertainty	Certainty
Hypotheses	Biases

some future outcome [5]. But belief and confidence about a treatment without the conclusive, objective support from a clinical trial become biases (see box). If that support existed, belief and confidence would be justified, and a clinical trial would be unnecessary.

Double-Blind Designs

Investigators who undertake drug trials often have pre-existing preferences for the new drug being tested, influenced by such things as favorable preclinical data, a strong belief in the biological basis of the therapy, and/or a professional/financial interest in the success of the drug [6]. To avoid biasing the trial, these preferences are neutralized by the double-blind trial design. First introduced in 1927, blinding (also called masking) aimed to minimize the error of inference that could result from a failure to separate the biological mechanisms of action of a drug from patient belief in the value of that drug. Treatment arms compared an active pill to a placebo pill that had a similar look, feel, and taste. These identical treatments made it possible to withhold information about which pill any particular patient received from the patient, the investigators, the research staff, the patient's medical provider, and most other entities in the trial.

The double-blind design creates design control for expectancy bias. First described by Sackett as therapeutic personality bias [7], and later by Chalmers and Matthews as optimism bias [8], expectancy bias occurs when the expectations and beliefs of investigators cause them to subconsciously influence behavior of the participants in a trial. In a double-blind design, neither the investigators, the staff, nor the participants

Expectancy Bias
A form of reactivity in which investigators' cognitive biases cause them to subconsciously influence participants in a trial. It can undercut the internal validity of a trial by triggering a placebo response, treatment contamination, ascertainment bias, and/or differential dropout or non-adherence.

know who is on active treatment and who is on placebo. This blinding prevents any pre-existing expectations, preferences, or beliefs about a particular treatment from affecting trial operations or participant participation. Trust among the patient, the provider, and the trial staff is maintained because they are all in the same boat of ignorance, becoming, in a sense, partners in a joint venture [9]. At its most fundamental level, this design control preserves scientific objectivity which is the hallmark of scientific inquiry.

This is not to say that double-blinding is perfect. Indeed, reviews of the success of blinding in double-blind, placebo-controlled randomized clinical trials have reported unsuccessful blinding in 23–60% of the trials that reported on blinding [5]. While not perfect, the double-blind placebo controlled trial is the best approach that exists in science for separating the active elements of a treatment from expectancy effects.

CHALLENGES FOR BEHAVIORAL TRIALS

Expectancy Bias

The exquisite design control that gives double-blind, placebo controlled drug trials their rigor is often impossible when the treatment is behavioral in nature. Because the treatments being compared often look quite different, participants, investigators, and staff often know which treatment any particular participant is receiving.

This difference is portrayed in the box at the right. In the double-blind trial, the treatments are pills that look identical. The investigator may have a clear preference for, and belief in, the active pill. But because neither the investigator nor anyone else knows which participants are on which pill, it is impossible for these preferences to influence trial operations. In contrast, the behavioral trial

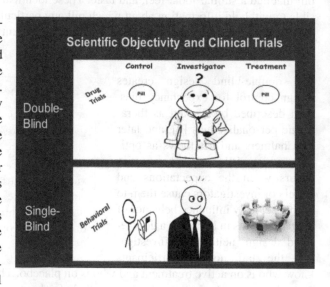

compares two treatments that are not identical but rather, in this example, mail-based or group-based. The investigator may have a clear preference for the group-based treatment. But articulating this preference when participants and staff know which treatment each participant is receiving enhances undesirable reactivity.

To preserve rigor despite the problem of non-identical treatments, behavioral trials are commonly designed as single-blind trials. Although the term "single blind" has no official definition, it has been described as keeping either the investigator or the participant blinded to participant treatment allocation [10]. In a behavioral trial, it is most often interpreted as keeping the outcomes assessors blinded to participant treatment allocation. This minimizes biased assessment which could result if an assessor, advertently or inadvertently, acted on a preference for a particular treatment by using different criteria to evaluate those randomized to the preferred arm relative to those randomized to the other. Blinding outcomes assessors has become a standard practice in behavioral trial methodology.

The challenge for behavioral trials is that limiting blinding to only the outcomes assessors may be necessary but not sufficient to prevent bias. Despite best efforts to keep assessors blinded to treatment allocation, it is often the case that interactions with participants reveal the arm to which they were allocated, even in the face of directives to participants to refrain from talking about their treatment arm.

But more importantly, there is an ethos, culture, atmosphere, or climate that develops in a trial which becomes more entrenched the longer the trial continues. It is in this ethos that preferences are revealed. They are revealed by the names used for trial arms: treatment (i.e., *"the new, exciting, potent innovation"*) vs. control (i.e., *"getting nothing"*). They are revealed in formal, casual, and spontaneous conversations among principal investigators, co-investigators, treating physicians, trial coordinators, research assistants, core lab staff, trial statisticians, adjudicators, and data monitoring committees [11]. They are revealed by descriptions of the trial presented to an array of professional and nonprofessional audiences including local media, institutional colleagues, local presentations, and presentations to recruiting colleagues. They travel indirectly through a variety of social networks.

Bias based upon preference and expectation operates more strongly when outcomes are subjective. But even seemingly objective outcomes such as blood pressure or the diagnosis of acute myocardial infarction can be affected by more indirect pathways. The impact of expectation bias on the outcome of trials is difficult to quantify, but there is some evidence from reviews and meta-analyses that unblinded studies overestimate treatment effects by somewhere between 17% and 64% [12, 13].

Complicating the problem for behavioral trialists is the often long-standing commitment they must make to the behavioral treatment they are testing. Without the multibillion dollar infrastructure support that exists for the development of new drugs, behavioral trialists often spend careers developing and refining behavioral treatments to ready them for rigorous testing in an efficacy or effectiveness trial. The more long-standing this commitment, the greater the likelihood that the behavioral trialist will hold strong beliefs about, and preferences for, the treatment's ultimate success.

Implications of Expectancy Bias

The combination of visible treatment status and visible expectations about treatments is lethal. It raises the possibility that participants will act on their pre-existing beliefs and be reluctant to be randomized. It also raises the possibility that participants will agree to random assignment but then be disappointed in the outcome either because of their pre-existing preferences, or preferences that are developed during the course of the trial. Any disappointment can translate into a disruption of the balance between arms when participants take differential, arm-specific actions that translate into biases and threaten the internal validity of the trial [8]. In a review of 105 clinical trials in hematological cancers conducted between 1955 and 1998, 71% were null trials, and expectancy bias was the major culprit leading to the null result [14].

The most important implications of expectancy bias in behavioral trials are described below.

Placebo Response

Expectations, beliefs, preferences, and prejudices about a treatment can become an unintended active treatment component that mobilizes a placebo or nocebo response and can result in a spurious judgment of treatment efficacy. Placebos and nocebos operate predominantly by producing symptomatic relief or exacerbation, rather than modifying the pathophysiology of disease [15]. In a classic 1955 paper, Beecher showed the power of the placebo response in a review of 15 trials where 35% of 1082 patients derived clinically significant benefit from a placebo arm across such diverse outcomes as pain, cough, mood, and the common cold [16]. More recent explorations of participants randomized to placebo arms in clinical trials have shown that between 19–20% report side

> ### Miracle or a Powerful Placebo Response?
>
> To be canonized as a saint, Mother Teresa needed evidence that she achieved two miracles. The first was achieved. The second occurred when a Brazilian man suffering from a viral brain infection and facing emergency surgery spontaneously recovered the morning of the surgery. His wife had been praying for months to Mother Teresa, but on the days preceding the emergency surgery, she, her family, and her priest intensified their prayers. A medical commission voted unanimously that the cure was inexplicable in light of present-day medical knowledge. A theological inquiry voted unanimously that there was a perfect connection between the cause–the intensified invocation of Mother Teresa–and the effect– the spontaneous healing. Absence of a medical explanation and contiguity in time between the prayers and the recovery was the evidence that led to the judgment that this was the second miracle.

effects, and 25% discontinue because of side effects [17]. Placebo response has known psychobiological pathways [17–19], has a greater impact on subjective than objective outcomes [15], operates even when subjects know that they are receiving a placebo [20], and can be sustained for as long at 2 years on both subjective and objective outcomes [21]. Expectation of benefit, or harm, a key psychological pathway, can be elicited by classical conditioning, experience of others, mass media reports, and even minor verbal or nonverbal cues [17, 19].

In a behavioral clinical trial, if participants in one arm develop more confidence in their treatment than participants in another arm, this differential confidence can serve as an unintended active treatment component, mobilize neurobiological and psychological pathways, and produce a spurious improvement in a primary outcome. This is a particularly dangerous problem when a treatment is being compared to a no-treatment control, and the perception of getting "something" vs. "nothing" is easily translated into participant confidence and the mobilization of a placebo or nocebo response.

Co-Intervention Bias

Co-intervention bias refers to the differential receipt of medications, therapies, or programs, after randomization, that alter the balance achieved at the time of randomization and change the risk of developing the outcome. For example, if medical providers have a preference for a particular treatment, they could more carefully evaluate patients in the preferred arm out of curiosity, or provide ancillary care to patients in the less preferred arm to make up for the perceived deficit. In the case of caregivers, preference for a treatment that was not received by the person in their care could promote interest in making up for the perceived deficit by encouraging adherence to drug therapy, commitment to lifestyle changes, attendance at scheduled appointments with their provider, and/or discontinuing participation in the trial. To the extent that participants in comparator conditions get more care or participants in treated conditions get more careful scrutiny, the direction of this bias is to dilute effect sizes.

Treatment Crossover/Contamination/"John Henry" Effect

If trial participants come to believe that they were unlucky enough to be randomized to "a control group," "standard treatment," or "no treatment," they could be inclined to pursue the favored "new" treatment offered in the other trial arm on their own. This effort to try harder to compensate for a perceived deficit is called the "John Henry" effect after the legendary American steel driver who, when he heard his output was being compared to that of a steam drill, worked so hard to outperform the machine that he died in the process. In the case of behavioral trials, treatment crossover or contamination occurs when participants pursue the "new" treatment on their own to make up for their unlucky allocation to a less preferred trial arm. Since participants in comparator conditions would now be getting the treatment under investigation or something comparable, the direction of the bias is toward a dilution of the effect size.

Ascertainment Bias

Outcomes assessors who have expectations about differential benefit from trial arms could inadvertently become unblinded during the process of outcome assessment. Despite instructions that participants not reveal details of their treatment to assessors, leaking of clues is more the rule than the exception. Preferences of outcomes assessors could appear as a differential tendency to assess side effects, quality of life, or ambiguous responses based upon the trial arm. This extends to research staff in charge of medical record adjudication who could inadvertently make decisions about whether or not to send a suspected case for endpoint adjudication based upon their knowledge of, and preference for, a particular treatment assignment. This bias is less important with a hard outcome such as death. But most other outcomes are susceptible, including cause of death, disease diagnosis, physical measurements, questionnaires, and patient-reported conditions [22].

Differential Dropout

A reasonable action for a participant to take if they develop an expectation that the arm to which they were assigned is unlikely to have any benefit is to drop out of the trial or to remain in the trial but be non-adherent to the treatment. Dropout rates are generally incorporated into sample size calculations because they undercut the power of the trial to detect hypothesized differences. But differential dropout, where the rate is higher in one arm than the other, triggers post-randomization imbalance between the arms and opens the door to confounding. It is common to adjust for missing data using such methods as multiple imputation. But most of these methods make conservative assumptions and, when differentially applied to a specific trial arm, can weaken the effect size.

OVERCOMING THESE CHALLENGES IN A BEHAVIORAL TRIAL

The dilemma for the behavioral trialist is how to achieve scientific rigor in the face of human emotions and convictions that could bias a trial conducted in a setting where double-blinding is not possible. Several strategies can help to resolve this dilemma.

Belief in Equipoise

Investigator equipoise is a state of genuine uncertainty regarding the comparative therapeutic merits of each arm of the trial [23]. It is motivated by a balance between interest in, and skepticism about, the possible benefit of a new treatment. It extends from the concept of clinical/community equipoise that refers to a general consensus in the expert medical community of uncertainty about the best treatment. Clinical equipoise is the fundamental reason for undertaking a clinical trial. Investigator equipoise is a fundamental element in obtaining a conclusive answer in that trial.

Equipoise Is Grounded in Reality

Belief in equipoise is not simply a mind game of restructuring cognitions. True uncertainty about the ultimate result of a trial is grounded in fact, despite convincing preliminary data.

The large majority of clinical trials produce in null findings. For example, recent evaluations of all clinical trials conducted by the US National Heart, Lung, and Blood Institute after 2000, with large budgets of >$500,000/year requiring pre-authorization, observed a

> **Equipoise and Reality**
>
> The odds are 1 in 5 of having a positive result from a big budget behavioral clinical trial [24].

significant benefit of the intervention on the primary outcome in only 8–18% of the trials [24–26]. When this evaluation was limited to the track record for big budget *behavioral* trials, a significant benefit on the primary outcome was observed in only 18% of the trials [24]. Thus, if history is a good predictor of the future, at best the odds are only 1 in 5 of having a positive result from a behavioral clinical trial. These odds must be considered in light of the fact that these large-budget trials were unlikely to be funded at such a high level without excellent preliminary evidence to support their potential efficacy.

Equipoise Is Grounded in Ethics

There must be sufficient doubt about a new treatment to permit withholding it from some. The key rationale for a clinical trial is community equipoise—uncertainty among the community of providers about whether or not a new treatment works. In agreeing to lead or participate in a trial, the individual investigator must be driven by community equipoise,

> **Equipoise and Ethics**
>
> *"On the moral compass of scientific research, equipoise points due north, providing a framework of ethical principles and research integrity beyond reproach."* [27]

agree to the merits of resolving it, and make the intellectually honest admission that the answer is not yet known. The ethical course of action, in the presence of community equipoise, is to get a conclusive answer.

It is ethical to be clear about facts, not beliefs. If an investigator is driven by getting a conclusive answer to the question posed, the fact is that the benefits of any arm are uncertain. This can and should be expressed to prospective participants in a way that is honest, simple, and understandable. Prospective participants must be helped to understand that by agreeing to random assignment they are not agreeing to get "something or nothing." Instead, they will get one of two or more conditions, and it is not known which one is the best. They will be partners in finding an answer. Sometimes a prospective participant agrees to be randomized to one of two conditions on the assumption that there is a 50% chance of getting a new treatment that will help them. In actuality, the prospective participant will get one of two arms, with limited information about whether either one will help them. Indeed, it has been the case that new treatments hypothesized to improve outcomes actually were associated with worse outcomes [28, 29].

Keep Preferences Private

A belief in equipoise is elegant in theory but elusive in reality [27]. Preferences for a treatment, preferences for a result, and confidence in a trial result are supported by academic incentives. In the high-stakes setting of medical research, influential studies that affect professional discourse are the milestones of prestige and success. They lead to academic advancement, success in grant funding and publishing, and financial rewards. The pull of these academic incentives is often stronger than any brakes imposed upon them by the ideals of equipoise. When the pull gets the upper hand, symptoms of preferences for, and confidence in, a specific trial result appear across a number of domains:

Language: *"I am going to prove this hypothesis."*

Reputation: Investigator is seen as a "true believer."

Choice of   Facilitates "spin" by assessing many outcomes and
Outcomes: claiming success from benefit obtained in only a few.

A translational science approach encourages positive expectations of benefit in early phases of treatment development. Positive expectations can foster the persistence needed to refine the treatment in the face of early failures. But movement from development to confirmation is associated with a transition away from preferences and toward objectivity. This is modeled by the principal investigator and evident throughout all trial operations. When the principal investigator believes in equipoise and seeks a conclusive answer to resolve it, all involved in the trial will follow suit and a culture of objectivity will be fostered. Similarly, when the principal investigator is confident that the preferred treatment will be supported by the trial, all involved in the trial will follow suit, and advertently or inadvertently bias will be fostered.

If a principal investigator has preferences for a particular result, they must have the discipline to keep them private. If this is not possible, the principal investigator's best role on the project is to supervise the intervention, not lead the trial. Leadership of the trial by an objective investigator will foster crucial objectivity. Leadership of the intervention by the passionate investigator will foster intervention strength. If the passionate investigator truly has confidence in the treatment being evaluated, there is no better way to act on this confidence than to do everything possible to get an objective, unbiased, and conclusive trial result.

Push to Extend the Blind

Double-blind designs use design control to neutralize investigator expectations. Behavioral clinical trials can make greater use of design control to neutralize investigator expectations by pushing to extend the blind. Rather than being locked into the restricted practice of blinding only the outcomes assessors, and the restricted label of a single-blind design, behavioral trial designs can push to extend blinding in as many ways, and to as many players, as possible in pursuit of neutralizing the adverse impact of expectations.

While it is impossible to create a general rule of thumb concerning who and how to blind that applies to all behavioral trials, some viable targets for extending the blind follow.

Blind to Hypotheses but Not to Aims

A particularly important, but often overlooked, target for blinding is the research hypothesis [30]. The hypothesis is a statement of a belief that will be tested. It reveals preferences. This is different from trial aims that reflect what is actually going to be done within each of the randomized arms. Ethics require a clear statement to prospective participants of what will be required in each arm if they agree to be randomized to the trial. Rigor requires a minimization of articulation of beliefs and preferences to minimize bias. Blinding to research hypotheses, but not to trial aims, is a way to achieve rigor without compromising ethics. A consent form could read like the following:

> *"We are comparing two treatments. Treatment A requires attendance at weekly group meetings. Treatment B requires reading educational tip sheets sent weekly in the mail. We do not know which of these treatments is more effective for your condition."*

This consent: (1) articulates the aims in the form of what the prospective participant is required to do within each treatment arm; (2) articulates the reality of the uncertainty about which is more effective; and (3) stops short of revealing the research hypothesis reflecting a tentative belief. The statement above should not be limited to interactions with participants. It should, in fact, reflect the way the trial is discussed within and across all entities. This makes it possible to blind a wide variety of investigators and staff to the research hypothesis under investigation.

Neutral Names for Trial Arms

Names for arms that do not reveal research hypotheses minimize expectancies. Names that are closely linked to the aims or the treatment are good choices. For example, a trial that compared a self-management skills training treatment to an education-only comparator could use the names "skills training" and "enhanced education." A trial that compared a self-management skills training treatment to enhanced usual care could use the names "skills training" and "enhanced care." In any trial, regardless of the choice of a comparator, participants receive enhanced care in the form of closer surveillance. Thus, use of the term "enhanced" is justified.

Blind to Outcomes

Blinding investigators to the primary outcome of a clinical trial until all data are collected and analyzed is standard in clinical trial methodology. The rationale for this is that if investigators, staff, and/or participants knew of the results of a trial before it ended, it could limit enthusiasm for completing the trial, encourage participants to seek out the better treatment, and result in dropouts, non-adherence, and treatment crossovers. After the last participant completes follow-up, investigators can be unblinded to the primary outcome, and papers focusing on the primary outcome can be published.

There is, however, debate on the wisdom of preparing interim reports on secondary outcomes before the trial has ended. Interim reports are common in medicine. A review of trials conducted between 2006 and 2015 with "interim" in the abstract reported that the majority of interim reports were in the areas of oncology, surgery, and cardiology, they were industry-sponsored, and they were not pre-specified in the protocol [31]. There is little information about interim reports in behavioral trials, but they appear to be equally, if not more, common. Since participants are aware of the particular behavioral treatment they are receiving, the risks of reactivity to an interim report are greater. Any interim reports should be carefully planned ahead of time with careful consideration of the risk of bias balanced against the importance of getting such reports out, approved by an independent monitoring committee, and pre-specified in the trial protocol.

A related question is whether or not interventionists should remain blinded to arm-specific, aggregated data on behavioral risk factor targets of treatment. For example, in a *Phase III* behavioral trial examining the impact of a treatment to reduce anger on blood pressure control, the behavioral risk factor is anger. If unblinding the interventionists to lower-than-expected changes in anger during the course of the trial motivates them to strengthen treatment delivery, it could improve the potency of the treatment. Alternatively, it could create undesired reactivity such as loss of interest. This question needs careful consideration by trial investigators since there are currently no guidelines for blinding to behavioral risk factor targets in *Phase III* behavioral efficacy trials.

Develop a Blinding Plan

A blinding plan can help investigators push to extend the blind to as many players as possible. Table 10.1 presents an example of a blinding plan using a matrix that describes potential players and potential blinding options. Within the matrix are examples of blinding (**B**) or unblinding (**U**) options. The goal of the plan is to seek as many "B's" as possible in pursuit of making a serious effort to extend the blind.

Table 10.1 Sample blinding plan

Players	Blinding Options					
	Trial Hypotheses	Trial Aims	Subject Treatment Assignment	Aggregate Outcomes	Treatment Fidelity	Intervention Protocols
Principal Investigator	U	U	B	B	U	U
Co-Investigators	B/U	U	B	B	U	B/U
Statistician	U	U	U	U	U	B
Project Director	B	U	B	B	U	U
Interventionists	B	U	U[a]	B	U[a]	U[a]
Research Assistants	B	U	B	B	U	B
Participants	B	U	U[a]	B	U[a]	U[a]
Participant Physicians	B	U	B	B	B	B
Outcome Assessors	B	U	B	B	B	B
Institutional Review Board	U[b]	U	B	B	B	U
Data Safety and Monitoring Board	U	U	U[c]	U	U	U

U = Unblinded, B = Blinded
[a]Unblinded only within own arm
[b]IRB Protocol unblinded; consent form blinded to hypotheses
[b]Unblinded in the aggregate only; blinded to individual participants

These are simply examples. Each trial is different in terms of its scope, resources, and goals. In planning a trial, investigators might consider developing their own matrix of players and options. The ultimate decision of who and how to blind depends upon the nature of the trial and the results of each of the decisions on ethical issues (i.e., safety), practicality (i.e., feasibility), bias (i.e., how serious the risk of bias is without blinding), and compromise (i.e., considering options for partial blinding) [32]. When objective digital outcomes assessment is used, it eliminates the human middleman and reduces the opportunity for human preferences to create bias. Consideration must also be made of where in the process of treatment development the program of research lies. In earlier phases of treatment development where resources are limited and the number of players is small, blinding options may be more limited.

Prevent and Detect Expectancy Bias

Differential preferences and absence of equipoise are subtle aspects of the culture of a clinical trial. They are difficult to document directly but can be inferred indirectly in a number of ways. In double-blind trials, a common practice is to ask participants to guess whether they were on active drug or placebo after the trial was completed. If participants are correct around 50% of the time in a two-arm trial, an inference of satisfactory blinding can be made [11]. This, of course, is not possible in a behavioral trial because all subjects know which treatment they are on. Here are some more feasible strategies for preventing and detecting risk of bias in a behavioral trial.

Prevent and Document Crossovers and Co-interventions
To prevent crossovers and co-interventions during the course of a trial, it is helpful to educate potential participants at baseline about how clinical trials work and how beginning new behavioral treatments and/or new lifestyle habits that are unrelated to the trial can undercut an ability to evaluate results. Once randomized, a thorough documentation of therapies, treatments, and lifestyle habits at baseline, and repeatedly throughout the follow-up, is advisable. This can help assess the possibility that differential expectations translated into differential co-interventions or crossovers creating a post-randomization imbalance between arms.

Conflict of Interest
Investigator conflict of interest can be an indirect indicator of preference or lack of equipoise. In biomedical research, conflicts have been associated with risk of bias [33] and statistically significant results [34]. In biomedical papers published in 2016, 20% reported a conflict, but prevalence increased to 32% in the subset of papers evaluating drug treatments [35]. Conflicts of interest are less common in behavioral trials but could occur when there are financial interests or a long-standing scientific commitment to a particular behavioral treatment. In the former case, transparency through disclosures and funding sources can help assess any influence on the integrity of a clinical trial. In the latter case, serious consideration of whether or not a long-standing interest in a particular behavioral treatment will compromise objectivity in the design, conduct, and analyses of trial data is essential.

Independent Monitoring
In *Phase III* efficacy trials, an independent data and safety monitoring board that monitors trial quality, and a data management center with independent authority to report on trial progress, provide objective and ongoing feedback to investigators concerning any evolving imbalances between arms. This maximizes the chance that such imbalances can be corrected earlier rather than later. For smaller projects, the principal investigator should work out a written agreement of independence with a statistician and data manager and report this in all publications as evidence of extending the blind. The practice of having the principal investigator who directs the

trial also analyze the data from the trial undercuts the objectivity of the results and should be avoided. This cannot be justified even by the smallest of budgets.

Assess the Risk of Bias

The Cochrane Collaboration has developed a Risk of Bias scale aimed at determining the extent of bias after the trial has been completed [36]. It assesses the risk of expectancy bias based upon metrics that are symptoms: treatment crossovers, differential co-interventions, differential attrition, and the subjectivity of the outcomes [30]. During the trial, use of this instrument can be helpful in the early detection and early remediation of any emerging biases triggered by differential expectations.

SELECTED EXPERIENCE FROM BEHAVIORAL TRIALS

"Something or Nothing" in a Multi-Site Behavioral Trial

The ENRICHD clinical trial tested the hypothesis that treatment for depression in those who were depressed after a new heart attack would reduce subsequent recurrent heart attacks or death [37]. The trial, conducted under the direction of the US National Heart, Lung, and Blood Institute, involved eight sites, a data coordinating center, a treatment fidelity center, and a data safety and monitoring board. A total of 2481 post-heart attack patients were randomized to either depression treatment or usual care. Those randomized to depression treatment received cognitive behavior therapy, supervised by experts at the Beck Institute where the treatment was developed. Those randomized to the comparator received usual care. For all patients, baseline scores on depression were sent to their primary care provider. Results on the primary endpoint of death or recurrent heart attack after 29 months showed no significant difference in event-free survival in usual care (75.9%) vs. depression treatment (75.8%). This was a null trial.

It is often said that "getting something" is better than "getting nothing." This is a rationale that drives many community-based studies to resist using randomized comparator groups. But in this trial, depressed patients who got a great deal of "something" (i.e., cognitive behavior therapy for depression supervised by experts) fared no better than getting "nothing" (i.e., usual care). Because the three authors of this book were all a part of this trial, we have inside knowledge of the mindsets of the investigators throughout the progression of the trial. Although the investigators were kept blinded to outcome data, symptoms of a lack of equipoise were present. For example, recruiters would come back to staff meetings and express great worry that a patient who was extremely depressed would end up in the usual care group. Upon conclusion of all data collection, an investigator unblinding session was scheduled.

This triggered discussions among the investigators about what the results might look like. There was not one of the approximately 40 investigators who thought this would be a null trial. Some measured their enthusiasm by speculating that the intervention would be more effective for recurrent heart attacks than for mortality. Others speculated that the intervention would prove to be more effective for those who were more severely depressed. But the predominant view was that getting something, especially a "something" that was a well-established, efficacious treatment for patients who needed it, would surely be better than getting nothing. It is safe to say that a null trial was an unexpected shock. It is also safe to say that this shock revealed a relatively hidden lack of equipoise on the part of the ENRICHD investigators.

The direction of bias in situations where there is a lack of equipoise is generally in favor of treatment. The treatment could prove to be superior because of a confound between its active ingredients and beliefs about its efficacy. In the case of ENRICHD, it is possible that any lack of equipoise did not translate into a spurious benefit for treatment because its effects were neutralized by the excellent operational procedures put in place by the independent data coordinating center. Early detection of differential expectancy in the form of monthly reports examining differential dropout and non-adherence by arm made it possible for early enhancement of retention strategies within specific subgroups.

Symptoms of Expectancy Bias in an Obesity Management Trial

POWeR+ was a behavioral clinical trial aimed at determining the effectiveness and cost-effectiveness of a web-based behavioral weight management intervention offered in conjunction with either face-to-face or remote nurse support for patients managed in primary care [38]. Eligible participants were obese (or overweight if they had co-morbid hypertension, hypercholesterolemia, or diabetes) who were recruited from 56 primary care practices in Central and South England. A total of 818 participants were assigned to one of three arms: a control group of web-based dietary advice plus 2 brief nurse contacts ($N = 279$), a web-based weight management program with face-to-face nurse contacts ($N = 269$), or a web-based weight management program with remote nurse contacts ($N = 270$). The clinically significant outcomes were weight loss averaged over 12 months and $\geq 5\%$ weight loss at 12 months.

At the 12-month follow-up, weight loss $\geq 5\%$ was achieved in 21% of the controls, 29% of the face-to-face group, and 32% in the remote group. Statistical significance was achieved between the control and remote group only. In a responder-only analysis, the controls underwent a clinically significant 3 kg of weight loss. By 12 months, 47% of the controls were taking part in a non-trial weight loss activity.

It is rare to see almost half of the participants in a control group in a weight management study opting to get weight loss treatment on their own. Widespread treatment crossover is a symptom of expectancy bias, but it is difficult to document because lack of equipoise and preference for a trial outcome is a subtle aspect of the trial culture. The long-standing interest the investigators had in internet-based programs such as POWeR+ supports the possibility that expectations prompted treatment crossover in the controls.

The corrective action of seeking weight management treatment on their own paid off for the controls in the form of a clinically significant weight loss. The controls in this trial underwent more weight reduction (3 kg) than they did in an earlier report (1.2 kg) [39]. But what was good for the controls was not necessarily good for the trial. Treatment crossovers weakened the effect size, undercut statistical power, and provided an alternative explanation for the failure to detect benefit in the face-to-face group.

The Dream of a "True Believer"

The Recurrent Coronary Prevention Project (RCPP) was one of the first behavioral clinical trials. Conducted in the 1980s, the hypothesis was that reducing Type A behavior in patients who had already had one heart attack would prevent a recurrent heart attack. The trial enrolled 862 post-heart attack patients and randomized them to group counseling to manage heart disease and reduce Type A behavior or to group counseling to manage heart disease alone. The primary endpoint was death or recurrent heart attack. At the 3-year follow-up, there was a 44% reduction in the primary endpoint in the Type A group [40], which was sustained through the next 8 years and more powerful than the 30% reduction in heart attack recurrence that was observed by beta blocker therapy, one of the most popular drugs prescribed after a heart attack.

This trial was among the first to demonstrate a connection between the mind and the body. It gave birth to the field of behavioral medicine because it showed that the mind could influence an objective physical condition in the body such as a recurrent heart attack. The principal investigator of the RCPP, Meyer Friedman, was an established cardiologist who had written a best-selling book, *Type A Behavior and Your Heart,* and the phrase "Type A behavior" was used to describe stress in everyday conversation. A trial of this importance deserved publication in a top medical journal such as *JAMA* or the *New England Journal of Medicine.* Indeed, it was Dr. Friedman's dream to get this trial published in one of these two journals. But the top journals rejected the paper. As the trial biostatistician, Dr. Powell (the first author of this book) scrutinized the reviews to identify fatal flaws, but they focused instead on small errors in presentation that were easily correctable. One could not help but believe that something else was going on. Ultimately, the papers were published in a less-visible journal. In the years following the RCPP, two other investigative teams conducted trials using group-based stress reduction treatments that were modeled after the RCPP and reported similar positive results [41, 42].

There are likely a variety of explanations for why Dr. Friedman's papers were not published in the top medical journals. Maybe he was ahead of the curve, and there was no community equipoise on the issue of whether or not stress contributed to recurrent heart attacks. But in addition, Dr. Friedman was widely perceived to be a "true believer" who had a financial and personal interest in showing that Type A behavior was a coronary-prone behavior. Were the RCPP to have been a null trial, publication problems in top journals may not have existed. But when findings were strong with important clinical implications that challenged the status quo for the optimum treatment of patients recovering from a myocardial infarction, an easy reason for disbelief among members of the medical community was that the trial was led by a "true believer" with a vested interest in producing positive results.

Extraordinary claims require extraordinary evidence. In retrospect, it may have been more convincing if the "true believer" handed over the leadership of the trial to another investigator who was an expert clinical trialist with no prior association with the field of Type A research. Rather than stepping away from the trial completely, ideal role for Dr. Friedman might have been to be the passionate supervisor of the Type A intervention arm.

RECOMMENDATIONS

The rigor of a behavioral clinical trial is based upon its strength in making an inference that a treatment, and not some extraneous confounder, caused an outcome. Random assignment balances arms at baseline which effectively balances both known and unknown confounders. But things can happen during the course of the trial that raise red flags about the continued equality of the randomized arms. This chapter has argued that one source of post-randomization imbalance is caused by differential expectations about the benefit of treatments being compared and a lack of equipoise about the expected trial result.

This is a serious problem for behavioral trials because the double-blind design, which effectively neutralizes the adverse effects of differential expectations, is generally not possible. Thus, the onus is on the behavioral trialist to maximize rigor by designing a trial and creating a culture that minimizes bias from differential expectations.

Investigator Discipline

The behavioral trialist faces a perfect storm of three challenges: academic advancement; long-standing commitment to a behavioral treatment; and the human longing for success. These powerful forces weigh heavily against a scientific mindset characterized by equipoise and freedom from prejudices.

Investigators must find the discipline to compartmentalize their mindset. Equipoise lives in the professional realm. A mindset of true uncertainty about the merits of any treatment, paired with a passion for a conclusive resolution of this uncertainty, should be evident in all trial interactions. Hope for a particular trial result is a private affair. It lives in the personal realm. When hope is brought to the worksite, it becomes bias. Passion for a trial result is the professional gratification of getting a conclusive answer to the question posed by the trial. It is reserved for the end of the road. It is the short leap after the long run.

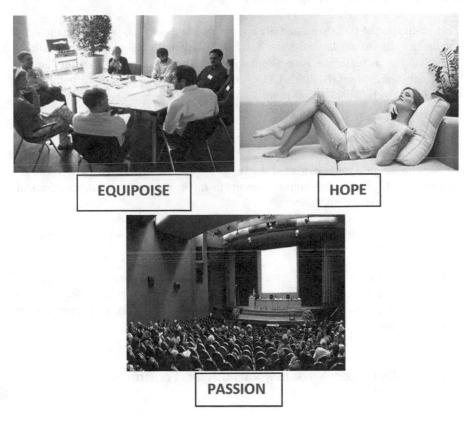

Such discipline and compartmentalization may be impossible for the trial leader. If the commitment to, and the passion for, a particular treatment is so strong and long-standing that a scientific mindset is not possible, the optimum role of such a "true believer" is to lead the treatment arm, not the trial. To serve as the passionate supervisor, trainer, and insurer of quality control in the treatment arm would have the greatest effect on the strength of the treatment and the quality of the trial. The emergence of clinical trial networks and national data coordinating centers makes it more feasible now than ever before to have a behavioral trial conducted with the highest quality without having to assume a leadership role.

Innovate to Extend the Blind

At least 20 scales exist to rate the quality of a clinical trial, and approximately half of them give points to double-blind designs [43]. The quality of blinding of both physicians and patients to therapy has been considered to be one of the most important aspects of any trial [44]. This means that behavioral clinical trials will always be rated as trials of lower quality based upon an uncontrollable factor inherent in the nature of the treatments being evaluated.

This motivates the push to extend the blind in as many ways as possible to make up for the inability to use double-blind designs. Behavioral clinical trial methodology is evolving to increase precision about what exactly is meant by "blinding" in any particular clinical trial. In 2001, CONSORT guidelines for reporting blinding in a clinical trial were dichotomous reports aimed at determining:

"Whether or not participants, those administering the interventions, and those assessing outcomes were blinded. If done, how the success of blinding was evaluated." [45]

In 2010, these guidelines extended the range of possible individuals who could be blinded and discarded dichotomous reports in favor of open-ended descriptions of how blinding was accomplished:

"If done, who was blinded after assignment to interventions (e.g., patients, care providers, those assessing outcomes) and how." [46]

A deep appreciation of the reality of equipoise and the adverse effects of preferences for a behavioral trial result can translate into innovations in finding ways to extend the blind in as many ways, and to as many individuals, as possible. Such innovations will go far in boosting the rigor of behavioral trials.

Placebo Response: Nuisance Variable or Treatment Component?

The literature on what constitutes a placebo response and the range of effects it can produce is evolving. It is now clear that the placebo response is a robust phenomenon that occurs in a variety of treatments for many diseases in diverse healthcare settings [47]. In drug trials, a placebo control disentangles improvement in biological dysfunction from any improvement triggered by the clinical encounter. An ability to make this distinction is consistent with the biomedical emphasis on the science, rather than the art, of medicine.

But when it comes to behavioral treatments, this distinction is less clear-cut. Soothing contextual factors such as attention, feeling cared for, and the ritual of administering the treatment are part of the art of healing and the reduction of symptoms [15, 19] with clear physiological benefits [18]. Thus, control for non-specific attention or intervention context may in actuality be overcontrol for an important component of a behavioral treatment.

It is an open question whether contextual factors produce a placebo response in need of control, or whether they serve as components of treatment which activate the "inner pharmacy" of self-healing [15, 48]. The status quo is to assume that these contextual factors are nuisance variables in need of control with appropriate comparators. A major step forward in behavioral clinical trial methodology would be taken by more in-depth consideration of what are, and what are not, active components of a behavioral treatment. This would make it considerably easier to choose an appropriate comparator for a behavioral trial.

REFERENCES

1. Howard DA, Giovanelli M (2019) Einstein's philosophy of science. In Zalta EN (ed) Stanford Encyclopedia of Philosophy. http://plato.stanford.edu/archives/fall2019/entries/einstein-philscience
2. Lakatos I (1977) Science and pseudoscience. Philos Pap 1:1–7
3. Cajal SR (1999) Advice for a young investigator. MIT Press, Cambridge
4. Wilson EO (2013) Letters to young scientist. Liveright, New York
5. Colagiuri B (2010) Participant expectancies in double-blind randomized placebo-controlled trials: potential limitations to trial validity. Clin Trials 7:246–255
6. Piantadosi S (2017) Clinical trials: a methodologic perspective, 3rd edn. Wiley, Hoboken
7. Sackett DL (1979) Bias in analytic research. J Chron Dis 32:51–63
8. Chalmers I, Matthews R (2006) What are the implications of optimism bias in clinical research? Lancet 367:449–450
9. Spodick DH (1979) Controlled trials: planned deception? Lancet 1:534–535
10. Altman DG (2005) What is a single blind trial? A rapid response to Al-Marzouki S, Evans S, Marshall T, Roberts T. Are these data real? Statistical methods for the detection of data fabrication in clinical trials. BMJ 331:267–270
11. Wang D, Bakhai A (2006) Clinical trials: a practical guide to design, analysis, and reporting. Remedica, London
12. Chalmers TC, Celano P, Sacks IIS, Smith II Jr (1983) Bias in treatment assignment in controlled clinical trials. N Engl J Med 309:1358–1361
13. Schulz KF, Chalmers I, Hayes RJ, Altman DG (1995) Empirical evidence of bias. Dimensions of methodological quality associated with estimates of treatment effects in controlled trials. JAMA 273:408–412
14. Magazin A, Kumar A, Soares H, Schell M, Hozo I, Djulbegovic B (2008) Expectation bias–the main culprit for large number of inconclusive randomized controlled trials in hematological malignancies. Blood 112:671. https://doi.org/10.1182/blood.V112.11.671.671
15. Miller FG, Colloca L, Kaptchuk TJ (2009) The placebo effect: illness and interpersonal healing. Perspect Biol Med 52:518–539
16. Beecher HK (1955) The powerful placebo. JAMA 159:1602–1606
17. Colloca L, Barsky AJ (2020) Placebo and nocebo effects. New Engl J Med 382:554–561
18. Benedetti F (2014) Placebo effects: understanding the mechanisms in health and disease, 2nd edn. Oxford University Press, Oxford
19. Finniss DG, Kaptchuk TJ, Miller F, Benedetti F (2010) Biological, clinical, and ethical advances of placebo effects. Lancet 375:686–696
20. Kaptchuk TJ, Friedlander E, Kelley JM, Sanchez MN, Kokkotou E, Singer JP, Kowalczykowski M, Miller FG, Kirsch I, Lembo AJ (2010) Placebos without deception: a randomized controlled trial in irritable bowel syndrome. PLoS One 5:e15591. https://doi.org/10.1371/journal.pone.0015591
21. Moseley JB, O'Malley K, Petersen NJ, Menke TJ, Brody BA, Kuykendall DH, Hollingsworth JC, Ashton CM, Wray NP (2002) A controlled trial of arthroscopic surgery for osteoarthritis of the knee. N Engl J Med 347:81–88
22. Hulley SB, Cummings SR, Browner WS, Grady DG, Newman TB (2013) Designing clinical research, 4th edn. Lippincott Williams & Wilkins, Philadelphia
23. Freedman B (1987) Equipoise and the ethics of clinical research. N Engl J Med 317:141–145
24. Irvin VL, Kaplan RM (2016) Effect sizes and primary outcomes in large-budget, cardiovascular-related behavioral randomized controlled trials funded by NIH since 1980. Ann Behav Med 50:130–146
25. Kaplan RM, Irvin VL (2015) Likelihood of null effects of large NHLBI clinical trials has increased over time. PLoS One 10:e0132382. https://doi.org/10.1371/journal.pone.0132382

26. Gordon D, Taddei-Peters W, Mascette A, Antman M, Kaufmann PG, Lauer MS (2013) Publication of trials funded by the National Heart, Lung, and Blood Institute. N Engl J Med 369:1926–1934
27. Chopra V, Davis M (2011) In search of equipoise. JAMA 305:1234–1235
28. Rossouw JE, Anderson GL, Prentice RL, LaCroix AZ, Kooperberg C, Stefanick ML, Jackson RD, Beresford SA, Howard BV, Johnson KC, Kotchen JM, Ockene J, Writing Group for the Women's Health Initiative Investigators (2002) Risks and benefits of estrogen plus progestin in healthy postmenopausal women: principal results from the Women's Health Initiative randomized controlled trial. JAMA 288:321–333
29. Frasure-Smith N, Lespérance F, Prince RH, Verrier P, Garber RA, Juneau M, Wolfson C, Bourassa MG (1997) Randomised trial of home-based psychosocial nursing intervention for patients recovering from myocardial infarction. Lancet 350:473–479
30. Boutron I, Ravaud P, Moher D (2012) Randomized clinical trials of nonpharmacological treatments. Chapman & Hall/CRC, Boca Raton
31. Woloshin S, Schwartz LM, Bagley PJ, Blunt HB, White B (2018) Characteristics of interim publications of randomized clinical trials and comparison with final publications. JAMA 319:404–406
32. Pocock SJ (1983) Clinical trials: a practical approach. Wiley, New York
33. Ahn R, Woodbridge A, Abraham A, Saba S, Korenstein D, Madden E, Boscardin WJ, Keyhani S (2017) Financial ties of principal investigators and randomized controlled trial outcomes: cross sectional study. BMJ 356:i6770. https://doi.org/10.1136/bmj.i6770
34. Friedman LS, Richter ED (2004) Relationship between conflicts of interest and research results. J Gen Intern Med 19:51–56
35. Grundy Q, Dunn AG, Bourgeois FT, Coiera E, Bero L (2018) Prevalence of disclosed conflicts of interest in biomedical research and associations with journal impact factors and altmetric scores. JAMA 319:408–409
36. Sterne JAC, Savovic J, Page MJ, Elbers RG, Blencowe NS, Boutron I, Cates CJ, Chen H-Y, Corbett MS, Eldridge SM, Emberson JR, Hernan MA, Hopewell S, Hrobjartsson A, Junqueira DR, Juni P, Kirkham JJ, Lasserson T, Li T, McAleenan A, Reeves BC, Shepperd S, Shrier I, Stewart LA, Tilling K, White IR, Whiting PF, Higgins JPT (2019) RoB2: a revised tool for assessing risk of bias in randomised trials. BMJ 366:l4898. https://doi.org/10.1136/bmj.d5928
37. Berkman LF, Blumenthal J, Burg M, Carney RM, Catellier D, Cowan MJ, Czajkowski SM, DeBusk R, Hosking J, Jaffe A, Kaufmann PG, Mitchell P, Norman J, Powell LH, Raczynski JM, Schneiderman N, the Enhancing Recovery in Coronary Heart Disease Patients Investigators (ENRICHD) (2003) Effects of treating depression and low perceived social support on clinical events after myocardial infarction: the Enhancing Recovery in Coronary Heart Disease Patients (ENRICHD) Randomized Trial. JAMA 289:3106–3116
38. Little P, Stuart B, Hobbs FR, Kelly J, Smith ER, Bradbury KJ, Hughes S, Smith PW, Moore MV, Lean ME, Margetts BM, Byrne CD, Griffin S, Davoudianfar M, Hooper J, Yao G, Zhu S, Raftery J, Yardley L (2016) An internet-based intervention with brief nurse support to manage obesity in primary care (POWeR+): a pragmatic, parallel-group, randomised controlled trial. Lancet Diabetes Endocrinol 4:821–828
39. Little P, Kelly J, Barnett J, Dorward M, Margetts B, Warm D (2004) Randomised controlled factorial trial of dietary advice for patients with a single high blood pressure reading in primary care. BMJ 328:1054. https://doi.org/10.1136/bmj.38037.435972.EE
40. Friedman M, Thoresen CE, Gill JJ, Powell LH, Ulmer D, Thompson L, Price VA, Rabin DD, Breall WS, Dixon T, Levy R, Bourg E (1984) Alteration of type A behavior and reduction in cardiac recurrences in postmyocardial infarction patients. Am Heart J 108:237–248
41. Andersen BL, Yang HC, Farrar WB, Golden-Kreutz DM, Emery CF, Thornton LM, Young DC, Carson WE 3rd (2008) Psychologic intervention improves survival for breast cancer patients: a randomized clinical trial. Cancer 113:3450–3458
42. Orth-Gomér K, Schneiderman N, Wang HX, Walldin C, Blom M, Jernberg T (2009) Stress reduction prolongs life in women with coronary disease: the Stockholm Women's Intervention Trial for Coronary Heart Disease (SWITCHD). Circ Cardiovasc Qual Outcomes 2:25–32

43. Olivo SA, Macedo LG, Gadotti IC, Fuentes J, Stanton T, Magee DJ (2008) Scales to assess the quality of randomized controlled trials: a systematic review. Phys Ther 88:156–175
44. Chalmers TC, Smith H Jr, Blackburn B, Silverman B, Schroeder B, Reitman D, Ambroz A (1981) A method for assessing the quality of a randomized control trial. Control Clin Trials 2:31–49
45. Moher D, Schultz KF, Altman D, CONSORT Group (2001) The CONSORT statement: revised recommendations for improving the quality of reports of parallel-group randomized trials. JAMA 285:1987–1991
46. Moher D, Hopewell S, Schultz K, Montori V, Gotzsche PC, Devereaux PJ, Elbourne D, Egger M, Altman DG (2010) CONSORT 2010 explanation and elaboration: updated guidelines for reporting parallel group randomised trials. BMJ 340:c869. https://doi.org/10.1136/bmj.c869
47. Colagiuri B, Schenk LA, Kessler MD, Dorsey SG, Colloca L (2015) The placebo effect: from concepts to genes. Neuroscience 307:171–190
48. Brody H, Brody D (2000) The placebo response: how you can release the body's inner pharmacy for better health. HarperCollins, New York

Chapter 11
The Future of Behavioral Randomized Clinical Trials

"It is difficult to make predictions, especially about the future."
Yogi Berra

Fundamental Point

Behavioral clinical trials will evolve in four areas in the future. They will be more rigorous, guided by the emergence of a metascience for behavioral trial methodology. They will benefit from stronger treatment effects resulting from precision targeting and tailoring to diverse risk profiles and from intervening simultaneously on multiple levels of ecological risk. They will be easier to implement using networks of investigators and drawing on big data to simplify approaches to recruitment, assessment, and intervention. They will be more relevant for improving healthcare delivery by strategic planning for dissemination at all stages of behavioral treatment development.

The chapter aims to predict the future of behavioral randomized trials in four key areas. The emergence of a metascience for behavioral clinical trials will replace the "one-size-fits all" approach to behavioral trial design with designs that feature a progression of questions, a progression of methods, and the use of guidelines to facilitate decision-making. Behavioral treatments will produce stronger effects with the emergence of precision lifestyle medicine that targets precisely those most likely to benefit and tailors precisely to diverse persons, settings, and time, and with multilevel trials that simultaneously intervene on more than one level of ecologic risk. Behavioral trials will be easier to implement using networks that collaborate on multi-site behavioral trials, leveraging data routinely collected in the healthcare system, and enhancing accessibility to trials using digital technology. The gap between trial results and implementation in practice will be narrowed by strategic planning for dissemination featuring outcomes in trials that are meaningful to clinicians and third-party payers, commitment to refine treatments that have failed, and a push toward influencing clinical practice guidelines with *Phase III* efficacy trials.

© Springer Nature Switzerland AG 2021
L. H. Powell et al., *Behavioral Clinical Trials for Chronic Diseases*,
https://doi.org/10.1007/978-3-030-39330-4_11

RANDOMIZED CLINICAL TRIALS WILL NOT BE OUTDATED

Are clinical trials becoming outdated? This question has been raised repeatedly by critics who have expressed a number of concerns. (1) Randomized trial data should not be prioritized over alternative ways of knowing whether a treatment works, such as observational studies, studies of mechanisms, uncontrolled case studies, and clinical experience. (2) Methodologic flaws in randomization procedures fail to create equality across treatment arms. (3) Limited external validity results from carefully selected target populations treated in artificial settings. (4) Group designs are unable to inform treatment response of an individual patient. (5) Priority is placed on whether a treatment works at the expense of understanding how it works [1].

Admittedly, clinical trials are not perfect. But they are widely accepted as the gold standard by which to determine whether or not a behavioral treatment works. There are several reasons for their primacy.

Randomized Clinical Trials Make the Strongest Causal Inferences

The argument that randomized trials should *not* be prioritized over other ways of knowing is a reflection of the "nirvana fallacy" of assuming that because they are imperfect, they are no better than other designs. This is an error in inference [1]. No other design is as successful in minimizing the error of inferring that a treatment, and not some factor related to that treatment, is responsible for benefit. No other design carries more weight in clinical practice guidelines, in third-party reimbursement, and, ultimately, in maximizing patient care. Clinical trials are a "crucial linchpin for evidence-based practice" [1].

An excellent example of their potency is with the question of the optimum diet to enhance health. Almost all nutritional variables are correlated with one another in the large, complex system of dietary intake. If one nutritional variable is correlated with an outcome, so too are many other nutritional variables. This problem of confounding is not solved by increasing the size of the dataset, now made possible by the advent of "big data." Nutritional variables will be intercorrelated similarly in datasets that are both large and small. Statistical adjustment for the influence of one dietary component on health over another in an observational study is challenging, if not impossible, due to this multicollinearity [2]. However, with a randomized trial, these intercorrelated dietary variables can be disentangled by randomizing participants to receive, or not receive, one single dietary component. This has often produced a dramatic difference in results from observational studies and clinical trials. For example, observational studies made a strong case for the benefit of omega-3 fish oil on vascular events in patients with diabetes. But the ASCEND trial found no such benefit [3]. The messy problem of confounding between intake of fish oil and the variety of dietary and socioeconomic factors that covary with it was solved by shifting the choice of ingesting omega-3 fish oil from the patient to a flip of a coin. No other way of knowing has such power in making a causal inference as random assignment.

Randomized Clinical Trials Can Have Strong Ecologic Validity

The argument that carefully controlled trials are limited because they are conducted in artificial settings which do not generalize to real-world contexts conflates ecological validity with internal validity. A treatment that is offered in a real-world context with high ecological validity can be evaluated using a randomized design with strong internal validity. An excellent example is a trial of blood pressure management that was conducted in black barbershops. Fifty-two black barbershops were randomly assigned to a treatment in which pharmacists prescribed blood pressure medication in the barbershop or to a comparator in which barbers provided lifestyle advice and encouragement to visit the doctor [4]. Retention was 95% in both arms and the trial showed a benefit from the pharmacist treatment. This was a randomized trial with strong internal validity that evaluated an ecologically valid intervention conducted in a real-world setting. This example can be easily extended to any pragmatic trial that uses a randomized design but brings the context closer to clinical or community reality.

Randomized Clinical Trials Are Essential to Translational Research

The argument that key patient subgroups are left out of clinical trials is not a problem of the randomized design but a problem with a "one fell swoop" approach to science that expects all questions to be answered in a single trial. Campbell has argued for the primacy of internal validity as a prerequisite for external validity based upon the premise that one cannot meaningfully generalize a finding unless it is a genuine finding [5]. A progressive program of translational research features a series of studies, each of which provides more information about a treatment and who would benefit from it. When results converge from case studies, clinical experience, observational studies, and studies of mechanisms, the case is strong for a definitive, confirmatory clinical trial where the inference of causality will be the strongest.

If the clinical trial shows benefit for the population selected to maximize internal validity, this opens the door to subsequent trials and other types of studies to *accumulate* evidence on external validity. Campbell and Stanley argued that external validity is accumulated over a series of studies. In their words:

"We learn about external validity only piece by piece through trial and error, typically over multiple studies that contain different kinds of persons, settings, treatments, and outcomes. Scientists do this by conducting a program of research." (p.86) [5]

Randomized clinical trials are a crucial part of the translational research enterprise that evolves through discovery, exploration, confirmation, and generalization, and moves from novel laboratory findings to the generation of robust evidence [6]. The place of the randomized trial in translational research is in confirmation. There may be other powerful ways to achieve randomization in the future. For example, Mendelian randomization compares outcomes in individuals who do, and do not, have gene variants linked to an exposure, such as physical activity. Because genes are free of environmental influences, randomly distributed, and thereby free of residual confounding, comparisons of outcomes in those with and without the gene provide a randomized natural experiment [7, 8]. There may be other ways to make convincing causal attributions. For example, the impact of policy-level changes using a time-lagged interrupted time series design which compares outcomes before and after serial implementations of policy may be a powerful, fast, efficient, and conclusive way to evaluate organizational change in a living healthcare system [9].

However, there is a general consensus that the future is less about abandoning randomized clinical trials and more about finding ways to improve them [10]. To draw on Bob Dylan's metaphor (see box), the behavioral clinical trial "wind is blowing" toward increased methodological rigor,

> *"You don't need a weather man to know which way the wind blows."*
>
> Bob Dylan
> Subterranean Homesick Blues, 1965
> Nobel Prize in Literature, 2016

stronger interventions, greater ease of implementation, and more relevant results.

BEHAVIORAL TRIALS WILL BE MORE RIGOROUS

Behavioral randomized clinical trial design has been stuck in a single mold. Most trials have been small and underpowered to detect improvements in clinically important outcomes and characterized by a multiplicity of outcomes [11, 12]. Successes tend to be left standing without replication, and failures are seldom refined and re-examined. Funders, publishers, societies, institutions, editors, reviewers, and authors all contribute to the cultural norms that support this status quo and the dysfunctional incentive system that sustains it [13].

These observations have fostered some soul-searching. This has translated into an emerging metascience for behavioral clinical trials that looks beyond a critique of any individual trial and focuses instead on the funda-mental processes of science that under-lie it. Metascience, the scientific study

> *"Stakeholders of science must not embrace the status quo, but instead pursue self-examination continuously for improvement and self-correction of the scientific process itself."*
>
> Munafò et al., 2017 [13]

of science itself [13], has been alive and well among the philosophers of science for more than two centuries. It is now gaining momentum in the behavioral clinical trial community [14–19].

Some of the highlights of the innovations that are emerging from the metascience movement in behavioral clinical trial methodology are the following:

- The goals of behavioral and social science research have been challenged to go beyond exploration and discovery and to be more applied and ori-ented toward solving practical problems [20, 21].

- The psychological side of science has shown the ways in which investiga-tors knowingly or unknowingly deceive themselves through the combina-tion of apophenia (the tendency to see patterns in random data), confirmation bias (the tendency to focus on evidence that is in line with expectations or favored explanations), and hindsight bias (the tendency to see an event as having been predictable only after it has occurred) [13].

- Progressive models for behavioral treatment development have been pro-posed that encourage the use of a variety of designs as questions about a treatment and the purpose of the study evolve [22].

- A systematic way to describe the nature of any behavioral intervention now exists [23].

- Guidelines have been developed for: choosing an appropriate comparator *(Chapter 6: Choice of a Comparator)*; conducting pilot, feasibility, and proof-of-concept studies *(Chapter 3: Behavioral Treatment Development; Chapter 7: Feasibility and Pilot Studies)*; framing research questions [24]; and reporting behavioral clinical trial results [25–28].

- The International Behavioural Trials Network (IBTN) (www.ibtnetwork. org) has been formed to provide an international network aimed at foster-ing methodological rigor in the development of interventions and in the conduct of behavioral clinical trials [29, 30].

- This book is essentially a metascience of behavioral randomized clinical trial methodology that applies principles of scientific inquiry to the devel-opment of behavioral treatments, and the design of behavioral clinical tri-als, over the spectrum of translational research.

The future of behavioral clinical trials will be one of enhanced methodological rigor shaped by these meta-scientific recommendations and guidelines. They will relieve the investigator from relying upon a "one-size-fits-all" status quo and foster instead a progressive approach characterized by an evolving understanding of a behavioral treatment, evolving questions that need to be answered, and a close link between evolving questions and evolving trial design. They will inspire pursuit of continuing education, networking, and training opportunities in this new metascience for investigators at all levels of their academic careers [13].

BEHAVIORAL TRIALS WILL TEST STRONGER INTERVENTIONS

Behavioral clinical trials often produce clinically insignificant effects on important clinical endpoints. Stronger behavioral treatments are needed. Momentum is building in two areas that offer promise for enhancing strength: precision lifestyle medicine and multilevel treatments.

Precision Lifestyle Medicine

Challenging the "one-size-fits-all" approach to behavioral treatment development, precision lifestyle medicine seeks to *target* subgroups most likely to benefit from a behavioral treatment and *tailor* treatments to diverse persons, settings, and time [31]. The vision is that a deeper understanding of the biological, psychological, social, and environmental mechanisms that facilitate behavior change will make it possible to design interventions that target those mechanisms precisely.

Target Subgroups Most Likely to Benefit
Genetic Predisposition. Medicine is personalized. The choice of a drug is based upon a match between the characteristics of the patient and the evidence that the drug will work for that patient. Precision medicine is an approach to treatment and prevention that takes into account individual variability in genes, environment, and lifestyle [32]. Its greatest success has been in the treatment of some types of cancer where advances in genome sequencing and biotechnology have made it possible to match treatment to the genetic characteristics of a particular tumor [33]. This success has fostered an interest in precision prevention [34] which seeks to use genetic markers of disease risk to personalize preventive interventions to reduce that risk.

At least two studies have posed a challenge to precision prevention. The first focused on the popular assumption that DNA is destiny and that lifestyle change is useless for those whose genetic risk is very high, and unnecessary for those whose genetic risk is very low. The study involved 55,685 participants who were assessed on 50 markers of genetic risk for coronary artery disease, and on healthy lifestyle, and then followed for approximately 19 years for incident coronary events. Results showed that a healthy lifestyle reduced risk within low, medium, and high tertiles of genetic risk, with the strongest benefits of lifestyle in those at highest genetic risk [35]. Everyone benefitted from healthy living, regardless of their genetic risk.

The second study was based upon the popular assumption that the optimum diet should be targeted to one's genetic weak link. This was a trial of 609 overweight or obese adults who were assessed for a low-fat-responsive and a low-carbohydrate-responsive genotype at baseline and then randomized to receive either a low-fat or low-carbohydrate diet [36]. It was hypothesized that those with a low-fat-responsive genotype would lose more weight when assigned to a low-fat diet and a parallel effect would be found for carbohydrates. However, no enhanced benefit for DNA and diet concordance was observed on weight loss at 1 year. Individuals in all sub-groups lost weight primarily because they improved overall diet quality. Everyone benefitted from a healthy diet, regardless of their genetic risk.

Thus, as far as healthy living goes, it appears that one size fits all. Healthy living provides benefits for all levels of genetic risk. This may be a robust finding given the fact that lifestyle is a root cause of most chronic diseases. Alternatively, it may be related to a limited understanding of the genetics of chronic diseases and metabolic factors. This field is exploding and more precise explorations into precision prevention are likely in the future.

Motivation. Generalizability of the benefits of a behavioral treatment to all patients with a target disease is widely viewed as a criterion for judging that treatment to be strong, persuasive, relevant, and exciting. But there are clearly sub-groups of patients with a disease who prefer drug management, or no management at all, over a commitment to change their lifestyle. Although this preference may be shaped by physical and social environments which could themselves be intervened upon, the need for individual agency and effort in many behavioral treatments suggests a misalignment between those with low motivation and those treatments. Persuading patients to enroll in a behavioral trial in pursuit of generalizability undermines patient respect and exposes a lack of investigator humility to accept that what is offered may not be what a patient wants. If they do end up in a trial, these patients require excessive attention and effort to achieve adherence and complete the trial. *(See Chapter 8: Protection of Random Assignment.)*

Precision lifestyle medicine reconsiders the target population for behavioral trials. Rather than targeting *all who have the disease*, a more precise target would be *all who have the disease and are motivated to change their behavior.* This shift is

consistent with recruitment approaches that reject the "hard sell," in favor of foster-
ing a clear understanding of the time and effort required, and a balanced consideration of the pros and cons [37, 38]. It is also consistent with efforts to identify
baseline predictors of treatment success. In a small study that examined the predictors of successful weight loss, a baseline question about self-efficacy in achieving
sustained exercise revealed that half of the cohort had low self-efficacy. If that half
had decided against participation, the rate of loss to follow-up would have decreased
from 30% to 17%, and the rate of successful weight loss would have increased from
51% to 80% [39].

Participants in behavioral trials who are not well aligned with the treatment offered
will vote with their feet, either before or, unfortunately for the trial, after they are
randomized. Stronger treatment effects can result from more precision in targeting
those most likely to benefit. Among the strategies to achieve this in future trials will
be a better understanding of true informed consent, a respect for patient preferences
for non-behavioral treatment options, a greater understanding of factors that influence motivation on a moment-to-moment basis, and a willingness to challenge cultural assumptions about ideal target populations.

Tailor Treatment to Patient Characteristics

Patient Preference. Patient preference designs provide the patient with the
opportunity to choose a preferred treatment while at the same time preserving the
randomized design. An excellent example of how this can be accomplished has been
offered by the HOMBRE trial of weight loss in overweight and obese Latino men
[40]. Participants were randomized to a culturally adapted intervention or a minimal
intensity comparator. Those randomized to the culturally adapted intervention could
choose from among three modes of administration: self-directed online videos,
coach-facilitated in-person groups, or coach-facilitated online groups. Those randomized to the minimal intensity comparator received online videos with coach
assistance, if needed. This design made it possible to determine whether the culturally
adapted intervention was better than the minimal intensity comparator—the basis of
the randomization. But the intention was to maximize the strength of the treatment by
giving participants the opportunity to choose their desired mode of receiving it.

In a review of patient preferences in clinical trials, 56% of participants had a preference for a particular treatment, but the range was wide (16–85%) and depended
upon the type of treatment [41]. The importance of this preference was unclear
because a match between preference and treatment produced only a modest benefit
[41, 42]. Future trials should assess baseline preference for the specific treatments
being evaluated so that understanding of the impact of preference on outcome can
be advanced.

Patient Response. Adaptive treatments go beyond tailoring to baseline characteristics by offering the potential to tailor a treatment based upon suboptimal early
response [43]. Drawing on the concept of drug titration where suboptimal response

to an initial drug is optimized by increasing the dose or adding another drug, behavioral treatments that do not achieve the desired response in a particular patient, or group of patients, can be optimized by such things as increasing the intensity of delivery or adding an additional treatment component. Adaptive treatments are developed from adaptive designs which feature randomization to various arms and inter-trial augmentations to produce empirically derived decision rules for the timing and nature of augmentation strategies. The resulting new adaptive treatment, with pre-determined algorithms for augmentation, can then be evaluated for efficacy in a traditional efficacy trial.

Neurobehavioral Mechanisms. The National Institutes of Health's Science of Behavior Change initiative (https://commonfund.nih.gov/behaviorchange/index; http://scienceofbehaviorchange.org/) sought to potentiate behavioral treatments by understanding how individuals achieve behavior change in three priority areas: self-regulation, stress response and resilience, and interpersonal relationships and processes. One innovative project in this initiative is the ENGAGE study, which aims to identify the neurological circuits of self-regulatory processes and then develop treatments to remediate any impairment in them [44]. Embedded within a larger trial of treatment of comorbid depression and obesity, ENGAGE is based upon the hypothesis that impaired self-regulation in emotion, cognition, and self-reflection neural circuits is implicated in everyday struggles to control behavior. By exploring interrelationships among these circuits, their relationship to depression and obesity, and their value in predicting response to treatment, relevant circuits can be identified, and patient-specific impairment in any of them can be assessed. The vision is to ultimately develop a "menu" of intervention strategies that can be aligned to an individual's unique profile of self-regulatory impairment to achieve a customized intervention with optimal potency.

This mechanism-focused experimental approach is new and evolving. Early efforts make big demands on the large amount of data collected, but they have been accompanied by conceptual and statistical innovations to ease the burden [45, 46]. The excitement, momentum, and NIH Common Fund support offers great potential for a new generation of brain-based behavioral interventions.

Multilevel Interventions

Theoretically, a behavioral treatment could be strengthened by targeting more than one of the web of causal factors for a particular chronic disease. There are several models that explain levels of causal factors. The "hub" model describes determinants of most chronic diseases as acting within complex networks made up of a small number of "hubs" that are extensively linked to relatively isolated determinants and are remarkably similar in structure and function at genetic, molecular, cellular, clinical, environmental, and societal levels [47]. The "ecologic" model conceptualizes risk behavior as embedded within an array of sources of influence going all of the way from genes, cells, and biology to neighborhood, social, and policy factors [48].

Considering this multiplicity of influences, it is reasonable to consider designing multilevel trials that simultaneously target two or more levels at once in pursuit of strengthening the effects of treatment on the outcome. Interest in the potential of this approach has evolved more rapidly than an understanding of methods for its design and analysis [49]. Some early examples include designs targeting simultaneously patients and their providers [50] or targeting simultaneously patients, providers, and the community [51].

The close link between multilevel causality of chronic diseases and multilevel clinical trials makes this a potentially fruitful and expanding area of research, particularly in public health. Although it is complex and evolving, its potential for strengthening the effects of behavioral treatments by intervening on more than one level of influence is enormous.

BEHAVIORAL TRIALS WILL BE EASIER TO IMPLEMENT

It has been suggested that expected effect sizes from clinical trials may be shrinking, given the background of effective therapies that are likely to exist in any comparator group [52]. Since the detection of modest effect sizes requires a large sample and generally a large number of investigators and clinical sites to achieve it, the cost and complexity of trials may be increasing. Thus, the Institute of Medicine has called for greater efficiency of clinical trials [53] while still preserving sensitivity to detect modest effects [52, 54]. To increase the efficiency of behavioral clinical trials, without sacrificing quality, two highlights deserve mention.

Behavioral Clinical Trial Networks

Ever since behavioral medicine emerged as a distinct field of research, the vast majority of studies have been conducted by individual investigators, or by small collaborative groups, at single sites or individual centers. This mode of scientific activity emphasizes the independence and creativity of individual investigators and research labs, and it has borne many fruits. Its downside is that it is not conducive to the large-scale efforts needed to address some of the most important and challenging questions in the field and needed to change clinical and public health practices and policies.

The game-changing studies tend to be large, multi-center, randomized *Phase III* efficacy trials conducted by well-organized research networks that follow carefully defined protocols with systematic training for interventionists and objective data collection methods. These networks make it feasible to enroll large and representative samples, evaluate treatment effects on clinically important outcomes, and draw on infrastructure support from clinical and data coordinating centers to insure quality. These features produce trials that far surpass what smaller, single-site trials, such as those that currently dominate the field of behavioral medicine, can accomplish.

For example, the Thrombolysis in Myocardial Infarction (TIMI) Study Group is a renowned cardiovascular research network that has conducted numerous multi-center trials since 1984. The TIMI Investigators have enrolled tens of thousands of patients in their studies at thousands of sites in over 50 countries. The results of their trials have transformed numerous areas of cardiovascular care. This impact could not have been accomplished without the benefits of rapid recruitment and economies of scale at the scientific and financial level. It could not have been accomplished single-handedly by individual investigators working as free agents.

Multidisciplinary, multi-site research networks have grown in many fields. Approximately 1145 English-language papers with research network corporate authorships were published between 2003 and 2007, and this number grew by 106% between 2008 and 2013, and by another 54% between 2013 and 2017. This parallels the rapid growth of multidisciplinary team science in health-related research [55, 56].

While some behavioral research networks are emerging and gaining traction (e.g., the International Behavioural Trials Network), relatively few currently exist, and fewer still are capable of, or intent on, conducting large, multi-center trials. A major step forward in developing a culture of multidisciplinary, collaborative behavioral networks has been presented by the formation of the Behavioral Medicine Research Council [57]. This Council is comprised of senior investigators from four of the leading behavioral medicine research organizations. Their initial mission is to identify strategic goals for applied behavioral medicine and then to promote multi-site collaborative efforts to achieve them. The ultimate aim is to improve health and quality of life through health behavior change. This effort has been described as behavioral medicine's "moon shot." The words of President Kennedy ring true to this effort.

> *"We engage in the goal not because it is easy, but because it is hard. . .*
> *because it takes the best of our energies and skills to achieve it."*
> President John F. Kennedy
> "Moon" Speech, September 12, 1962

Multi-site trials require effective leadership and elaborate organizational structures. The participating research teams must also be able to collaborate, despite scientific differences and geographically dispersed locations. Experience is the glue that holds all of this together. The more experience the leadership has with multi-site, multidisciplinary research, and the more experience the network has with working together, the more likely they will be successful in meeting the complex challenges of conducting multi-site trials.

Early- and mid-career investigators step into the future when they get involved in existing research networks (e.g., International Behavioural Trials Network: www.ibtnetwork.org; the Behavioral Medicine Research Council) and participate in ongoing multi-site trials. By so doing, they gain the expertise that the next generation of multi-site behavioral trial leaders will need.

Big Data in Behavioral Clinical Trials

Large, confirmatory clinical trials must be more efficient. They must be conducted with smaller budgets, but without a loss of quality. Methods are needed to: (1) minimize specialized trial infrastructure; (2) minimize trial-related visits; and (3) employ low-cost methods for obtaining informed consent and monitoring trial progress [10].

Technology offers promise for the achievement of these objectives. Electronic medical records and registries are disruptive technologies that can be leveraged to conduct clinical trials more efficiently [10]. Hybrid trials use a combination of existing data and newly collected trial data. Existing data in electronic medical records makes it possible to create algorithms that identify potential participants for a clinical trial quickly and efficiently. In the nonclinical setting, web-based recruitment uses a variety of general and disease-specific platforms to identify and attract potential participants for a trial. Web-based eligibility and baseline assessment streamline the process of randomization into a trial. Once in, web-based outcome assessment further improves efficiency.

However, this efficiency cannot be achieved by sacrificing data quality. Concerns have been raised about: (1) the completeness of data when it is not systematically entered because it is not relevant for managing a specific patient; (2) the validity of data where definitions and semantics vary across providers and healthcare organizations; and (3) the adequacy of data for a particular trial when the point of time at which an assessment is made in an electronic record is inconsistent with the timing of assessment in the trial protocol [58].

A glimpse into the future overcomes these quality concerns with randomized registry trials embedded into learning healthcare systems. An excellent example is provided by the PCORI-funded Scalable Collaborative Infrastructure for a Learning Healthcare System [59]. Ten healthcare systems covering more than eight million patients harmonized their informatics infrastructure, data models, regulatory processes, policies, and patient identification systems. The resulting learning healthcare system has, among other things, fostered high-quality and efficient clinical trial methods in such areas as consent, enrollment, randomization, and outcome assessments.

Opportunities are not limited to trial operations but also include potential to simplify intervention delivery and surveillance. Internet and eHealth interventions are still in their youth but are accelerating in development, particularly in response to the COVID pandemic. Between 2009 and 2012, there were 31 published reviews of eHealth interventions, defined as the delivery of personalized healthcare at a distance through the use of technology [60]. Of these reviews, 7 (23%) reported effective and cost-effective results, and 13 (42%) reported promising results. Telehealth, the most successful of the remote interventions, has been associated with lower mortality and fewer emergency room admissions in patients with diabetes, heart failure, and chronic obstructive pulmonary disease [61]. eHealth behavioral interventions make it possible to intervene efficiently without ever needing face-to-face contact with participants. An accurate understanding of the strengths and limitations of eHealth has been facilitated by the development of uniform reporting guidelines [62]. This is an exploding area of research which is appealing because it offers the possibility that remote delivery of behavioral treatments will reduce their cost, preserve their efficacy, and shift the cost-effectiveness balance.

In summary, it is not much of a leap of faith to envision a future for behavioral clinical trials in which every part of the trial is conducted on laptops or tablet computers. The vast and expanding amount of data collected digitally in the healthcare system is creating a future in which big data is transformed from "refuse to riches," [63] particularly when they are used to make clinical trials more efficient [10, 52, 54, 63, 64]. To achieve this future, expansion of the breadth and quality of behavioral variables included in electronic health records, and federal guidelines that promote quality and uniformity in data collection procedures are needed. Sweden provides an excellent model for how federal investment in a national infrastructure can promote high-quality and efficient clinical trials [65].

BEHAVIORAL TRIALS WILL BE MORE RELEVANT

There is a gap between positive results from a definitive *Phase III* behavioral clinical trial and uptake of that behavioral treatment into clinical practice. Although there are a variety of reasons for this gap, one important reason is the fragmentation that exists between the world of behavioral clinical trials and the worlds of medical practice and third-party payers. In the future, this gap can close with a greater commitment to strategic planning where long-term goals figure heavily into behavioral trial design decisions made in the present. Two directions are especially noteworthy.

Strategic Planning for Dissemination and Implementation

Uptake of positive results from behavioral clinical trials is enhanced when those results solve a problem in clinical practice or show a reduction in healthcare costs. Many of the outcomes in behavioral trials, such as self-efficacy or health beliefs, are meaningless to medical gatekeepers or third-party payers.

Medical practitioners follow clinical practice guidelines. These guidelines are shaped most strongly by rigorous *Phase III* trials. *(See Chapter 2: Quality of a Clinical Trial.)* Third-party payers support programs that provide rigorous evidence that they can cut the immediate and escalating costs of procedures and therapies. Planning for dissemination and implementation includes a push toward a *Phase III* efficacy trial with an eye to influencing clinical practice guidelines. Planning for dissemination and implementation also includes greater sensitivity to concerns of third-party payers. If their concern is about the escalating cost of a drug for a particular condition, use of this drug should be part of the assessment battery at every stage of the development of a behavioral treatment for patients with that condition.

Strategic Planning for Failure

Reverse translation refers to the process of reversing the translational process of bench to bedside, to the process of bedside to bench [66]. One of its targets is the diversity of patient response in a clinical trial and working backward to uncover the basis for that response. To many, a failed intervention in a clinical trial is a feared outcome. But in reverse translation, failure becomes an opportunity. Unexpected responses can stimulate interest in looking back to evaluate what went wrong.

> **Reverse Translation**
>
> *"The beauty of reverse translation is that there is no such thing as a failed clinical trial. There is only expected and unexpected outcomes and the inevitable variability in human response that needs further explanation and exploration. . . A failure is really an opportunity."*
>
> Shakhnovich, 2018 [66]

To accept failure without understanding it, condemns us to go from one failure to another without ever learning from it [67].

This idea is not new. It is part of the foundation of Karl Popper's philosophy that science proceeds by posing hypotheses and then welcoming falsification as a way to advance knowledge [68]. What is new, however, is that biomedical science is beginning to welcome treatment failures as opportunities to fine-tune therapeutics for individual patients and advance personalized medicine [69]. What is also new is the "science of science" study of scholarly failures and successes. Given that scientists fail more often than they succeed, knowing when, why, and how an idea fails is an essential focus for improving the scientific process [56].

Behavioral trials of the future will get into the reverse translation game. They will plan for treatment failure and the opportunity it provides to fine-tune the treatment. They will be able to dissect unexpected variability in response with the use of a hypothesized pathway which quantifies each step of the path by which a treatment is expected to benefit an outcome. *(See Chapter 4: Hypothesized Pathway and Bias.)* If blood samples included in assessment batteries are stored, behavioral trials of the future will be able to capitalize on the explosion of knowledge in genomics, proteomics, and other technologies to improve understanding of the genetic determinants of patient success or failure. As knowledge increases, these stored samples can get behavioral trials into the big money, biomedical game of personalized medicine.

Strategic planning for dissemination and implementation, and decision-making in the face of failure, are now becoming an accepted part of the biomedical translational process [70]. In the future, the behavioral translational process will follow suit.

SUMMARY

Randomized behavioral clinical trials will remain the gold standard for assessing whether or not a treatment works or how well it works compared to a clinically relevant alternative. They are not perfect. But there is simply no other design that is as powerful at making causal inferences. Behavioral trial methods will evolve to become more rigorous, targeted, efficient, and relevant. Behavioral trialists will become more collaborative, united by a common vision to conduct the type of rigorous multi-site behavioral trials that will have a transformative impact on healthcare systems.

REFERENCES

1. Lillenfeld SO, McKay D, Hollan SD (2018) Why randomised controlled trials of psychological treatments are still essential. Lancet 5:536–538
2. Ioannidis JP, Fanelli D, Dunne DD, Goodman SN (2015) Meta-research: evaluation and improvement of research methods and practices. PLoS Biol 13:e1002264. https://doi.org/10.1371/journal.pbio.1002264
3. ASCEND Study Collaborative Group, Bowman L, Mafham M, Wallendszus K, Stevens W, Buck G, Barton J, Murphy K, Aung T, Haynes R, Cox J, Murawska A, Young A, Lay M, Chen F, Sammons E, Waters E, Adler A, Bodansky J, Farmer A, McPherson R, Neil A, Simpson D, Peto R, Baigent C, Collins R, Parish S, Armitage J (2018) Effects of n-3 fatty acid supplements in diabetes mellitus. N Engl J Med 379:1540–1550
4. Victor RG, Lynch K, Li N, Blyler C, Muhammad E, Handler J, Brettler J, Rashid M, Hsu B, Foxx-Drew D, Moy N, Reid AE, Elashoff RM (2018) A cluster-randomized trial of blood-pressure reduction in black barbershops. N Engl J Med 378:1291–1301
5. Shadish WR, Cook TD, Campbell DT (2002) Experimental and quasi-experimental designs for generalized causal inference. Houghton Mifflin, Boston
6. Hudson KL, Lauer MS, Collins FS (2016) Toward a new era of trust and transparency in clinical trials. JAMA 316:1353–1354
7. Choi KW, Chen CY, Stein MB, Klimentidis YC, Wang MJ, Koenen KC, Smoller JW, Major Depressive Disorder Working Group of the Psychiatric Genomics Consortium (2019) Assessment of bidirectional relationships between physical activity and depression among adults: a 2-sample mendelian randomization study. JAMA Psychiat 76:399–408
8. Byrne EM, Yang J, Wray NR (2017) Inference in psychiatry via 2-sample mendelian randomization–From association to causal pathway? JAMA Psychiat 74:1191–1192
9. Institute of Medicine (2007) The learning healthcare system: workshop summary. National Academies Press, Washington DC. https://doi.org/10.17226/11903
10. Lauer MS, Bonds D (2014) Eliminating the "expensive" adjective for clinical trials. Am Heart J 167:419–420
11. Naci H, Ioannidis JPA (2015) Evaluation of wellness determinants and interventions by citizen scientists. JAMA 314:121–122
12. Ioannidis JPA (2005) Why most published research findings are false. PLoS Med 2:e124. https://doi.org/10.1371/journal.pmed.0020124
13. Munafò MR, Nosek BA, Bishop DVM, Button KS, Chambers CD, du Sert NP, Simonsohn U, Wagenmakers EJ, Ware JJ, Ioannidis JPA (2017) A manifesto for reproducible science. Nat Hum Behav 1:0021. https://doi.org/10.1038/s41562-016-0021
14. Button KS, Ioannidis JPA, Mokrysz C, Nosek BA, Flint J, Robinson ES, Munafò MR (2013) Power failure: why small sample size undermines the reliability of neuroscience. Nat Rev Neurosci 5:365–376
15. Fanelli D (2010) "Positive" results increase down the hierarchy of the sciences. PLoS One 5:e10068. https://doi.org/10.1371/journal.pone.0010068
16. John LK, Loewenstein G, Prelec D (2012) Measuring the prevalence of questionable research practices with incentives for truth telling. Psychol Sci 23:524–532
17. Makel MC, Plucker JA, Hegarty B (2012) Replications in psychology research: how often do they really occur? Perspect Psychol Sci 7:537–542
18. Wicherts JM, Borsboom D, Kats J, Molenaar D (2006) The poor availability of psychological research data for reanalysis. Am Psychol 61:726–728
19. Kerr NL (1998) HARKing: hypothesizing after the results are known. Pers Soc Psychol Rev 2:196–217
20. Watts DJ (2017) Should social science be more solution-oriented? Nat Hum Behav 1:0015. https://doi.org/10.1038/s41562-016-0015
21. Freedland KE (2017) A new era for Health Psychology. Health Psychol 36:1–4

22. Czajkowski SM, Powell LH, Adler N, Naar-King S, Reynolds KD, Hunter CM, Laraia B, Olster DH, Perna FM, Peterson JC, Epel E, Charlson M (2015) From ideas to efficacy: the ORBIT model for developing behavioral treatments for chronic diseases. Health Psychol 34:971–982

23. Michie S, Richardson M, Johnston M, Abraham C, Francis J, Hardeman W, Eccles MP, Cane J, Wood CE (2013) The behavior change technique taxonomy (v1) of 93 hierarchically clustered techniques: building an international consensus for the reporting of behavior change interventions. Ann Behav Med 46:81–95

24. Thabane L, Thomas T, Ye C, Paul J (2009) Posing the research question: not so simple. Can J Anaesth 56:71–79

25. Schulz KF, Altman DG, Moher D, CONSORT Group (2010) CONSORT 2010 statement: updated guidelines for reporting parallel group randomised trials. Ann Intern Med 152:726–732

26. Boutron I, Moher D, Altman DG, Schulz KF, Ravaud P, CONSORT Group (2008) Extending the CONSORT statement to randomized trials of nonpharmacologic treatment: explanation and elaboration. Ann Intern Med 148:295–309

27. Montgomery P, Grant S, Hopewell S, Macdonald G, Moher D, Michie S, Mayo-Wilson E (2013) Protocol for CONSORT-SPI: an extension for social and psychological interventions. Implement Sci 8:99. https://doi.org/10.1186/1748-5908-88-99

28. Chan AW, Tetzlaff JM, Gøtzsche PC, Altman DG, Mann H, Berlin JA, Dickersin K, Hróbjartsson A, Schulz KF, Parulekar WR, Krleza-Jeric K, Laupacis A, Moher D (2013) SPIRIT 2013 explanation and elaboration: guidance for protocols of clinical trials. BMJ 346:e7586. https://doi.org/10.1136/bmj.e7586

29. Bacon SL, Lavoie KL, Ninot G, Czajkowski S, Freedland KE, Michie S, Montgomery P, Powell LH, Spring B (2015) An international perspective on improving the quality and potential of behavioral clinical trials. Curr Cardiovasc Risk Rep 9:427. https://doi.org/10.1007/s12170-014-0427-0

30. Lavoie KL, Powell LH, Ninot G, Bacon SL, on behalf of the Faculty of the 2nd IBTN Meeting (2019) Proceedings from IBTN 2018: It's time for a culture change in behavioral medicine. Ann Behav Med 53:296–298

31. Ma J, Rosas LG, Lv N (2016) Precision lifestyle medicine: a new frontier in the science of behavior change and population health. Am J Prev Med 50:395–397

32. US National Library of Medicine (2018) What is precision medicine? https://ghr.nlm.nih.gov/primer/precisionmedicine/definition

33. Ashley EA (2015) The precision medicine initiative: a new national effort. JAMA 313:2119–2120

34. Khoury MJ, Evans JP (2015) A public health perspective on a national precision medicine cohort: balancing long-term knowledge generation with early health benefit. JAMA 313:2117–2118

35. Khera AV, Emdin CA, Drake I, Natarajan P, Bick AG, Cook NR, Chasman DI, Baber U, Mehran R, Rader DJ, Fuster V, Boerwinkle E, Melander O, Orho-Melander M, Ridker PM, Kathiresan S (2016) Genetic risk, adherence to a healthy lifestyle, and coronary disease. N Engl J Med 375:2349–2358

36. Gardner CD, Trepanowski JF, Del Gobbo LC, Hauser ME, Rigdon J, Ioannidis JPA, Desai M, King AC (2018) Effect of low-fat vs low-carbohydrate diet on 12-month weight loss in overweight adults and the association with genotype pattern or insulin secretion: the DIETFITS randomized clinical trial. JAMA 319:667–679

37. Goldberg JH, Kiernan M (2005) Innovative techniques to address retention in a behavioral weight-loss trial. Health Educ Res 20:439–447

38. Kiernan M, Oppezzo MA, Resnicow K, Alexander GL (2018) Effects of a methodological infographic on research participants' knowledge, transparency, and trust. Health Psychol 37:782–786

39. Kong W, Langlois MF, Kamga-Ngandé C, Gagnon C, Brown C, Baillargeon JP (2010) Predictors of success to weight-loss intervention program in individuals at high risk for type 2 diabetes. Diab Res Clin Pract 90:147–153
40. Rosas LG, Lv N, Azar KMJ, Xiao L, Hooker SP, Lewis MA, Zavella P, Venditti EM, Ma J (2018) HOMBRE: a randomized controlled trial to compare two approaches to weight loss for overweight and obese Latino men (Hombres con Opciones para Mejorar el Bienestar y bajar el Riesgo de Enfermedades crónicas; men with choices to improve well-being and decrease chronic disease risk). Contemp Clin Trials 68:23–34
41. Preference Collaborative Review Group (2008) Patients' preferences with randomised trials: systematic review and patient level meta-analysis. BMJ 337:a1864. https://doi.org/10.1136/bmj.a1864
42. King M, Nazareth I, Lampe F, Bower P, Chandler M, Morou M, Sibbald B, Lai R (2005) Impact of participant and physician intervention preferences on randomized trials: a systematic review. JAMA 293:1089–1099
43. Almirall D, Nahum-Shani I, Sherwood NE, Murphy SA (2014) Introduction to SMART designs for the development of adaptive interventions: with application to weight loss research. Transl Behav Med 4:260–274
44. Williams LM, Pines A, Goldstein-Piekarski AN, Rosas LG, Kullar M, Sacchet MD, Gevaert O, Bailenson J, Lavori PW, Dagum P, Wandell B, Correa C, Greenleaf W, Suppes T, Perry LM, Smyth JM, Lewis MA, Venditti EM, Snowden M, Simmons JM, Ma J (2018) The ENGAGE study: integrating neuroimaging, virtual reality and smartphone sensing to understand self-regulation for managing depression and obesity in a precision medicine model. Behav Res Ther 101:58–70
45. Hellhammer D, Meinlschmidt G, Pruessner JC (2018) Conceptual endophenotypes: a strategy to advance the impact of psychoneuroendocrinology in precision medicine. Psychoneuroendocrinology 89:147–160
46. Lamont A, Lyons MD, Jaki T, Stuart E, Feaster DJ, Tharmaratnam K, Oberski D, Ishwaran H, Wilson DK, Van Horn ML (2018) Identification of predicted individual treatment effects in randomized clinical trials. Stat Methods Med Res 27:142–157
47. Barabási A-L (2007) Network medicine--from obesity to the "diseasome". N Engl J Med 357:404–407
48. Institute of Medicine Committee on Understanding Eliminating Racial and Ethnic Disparities in Health Care, Smedley BD, Stith SY, Nelson AR (eds) (2003) Unequal treatment: confronting racial and ethnic disparities in health care. National Academies Press, Washington DC
49. Gorin SS, Badr H, Krebs P, Prabhu Das I (2012) Multilevel interventions and racial/ethnic health disparities. J Natl Cancer Inst Monogr 44:100–111
50. Mangla A, Doukky R, Richardson D, Avery EF, Dawar R, Calvin JE Jr, Powell LH (2018) Design of a bilevel clinical trial targeting adherence in heart failure patients and their providers: the Congestive Heart Failure Adherence Redesign Trial (CHART). Am Heart J 195:139–150
51. Stevens J, Pratt C, Boyington J, Nelson C, Truesdale KP, Ward DS, Lytle L, Sherwood NE, Robinson TN, Moore S, Barkin S, Cheung YK, Murray DM (2017) Multilevel interventions targeting obesity: research recommendations for vulnerable populations. Am J Prev Med 52:115–124
52. Eapen ZJ, Lauer MS, Temple RJ (2014) The imperative of overcoming barriers to the conduct of large, simple trials. JAMA 311:1397–1398
53. Institute of Medicine Forum on Drug Discovery, Development, and Translation (2010) Transforming clinical research in the United States. Challenges and opportunities: workshop summary. National Academies Press, Washington DC
54. Antman EM, Harrington RA (2012) Transforming clinical trials in cardiovascular disease: mission critical for health and economic well-being. JAMA 308:1743–1744

55. National Research Council Committee on the Science of Team Science, Cooke NJ, Hilton ML (eds) (2015) Enhancing the effectiveness of team science, National Academies Press, Washington DC.

56. Fortunato S, Bergstrom CT, Börner K, Evans J, Helbing D, Milojević S, Petersen AM, Radicchi F, Sinatra R, Uzzi B, Vespignani A, Waltman L, Wang D, Barabási A-L (2018) Science of science. Science 359:eaao0185. https://doi.org/10.1126/science.aao0185

57. Freedland KE (2019) The Behavioral Medicine Research Council: its origins, mission, and methods. Health Psychol 38:277–289

58. Opmeer BC (2016) Electronic health records as sources of research data. JAMA 315:201–202

59. Mandl KD, Kohane IS, McFadden D, Weber GM, Natter M, Mandel J, Schneeweiss S, Weiler S, Klann JG, Bickel J, Adams WG, Ge Y, Zhou X, Perkins J, Marsolo K, Bernstam E, Showalter J, Quarshie A, Ofili E, Hripcsak G, Murphy SN (2014) Scalable Collaborative Infrastructure for a Learning Healthcare System (SCILHS): architecture. J Am Med Inform Assoc 21:615–620

60. Elbert NJ, van Os-Medendorp H, van Renselaar W, Ekeland AG, Hakkaart-van Roijen L, Raat H, Nijsten TE, Pasmans SG (2014) Effectiveness and cost-effectiveness of ehealth interventions in somatic diseases: a systematic review of systematic reviews and meta-analyses. J Med Internet Res 16:e110. https://doi.org/10.2196/jmir.2790

61. Steventon A, Bardsley M, Billings J, Dixon J, Doll H, Hirani S, Cartwright M, Rixon L, Knapp M, Henderson C, Rogers A, Fitzpatrick R, Hendy J, Newman S, Whole System Demonstrator Evaluation Team (2012) Effect of telehealth on use of secondary care and mortality: findings from the Whole System Demonstrator cluster randomised trial. BMJ 344:e3874. https://doi.org/10.1136/bmj.e3874

62. Eysenbach G, CONSORT-EHEALTH Group (2011) CONSORT-EHEALTH: improving and standardizing evaluation reports of web-based and mobile health interventions. J Med Internet Res 13:e126. https://doi.org/10.2196/jmir.1923

63. Murdoch TB, Detsky AS (2013) The inevitable application of big data to health care. JAMA 309:1351–1352

64. Lauer MS (2012) Time for a creative transformation of epidemiology in the United States. JAMA 308:1804–1805

65. Nyberg K, Hedman P (2019) Swedish guidelines for registry-based randomized clinical trials. Ups J Med Sci 124:33–36

66. Shakhnovich V (2018) It's time to reverse our thinking: the reverse translation research paradigm. Clin Transl Sci 11:98–99

67. Ledford H (2008) Translational research: the full cycle. Nature 453:843–845

68. Popper KR (1959) The logic of scientific discovery. Basic Books, New York

69. Murphy J (2019) Reverse translational medicine: the promising future of failure. BioProcess Intl. https://bioprocessintl.com/business/pre-clinical-and-clinical-trials/elucidation-on-reverse-translational-medicine-the-promising-future-of-failure

70. Collins FS (2011) Reengineering translational science: the time is right. Sci Transl Med 3:90cm17. https://doi.org/10.1126/scitranslmed.3002747

Chapter 12
Epilogue

"As the present now
Will later be past
The order is rapidly fadin'
And the first one now
Will later be last
For the times they are a-changin'"

Bob Dylan
The Times They Are A-Changin', 1964
Nobel Prize in Literature, 2016

There is a gap between the identification of effective behavioral strategies for managing chronic diseases and their uptake in clinical practice. This is an important limitation of the healthcare system, not only because behavior is a root cause of most chronic diseases but because those strategies can reduce healthcare costs. There are many reasons for this gap. The one most relevant here is that medical practitioners and third-party payers use more stringent criteria for evaluating efficacy than criteria reflected in the literature of many trials of behavioral interventions. Thus, one way to enhance uptake of behavioral treatments into clinical practice is to increase the rigor of behavioral treatment development and evaluation; that is, to speak the language of medicine.

This has led to the emergence of a translational behavioral science cultural movement. It is a movement that has, as a basic underpinning, the application of a progressive, translational approach to behavioral treatment development and evaluation, going all of the way from basic science discovery through rigorous *Phase III* efficacy and *Phase IV* effectiveness trials.

This movement has run up against a cultural divide. This divide is between those who explore and discover and those who confirm and apply. Coller [1] has made

© Springer Nature Switzerland AG 2021
L. H. Powell et al., *Behavioral Clinical Trials for Chronic Diseases*,
https://doi.org/10.1007/978-3-030-39330-4_12

Table 12.1 Comparison of the cultures of basic science discovery and applied clinical medicine

Variable	Basic Science Discovery	Applied Clinical Medicine
Mission	New knowledge	Better health
Strategy	Test models	Solve health problem
Goal	Progress science	Progress translation
Values	Freedom to explore	Responsibility to patients
Dress code	Jeans and tee shirts	Suits
Perceptions of the Other	Impatient, concrete, conservative, superficial	Overly skeptical, indecisive, divorced from reality

these differences visible within the context of clinical medicine (Table 12.1). The "jeans and tee shirt" basic scientist is driven to discover new knowledge, to test models, and to explore freely, while the "suited" applied scientist is driven to improve health, improve patient care, and solve clinical problems. The basic scientist sees the clinician as concrete and conservative, while the clinician sees the basic scientist as divorced from reality. They may not understand each other very well, and may have little interest in so doing. It is not difficult to see how these two worlds could become fragmented and isolated from one another. The translational science movement aims to integrate the worlds of basic and applied science. This integration is essential for making the multidisciplinary case for the strength and necessity of a behavioral treatment.

The movement has also run up against a long-standing status quo. Methods used to develop and evaluate behavioral treatments for chronic diseases are dominated by the basic science culture of experimentation and discovery. This dominance exists regardless of where a treatment falls on the translational spectrum. Experiments and clinical trials certainly share a randomized design. But their questions and methods for answering them diverge.

Translational research encourages progression through a full range of questions and methods when developing and evaluating the effectiveness of a behavioral treatment. Without this progression, there is risk for a mismatch between the aim of a trial and its design, an underappreciation of the value of various translational steps, mistaken priority setting, inappropriate allocation of resources, missed opportunities for promising treatments, and investigator frustration [1].

By default, the cultural divide and the status quo endure, sustained by the academic incentive system which has been described succinctly by Watts [2].

"Although our work is ostensibly motivated by a desire to understand, explain, and possibly intervene, neither the training nor the structure of incentives in academia are specifically designed for this purpose. Rather social scientists are raised inside disciplinary environments where they are immersed in particular theoretical and methodological frameworks. They are then encouraged to take the framework they have absorbed and apply it to every problem they work on. Journals value novel, counterintuitive, or otherwise interesting results over steady cumulative advances in knowledge." [2]

Thus, a movement to break down the cultural divide and challenge the status quo is needed. This movement seeks to transform an invisible culture into one that is visible [2–4]. It seeks to replace isolation and fragmentation with integration. It seeks to integrate the visions of advancing new knowledge with those of improving health. It seeks to augment professional training in experimental design [5] with training in clinical trial methodology [6, 7]. It seeks to close the gap between efficacy and clinical practice with a strategic plan of action [8]. It seeks to change the incentive system that sustains the status quo [3].

But most of all, it is motivated by a commitment to make effective behavioral treatments available to the patients who need them. Without this, the healthcare system will continue to be limited and costly, and the patients will finish last.

We have yet to realize the full power of behavioral treatments in the clinical management of patients with chronic diseases. We have yet to realize the full power of behavioral clinical trials to make this case. We move closer to this power when we are willing to break down barriers, rethink the status quo, and challenge it where it is found to be lacking.

This was the inspiration for this book.

REFERENCES

1. Coller BS (2008) Translational research: forging a new cultural identity. Mt Sinai J Med 75:478–487
2. Watts DJ (2017) Should social science be more solution-oriented? Nat Hum Beh 1:0015. https://doi.org/10.1038/s41562-016-0015
3. Freedland KE (2017) A new era for Health Psychology. Health Psychol 36:1–4
4. Lavoie KL, Powell LH, Ninot G, Bacon SL, on behalf of the Faculty of the 2nd IBTN Meeting (2019) Proceedings from IBTN 2018: It's time for a culture change in behavioral medicine. Ann Behav Med 53:296–298
5. Shadish WR, Cook TD, Campbell DT (2002) Experimental and quasi-experimental designs for generalized causal inference. Houghton Mifflin, Boston
6. Friedman LM, Furberg CD, DeMets D, Reboussin DM, Granger CB (2015) Fundamentals of clinical trials, 5th edn. Springer, Cham
7. Powell LH, Freedland KE, Kaufmann PG (2021) Behavioral clinical trials for chronic diseases. Scientific foundations. Springer, New York, IBSN 978-3-030-39328.1
8. Freedland KE (2019) The behavioral medicine research council: its origins, mission, and methods. Health Psychol 38:277–289

APPENDIX
Books on Clinical Trials

There is a large number of books on clinical trial methods. This list is a subset of those that are recommended for investigators with interests in behavioral clinical trials for chronic diseases. They provide the foundation for the widely accepted "rules" of clinical trial methodology that have been developed over the past 40 years in medicine and epidemiology.

Schwartz D, Flamant R, Lellouch J (1980) Clinical trials. Academic Press, New York
This is a practical guide for clinicians and medical statisticians who are engaged in the planning, analysis, and interpretation of clinical trials. Emphasis is placed on practical problems such as the determination of the appropriate number of subjects, the details of treatment allocation, and the meaning to be attached to the results of statistical analysis. A distinction is made between two objectives a clinical trial can have: pragmatic (to reach a practical decision on the most appropriate treatment) or explanatory (to increase scientific knowledge). This fundamental difference radically influences every stage of a trial. [Author Note: Differences between confirmatory and exploratory clinical trials are a fundamental concept in progressive translational research. This is the first time these differences were identified.]

Pocock SJ (1983) Clinical trials: a practical approach. Wiley, New York
This is a comprehensive text on the principles, practice, and conduct of clinical trials. It describes design, analysis, and interpretation of clinical trials in a non-technical manner and provides a general perspective on their historical development, current status, and future strategies, featuring examples derived from the author's personal experience. [Author Note: Written by a highly respected expert and leader in the development of clinical trial methodology.]

© Springer Nature Switzerland AG 2021
L. H. Powell et al., *Behavioral Clinical Trials for Chronic Diseases*,
https://doi.org/10.1007/978-3-030-39330-4

Spiegelhalter DJ, Abrams KR, Myles JP (2004) Bayesian approaches to clinical trials and health-care evaluation. John Wiley & Sons, Chichester
The Bayesian approach goes beyond sole reliance upon inferential statistics and involves synthesizing data and judgment to reach conclusions about unknown quantities and make predictions. Despite the popularity of Bayesian approaches, there are few books available that cover clinical trials and biostatistical applications. This book provides an overview of this rapidly evolving field, including basic Bayesian ideas, prior disributions, clinical trials, and cost-effectiveness analyses. This book includes case studies and exercises in each chapter and an accompanying website. [Author Note: A fellow in the Royal Society and member of the Medical Research Council, the author desribes the use of Bayesian approaches to judge clinically significant benefit of a treatment.]

DeMets DL, Furberg CD, Friedman LM (2005) Data monitoring in clinical trials: a case studies approach, 2006 edn. Springer, New York
A fundamental principle of clinical trials is that they should not continue longer than necessary to reach their objectives. Therefore, trials must be moitored for recruitment progress, quality of data, adherence to treatment, and early evidence of benefit or harm. Frequently a group of external experts, independent from the investigators and trial sponsor, is charged with this monitoring responsibility. Through a series of 29 case studies described by 70 distinguished clinical trial experts, an overview of this process, its complexity, and lessons learned are presented. [Author Note: The authors of a highly respected book on fundamentals of clinical trials, describe the essential function of independent monitoring of trial progress.]

Wang D, Bakhai A (2006) Clinical trials: a practical guide to design, analysis, and reporting. Remedica, London
The author takes a back-to-basics approach to explaining statistics specifically for a medically literate audience. Topics include background, rationale, and when and how specific procedures should be applied. Readers will gain not only an understanding of the basics of medical statistics but also a critical insight into how to review and evaluate clinical trial evidence. [Author Note: Excellent description of basic statistical approaches to clinical trials intended for investigators who are not statisticians.]

Jadad AR, Enkin MW (2007) Randomized controlled trials. Questions, answers, musings, 2nd edn. Blackwell/BMJ, Malden
This book is a convenient and accessible description of the underlying principles and practice of randomized controlled trials and their role in clinical decision-making. Structured in a jargon-free question-and-answer format, each chapter provides concise and understandable information on a different aspect of randomized controlled trials including the basics of design and terminology, ethics, implications for evidence-based medicine, and a debate on strengths and limitations of trial data. Each chapter ends with musings drawing on extensive personal experience with clinical trials. [Author Note: The musings are the "gems" of this book. They present invaluable information known by experienced trialists but rarely found in more formal books and papers.]

Matthews JNS (2008) Introduction to randomized controlled clinical trials, 2nd edn. Chapman & Hall/CRC, Boca Raton
Statistical methods play a key role in all stages of clinical trials, including their justification, design, and analysis. This book provides a concise presentation of the principles, concepts behind randomization, methods for designing and analyzing trials, meta-analysis, and specialized designs such as cross-over trials, cluster-randomized designs, and equivalence studies. This book is geared toward a statistically conversant audience and each chapter focuses on a key analytic challenge and its associated statistical implications. [Author Note: Useful for biostatisticians who are beginning to work in clinical trials.]

Domanski M, McKinlay S (2009) Successful randomized trials. A handbook for the 21st century. Lippincott Williams & Wilkins, Philadelphia
This is a reference on the theory and operation of modern, large, multicenter, randomized clinical trials that have come to be the basis of evidence-based medicine. Written in a concise, engaging style geared to physicians, the book explains the rationale and theoretical foundations for clinical trials, the components of modern clinical trials including their functions and interactions, practical considerations in design and implementation, and an introduction to the economics and business aspects. [Author Note: This is an excellent overview of modern multicenter trials written by experts with considerable experience leading data coordinating centers.]

Hackshaw AK (2009) A concise guide to clinical trials. Wiley Blackwell/ BMJ, Hoboken
This is a comprehensive yet easy-to-read overview of the design, conduct, and analysis of trials. It requires no prior knowledge on the subject and is useful in isolating those concepts that are most important. Chapters include the different types of trials, systematic reviews, health-related quality of life, health economic evaluation, and ethical and legal requirements in setting up a clinical trial. [Author Note: This is a good reference for someone who is new to the field of clinical trials.]

Julious SA (2009) Sample sizes for clinical trials. Chapman & Hall/CRC, Boca Raton
This book takes readers through the process of calculating sample sizes for a variety of types of clinical trials with a practical emphasis. It uses extensive examples that focus on normal, binary, ordinal, and survival data, drawing on a range of trials including superiority, equivalence, non-inferiority for parallel group, and crossover designs. Included are hints, tips, advice, and opinions that are highly relevant coming from an experienced trialist. [Author Note: Written by a biostatistician, for biostatisticians, this book provides details of the variety of considerations needed to arrive at an appropriate sample size for a clinical trial.]

Machin D, Fayers PM (2010) Randomized clinical trials: design, practice and reporting. Wiley-Blackwell, Hoboken
Using examples and case studies from industry, academia, and research literature, this book provides a detailed overview of the key issues involved in designing, conducting, analyzing, and reporting randomized clinical trials. It examines the methodology for conducting *Phase III* clinical trials, developing the protocols, capturing, measuring, and analyzing the resulting clinical data, and subsequent reporting. Emphasis is placed on the importance of clinical trials in the determination of relative efficacy and safety of alternative treatments and the key evidence needed for regulatory approval. [Author Note: This book provides insight into the strength of the data needed for regulatory approval of a new drug and how these criteria align with clinical trial design.]

Chin R, Bairu M (2011) Global clinical trials. Effective implementation and management. Academic Press, Cambridge
This book explores the opportunities and challenges that exist in conducting clinical trials in developing countries. By examining the various regulations specific to the major players and providing insight into logistical challenges including language barriers, this book provides a working tool for clinical researchers and administrators to navigate the intricacies of clinical trials in developing countries. Ethical issues highlight the significant differences in conducting this work in various jurisdictions, including a comprehensive guide to the ins and outs of clinical trials in various countries to maximize their effectiveness. [Author Note: This is an excellent resource for those with interests in cross-cultural clinical trials.]

Ezekiel EJ, Grady CC, Crouch RA, Lie RK, Miller FG, Wendler DD (2011) The Oxford textbook of clinical research ethics, reprint edn. Oxford University Press, New York
This is the first comprehensive and systematic reference on clinical research ethics, presented as 73 chapters written by experts from the US National Institutes of Health. Chapters include the history of research on humans, ethical guidance from codes and declarations, value of clinical trials, importance of equipoise, incentives for participation, special populations, informed consent, independent review, investigator conflict of interest, and respect. [Author Note: This is an excellent and comprehensive "must-read" for developing sophistication in the ethics of clinical trials.]

Lui K-J (2011) Binary data analysis of randomized clinical trials with noncompliance. John Wiley & Sons, New York.
Non-compliance in clinical trials is common and often occurs non-randomly. Common approaches to achieve an unbiased inference about treatment efficacy include intent-to-treat and per-protocol analyses. This book provides a systematic approach to analyzing trials with noncompliance under the most frequently encountered situations and presents the advantages and biases associated with each of them. Real-life examples, exercises, computer-simulated data, and SAS programs enhance comprehension. [Author Note: This book tackles noncompliance in a clinical trial, the tension between intent-to-treat and per-protocol analyses, and statistical approaches to noncompliance when it is not missing at random. It is pitched toward biostatisticians and clinical trial experts.]

Tal J (2011) Strategy and statistics in clinical trials. A non-statisticians guide to thinking, designing and executing. Academic Press, Cambridge
The focus is on the research process and the role of statistics in these processes. It describes the statistical building blocks and concepts of clinical trials and promotes effective cooperation between statisticians and other important parties. Topics include the link between research objectives and statistical thinking, estimation, testing procedures, statistical significance, explanation, and prediction. It distinguishes between exploratory and confirmatory trials, describes the tension between hypothesis testing and multiplicity, and outlines basic elements of clinical trials, choice of endpoints, and determination of sample size. [Author Note: Useful for any non-statistician who is interested in obtaining a better basic understanding of how statistics are applied to clinical trials.]

Browner WS (2012) Publishing & presenting clinical research, 3rd edn. Lippincott Williams & Wilkins, Philadelphia
This book explains the essentials of clinical trials and and how to publish them. It is perfect for investigators who seek information on how to organize, deliver, and publish the outcomes of their trials in the most effective way. It includes topics on how to make clear oral presentations and details on how to prepare manuscripts, tables, and abstracts for publication. [Author Note: The unique focus of this book is on publication and presentation of clinical trial results, an important but neglected area in clinical trial methods.]

Harrington D (2012) Designs for clinical trials. Perspectives on current issues. Springer, New York
This edited volume is an examination of current issues and controversies in the design of clinical trials, including topics in adaptive and sequential designs, the design of correlative genomic studies, the design of studies in which missing data are anticipated, and interim monitoring for futility. As a collection, the chapters serve as guidance for statisticians designing clinical trials. [Author Note: The book is written by a biostatistician who is a recognized and respected leader in statistical methods for clinical trials and an expert in data coordinating centers.]

Meinert CL (2012) Clinical trials dictionary: terminology and usage recommendations, 2nd edn. Wiley, Hoboken
This book provides clear, precise, and detailed entries on all aspects of modern-day clinical trials, incorporating the disciplines of medicine, statistics, epidemiology, computer science, and bioethics. It supplies readers with A–Z terminology needed to design, conduct, and analyze trials. It features historical figures and institutions in the field, and an extensive bibliography for additional resources. [Author Note: This book is written by one of the world's leading clinical trialists and is a valuable resource for developing a comprehensive understanding of trial terminology and the range of considerations needed to maximize the strength of a clinical trial.]

van Belle G, Kerr KF (2012) Design and analysis of experiments in the health sciences. Wiley, Hoboken
This book advances the idea that design drives analysis and analysis reveals the design. It explains how to apply design and analysis principles in animal, human, and laboratory experiments while illustrating topics with examples from randomized clinical trials. The authors focus on five types of designs that form the basis of most experimental structures: completely randomized designs, randomized block designs, factorial designs, multilevel experiments, and repeated measures designs. A website features data sets that are used throughout the book and allow readers hands-on applications, and an extensive bibliography outlines additional resources for further study. [Author Note: The theme of this book is the intimate connection between design and analysis. The five designs presented are the most common designs in clinical trials.]

Hulley SB, Cummings SR, Browner WS, Grady DG, Newman TB (2013) Designing clinical research, 4th edn. Lippincott Williams & Wilkins, Philadelphia
This book continues to set the standard as a practical guide for doctors, nurses, pharmacists, and other health professionals involved in all forms of clinical, translational, and public health research. It presents advanced epidemiologic concepts in a reader-friendly way and provides common sense approaches to the challenging judgments involved in designing, funding, and implementing a clinical trial. [Author Note: This book integrates epidemiological concepts with clinical trial methodology. It is among the top books on clinical trials, written by a leader of, and commentator on, some of the most influential behavioral efficacy trials to date.]

Meinert CL (2013) Clinical trials handbook. Design and conduct. Wiley, Hoboken
The success or failure of clinical trials hinges on hundreds of details that need to be developed, often under less than ideal conditions. This is a systematic approach to all aspects of designing clinical trials, with a focus on simplifying the process and avoiding costly mistakes. Topics include masking, randomization, consent, enrollment, eligibility, sample size, data collection, working with study centers and research staff, monitoring, and data analysis. [Author Note: This book is written by one of the world's leading trialists as a companion to the Clinical Trials Dictionary. It provides insights from an experienced expert into the complexity and range of decisions needed in a clinical trial and how to make them.]

Friedman LM, Furberg CD, DeMets D, Reboussin DM, Granger CB (2015) Fundamentals of clinical trials, 5th edn. Springer, Cham

The clinical trial is the most definitive tool for comparing the potential for alternative treatments to improve health, improve the quality of health care, and control costs. It has been called "the gold standard" against which all other clinical research works are measured. Although many clinical trials are of high quality, a careful reader of the medical literature will notice a large number of deficiencies in design, conduct, analysis, presentation, and/or interpretation of results. Improvements have occurred over the past few decades, but too many trials are still conducted without adequate attention to the fundamental principles, suggesting that attention to these fundamentals is needed. The fifth edition adds two new authors, a chapter on regulatory issues, more detail on data monitoring, contemporary clinical trial examples, and new material on adverse events, adherence, analysis, electronic data sharing, and international trials. [Author Note: This is the best book on fundamentals of clinical trials to date. It is a must-read for a behavioral clinical trialist who follows a progressive translational model, pushes toward a *Phase III* efficacy trial, and wants a firm foundation in clinical trials fundamentals.]

George TC (2016) Investigator initiated trials (IITs) simplified. A practical guide for clinical trial investigators to conduct IITs. Sunshine Press, Edison

This book is designed to serve as a guide for the clinical trial investigator who is willing to initiate a trial on their own. The chapters include basics of IITs, regulation, association with industry, protocol design, budget preparation, case report forms, informed consent, reporting, clinical trial registration, conduct, monitoring, and data management. [Author Note: This book focuses on the operational side of clinical trials.]

Rosenberger WF, Lachin JM (2016) Randomization in clinical trials. Theory and practice, 2nd edn. Wiley, Hoboken

This is a go-to guide for biostatisticians that features a unique combination of the applied aspects of randomization in clinical trials with a nonparametric approach to inference. [Author Note: This is everything you wanted to know about random assignment.]

Shih WJ, Aisner J (2016) Statistical design and analysis of clinical trials: principles and methods. Chapman & Hall/CRC, Boca Raton

This book concentrates on the biostatistics component of clinical trials. Developed from the authors' courses taught to public health and medical students, residents, and fellows during the past 15 years, the text shows how biostatistics in clinical trials is an integration of many fundamental scientific principles and statistical methods. [Author Note: Drawing on extensive teaching experience, this book makes statistical analyses of clinical trials easy and accessible.]

Wassmer G, Brannath W (2016) Group sequential and confirmatory adaptive designs in clinical trials. Springer International, Switzerland
This book provides a review of the general principles of, and techniques for, confirmatory adaptive designs. In these designs, interim analyses are performed with control for the type I error rate and a data-driven change in aspects of the design at interim stages is permitted, including sample-size reassessment, treatment arm selection, and selection of a prespecified population. Adaptive design methodology is introduced at an elementary level and is appropriate for applied statisticians with a sound statistical background. [Author Note: The focus of this book is on the meaning of an adaptive design for a clinical trial in the statistical literature.]

Pfeiffer J, Wells C (2017) A practical guide to managing clinical trials. CRC Press, Boca Raton
This is a basic, comprehensive guide to the operational side of clinical trials. This user-friendly reference guides the reader through each step of the clinical trial process from site selection to site setup, subject recruitment, trial visits, and trial closeout. Topics include staff roles/responsibilities/training, budget and contract review and management, subject study visits, data and document management, event reporting, research ethics, audits and inspections, consent processes, IRB and FDA regulations, and good clinical practices. [Author Note: This excellent book is focused on trial operations and will be of considerable value to research staff.]

Piantadosi S (2017) Clinical trials: a methodologic perspective, 3rd edn. Wiley, Hoboken
This is a straightforward, detailed, and authoritative presentation of quantitative methods for clinical trials. Readers will encounter the principles of design for various types of clinical trials and are then guided through the complete process of planning the experiment, assembling a study cohort, assessing data, and reporting results. Throughout the process, readers are alerted to the problems that may arise and are offered common sense solutions. [Author Note: This book is written by one of the world's leading experts in the design and analysis of clinical trials in cancer.]

Rauch G, Schüler S, Kieser M (2017) Planning and analyzing clinical trials with composite endpoints. Springer, New York
This book addresses the planning and evaluation of clinical trials with composite primary endpoints so that clinically meaningful and valid interpretations result. Composite endpoints combine several variables of interest within a single composite measure and, as a result, all variables that are of major clinical relevance can be considered in the primary analysis without the need to adjust for multiplicity. Composite endpoints can increase the size of the expected effects thus making clinical trials more powerful. [Author Note: This book provides details on the pros and cons of using composite endpoints to maximize efficiency without losing clinical or statistical significance.]

National Academies of Sciences, Engineering, and Medicine (2019) Virtual clinical trials: challenges and opportunities: Proceedings of a workshop. National Academies Press, Washington, DC
The current model for clinical trials is outdated, inefficient, and costly. Clinical trials are limited by small sample sizes that do not reflect diversity, financial burdens on participants, slow processes, and, as a result, disconnect between research and practice. This workshop was convened to explore benefits and challenges to implementing virtual clinical trials as an enhanced alternative for the future. [Author Note: Virtual clinical trials are the wave of the future but are not without challenges. This book presents the current state of the art and balances the opportunities against the challenges.]

Pawlik TM, Sosa JA (2020) Clinical trials, 2nd edn. Springer, Cham
This is a comprehensive book on clinical trials covering history, ethics, design, types of trials (pragmatic, cooperative, international), data handling, statistics, budget, publishing, and patient-reported outcomes. The focus is on trials in surgery but the topics reflect recent developments in basic clinical trial methodology that apply to a variety of outcomes. [Author Note: Surgical trials tend to be unblinded and, as such, face challenges that are similar to those of behavioral trials. It is instructive to see how similar challenges are being met across different disciplines.]

APPENDIX
Books on Behavioral Clinical Trials

These books represent the emerging literature on behavioral clinical trial methodology. They are a reflection of the relatively recent realization that trials testing behavioral treatments face unique challenges seldom seen in double-blind drug trials.

Nezu AM, Nezu CM (2008) Evidence-based outcome research: a practical guide to conducting randomized controlled trials for psychosocial interventions. Oxford University Press, New York
This edited volume provides both conceptual and practical information for conducting and evaluating evidence-based outcome studies. It encompasses psychotherapy research for traditional mental health disorders, such as depression and anxiety, and psychosocial-based treatments provided to medical patients to influence such disease processes as pain and cardiovascular risk or to improve quality of life. This is a hands-on book with an emphasis on the practical nuts-and-bolts implementation of psychosocial-based randomized trials from conception to completion. [Author Note: This book emphasizes psychotherapy for mental health disorders and features excellent chapters on treatment manuals, training therapists, and treatment fidelity. Written by leading researchers and statisticians, chapters are organized around conceptual, assessment, design, and data analysis issues.]

Torgerson DJ, Torgerson CJ (2008) Designing randomised trials in health, education and the social sciences. An introduction. Palgrave Macmillan, New York
This book focuses on the design of rigorous trials rather than their statistical underpinnings. It features chapters on pragmatic designs, placebo controls, preference designs, unequal allocation, economic evaluation, analytical approaches, and randomization methods. [Author Note: This book provides an introduction to the design of randomized trials in the social sciences. It features excellent descriptions of factorial designs, cluster randomized designs, pragmatic trials, and explanatory trials.]

© Springer Nature Switzerland AG 2021
L. H. Powell et al., *Behavioral Clinical Trials for Chronic Diseases*,
https://doi.org/10.1007/978-3-030-39330-4

Boutron I, Ravaud P, Moher D (2012) Randomized clinical trials of nonpharmacological treatments. Chapman & Hall/CRC, Boca Raton
Nonpharmacological treatments include a wide variety of treatments such as surgery, technical procedures, implantable and non-implantable devices, rehabilitation, psychotherapy, and behavioral interventions. Unlike pharmacological treatments, these have no specific requirements for approval and consequently can be widely proposed in clinical practice but inadequately evaluated. This situation is an important barrier for the evaluation of the beneficial effects of these treatments and the conduct of clinical trials. This edited book focuses on the methods for assessing nonpharmacological treatments, highlighting specific issues and trial designs. [Author Note: Edited by leaders in the CONSORT collaboration, this book includes excellent chapters on blinding, placebos, external validity, cluster randomized designs, patient preference designs, and reporting guidelines.]

Areán PA, Kraemer HC (2013) High-quality psychotherapy research: From conception to piloting to national trials. Oxford University Press, New York
Although psychotherapy research shares many of the same methodological issues that pharmacology trials do, psychotherapy research poses unique challenges, including the difficulty of keeping participants blind to treatment assignment, the need for a replicable treatment manual and therapist training procedure, the importance of outside observation of therapy quality ratings, and the problems researchers face in measuring the active ingredients of psychotherapy. Organized developmentally, this book explains the conceptualization of the trial, the pilot study, the large-scale study, and the multi-site trial. Topics include innovations in data analysis, the operation of a multi-site psychotherapy trial, mediation of treatment outcomes, translation to community practice, training community providers to be study therapists, and recruiting hard-to-reach populations. This is a practical book appropriate for a broad range of readers, from junior investigators developing their first study idea to seasoned investigators who wish to take their research to a larger-scale level. [Author Note: This book is co-authored by a leader in behavioral clinical trial methodology who has published extensively on methodological innovation. The book is organized using a progressive translational model and features excellent chapters on treatment manuals, interventionist training, and fidelity assessment. Highly recommended for behavioral trialists with or without interests in psychotherapy treatments.]

Tohen M, Bowden CL, Nierenberg AA, Geddess JR (2015) Clinical trial design challenges in mood disorders. Academic Press, Cambridge
Poor clinical trial designs result in failed studies, wasted research funds, and limited advancement of cures for disorders. This edited book outlines classic problems researchers face in designing clinical trials for mood disorder treatments and discusses how to address them for the most definitive and generalizable results. Topics include the placebo response, the generalizability of studies conducted in the developing world, maintenance studies, and the application of findings to clinical practice. With international contributors from academia, industry, regulatory agencies, and advocacy groups, this book will contribute to improved clinical trial design and valid, precise, and reliable answers about what works better and faster for patients. [Author Note: This book focuses on clinical trials for patients with mood and bipolar disorders. It is a comprehensive description of the most problematic methodological issues that emerge when a treatment is aimed at alleviating mental health disorders.]

Gitlin LN, Czaja SJ (2016) Behavioral intervention research. Designing, evaluating, and implementing. Springer, New York
This unique text provides comprehensive coverage of one of the most neglected, yet vitally important, areas of public health research: developing, evaluating, and implementing novel behavioral interventions in service and practice settings. Written for novice and expert researchers, this book examines the most critical issues needed to successfully implement current and future evidence-based protocols in practice settings. Topics include ways to develop and advance an intervention, hybrid trial designs, theories and models for integrating behavioral interventions with implementation science, recruitment and retention strategies for diverse samples, research designs for different stages of intervention development, treatment fidelity models and measures, novel measurement and analytic strategies, cost analyses, selection of control groups, use of mixed methodology, ethics and informed consent, technology-based intervention approaches, and professional considerations. Abundant case examples from successful national and international behavioral intervention trials illustrate key concepts. [Author Note: This edited book focuses on the practical side of designing and implementing behavioral clinical trials. It includes excellent chapters on implementation/dissemination, grant writing, publishing, and the importance of assembling the right team.]

Robertson CT, Kesselheim AS (2016) Blinding as a solution to bias. Strengthening biomedical science, forensic science, and law. Academic Press, Cambridge

What information should jurors have during court proceedings to render a just decision? Should politicians know who is donating money to their campaigns? Will scientists draw biased conclusions about drug efficacy when they know more about the patient or study population? The potential for bias in decision-making by physicians, lawyers, politicians, and scientists has been recognized for hundreds of years and drawn attention from media and scholars seeking to understand the role that conflicts of interest and other psychological processes play. However, commonly proposed solutions to biased decision-making, such as transparency (disclosing conflicts) or exclusion (avoiding conflicts), do not directly solve the underlying problem of bias and may have unintended consequences. [Author Note: Behavioral clinical trials often preclude the ability to double-blind to treatments. This book is a deep dive into blinding, the consequences that result when it is not protected, and its central role in producing a conclusive result in a behavioral trial. It is recommended for those with serious interests in pushing toward confirmatory behavioral clinical trials.]

Leigh A (2018) Randomistas. How radical researchers changed our world. Yale University Press, New Haven

Across medicine, business and government, there's no simpler or more powerful tool for finding out what works than a randomised experiment. Investigating everything from jails to ad compaigns, philanthropy, teaching, and crime, the randomistas build evidence and bust myths. Andrew Leigh is an economist who tells the stories of the radical researchers who overturned conventional wisdom in medicine, politics, economics, and law enforcement. From finding the cure to scurvy to discovering what policies really improve literacy rates, randomistas have shaped life as we know it—but they often had to fight to conduct their trials and have their findings implemented. [Author Note: This book features an engaging set of stories about how random assignment has led to the debunking of myths and discovery of truth. It is fun to read and in the process produces an in-depth understanding of the value of randomization: the sine qua non of clinical trials.]

APPENDIX
Chapter Reviewers

Walter Ambrosius, PhD
Department of Biostatistical Sciences
Division of Public Health Sciences
Wake Forest University Health Sciences
VINE, 4529
Medical Center Boulevard
Winston-Salem, NC 27157

Simon L. Bacon, PhD, FTOS, FCCS,
FABMR
Department of Health, Kinesiology, and
  Applied Physiology
Concordia University
7141 Sherbrooke St. West, L-SP 165 35
Montreal, Quebec, H4B 1R6
Canada

Rogelio A. Coronado, PhD
Department of Orthopaedic Surgery and
  Rehabilitation
Vanderbilt University Medical Center
Nashville, TN 37232

Susan M. Czajkowski, PhD
Health Behaviors Research Branch
Behavioral Research Program
Division of Cancer Control
  and Population Sciences
National Cancer Institute
National Institutes of Health
9609 Medical Center Drive
BG 9609 MSC 9760
Bethesda, MD 20892

Bradley Appelhans, PhD
Department of Preventive Medicine
Rush University Medical Center
1700 W. Van Buren St., Suite 470
Chicago, IL 60612

Kelly Glazer Baron, PhD, MPH, DBSM
Division of Public Health
Department of Family and Preventive Medicine
University of Utah
Salt Lake City, UT 84132

Melissa Crane, PhD
Department of Preventive Medicine
Rush University Medical Center
1700 W. Van Buren St., Suite 470
Chicago, IL 60612

Bradley Efron, PhD
Department of Statistics
390 Serra Mall
Stanford University
Stanford, CA 94305

© Springer Nature Switzerland AG 2021
L. H. Powell et al., *Behavioral Clinical Trials for Chronic Diseases*,
https://doi.org/10.1007/978-3-030-39330-4

Angela Fidler Pfammatter, PhD, MS
Department of Preventive Medicine
Northwestern University Feinberg School of
    Medicine
680 N. Lake Shore Drive, Suite 1400
Chicago, IL 60611

Robert M. Kaplan, PhD
Clinical Excellence Research Center (CERC)
Littlefield Center, Room 337
365 Lasuen Street
Stanford University
Stanford, CA 94305

Emily Kuschner, PhD
Perelman School of Medicine
University of Pennsylvania
Department of Radiology
2716 South St., Rm 5251
Philadelphia, PA 19146

Kim Lavoie, PhD
Montreal Behavioral Medicine Center
Department of Psychology
University of Quebec at Montreal
CP 8888, Succursale Centre-Ville,
Montreal, Quebec, H3C 3P8
Canada

Jun Ma, MD, PhD
Institute for Health Research and Policy
University of Illinois at Chicago
586 Westside Research Office Bldg.
    (MC 275)
1747 West Roosevelt Road
Chicago, IL 60608

Amanda R. Mathew, PhD
Department of Preventive Medicine
Rush University Medical Center
1700 W. Van Buren St., Suite 470
Chicago, IL 60612

Ty A. Ridenour, PhD, MPE
Division of Behavioral Health and Criminal
Justice Research
RTI, International
Research Triangle Park
PO Box 1219
3040 Cornwallis Rd
Durham, NC 27709

Celeste Fraser, MA
Senior Editor, Scott Foresman Co. (retired)
Education Specialist, Chicago Children's
    Museum (retired)
Estes Park, Colorado 80517

Michaela Kiernan, PhD
Stanford Prevention Research Center
Stanford University School of Medicine
MSOB 1265 Welch Road X342
Stanford, CA 94305

Brittney Lange-Maia, PhD
Department of Preventive Medicine
Rush University Medical Center
1700 W. Van Buren St., Suite 470
Chicago, IL 60612

Philip Liebson, MD
Department of Preventive Medicine
Rush University Medical Center
1700 W. Van Buren St., Suite 470
Chicago, IL 60612

Kevin S. Masters, PhD
Director, Clinical Health Psychology
Department of Psychology
PO Box 173364
University of Colorado, Denver
Denver, CO 80217

Kei Ouchi, MD, MPH
Division of Health Policy Research and
    Translation
Department of Emergency Medicine
Brigham and Women's Hospital/Harvard
    Medical School
75 Francis St.
Boston, MA 02115

Catherine M. Stoney, PhD
Division of Cardiovascular Sciences
National Heart, Lung, and Blood Institute
National Institutes of Health
6701 Rockledge Drive
Bethesda, MD 20892

Christine Vinci, PhD
Tobacco Research & Prevention Program
Moffitt Cancer Center
Morsani College of Medicine
University of South Florida
4115 E. Fowler Avenue
Tampa, FL 33617

Rachel Wu, PhD, MS
Department of Psychology
University of California, Riverside
900 University Avenue
Riverside, CA 92521

Index

© Springer Nature Switzerland AG 2021
L. H. Powell et al., *Behavioral Clinical Trials for Chronic Diseases*,
https://doi.org/10.1007/978-3-030-39330-4